Bile, Bile Acids, Gallstones, and Gallstone Dissolution

Bile, Bile Acids, Gallstones, and Gallstone Dissolution

A bibliography of relevant articles, abstracts, and editorials

Compiled and Indexed by

Alan F. Hofmann MD
University of California, San Diego

with assistance of
Vicky L. Huebner
and
Joseph H. Steinbach PhD

A new bibliography of publications dealing with bile formation and secretion; bile acid biology, chemistry, and physiology; and gallstone epidemiology, pathogenesis, and medical treatment. With a complete author and subject index.

MTP PRESS LIMITED · LANCASTER · BOSTON · THE HAGUE
International Medical Publishers

Published in the UK and Europe by
MTP Press Limited
Falcon House
Lancaster, England

Published in the USA by
MTP Press
A division of Kluwer Boston Inc
190 Old Derby Street
Hingham, MA 02043, USA

British Library Cataloguing in Publication Data

Hofmann, Alan F.
Bile, bile acids, gallstones and gallstone dissolution
1. Calculi, Biliary – Bibliography
2. Chenodeoxycholic acid – Therapeutic use – Bibliography
I. Title II. Huebner, Vicky L.
III. Steinbach, Joseph H.
016.6163'65 Z6664.C1

ISBN 0-85200-497-4

Printed in Great Britain

Foreword

This is an updated version of my previous bibliography. The title has been changed to reflect its scope. When the previous edition was issued, I was quite certain there were few important omissions; this time I have no certainty whatsoever, because of the high rate of publication in this field. Indeed, I have already discovered more key omissions than I care to admit.

The selection of articles continues to be arbitrary, reflecting scientific, personal, and even political considerations. The literature of gallstone formation and treatment does not suffer from a lack of redundancy of content!! If you feel your article belongs here, please write me; and I will consider it for the next edition--if such occurs.

I believe the accompanying subject index justifies the issuance of such a bibliography. Computerized indices are improving greatly, and it is unclear that manual indexing will be necessary in the future if each article is accompanied by an appropriate list of key or index words. Part of the difficulty of recording the bile acid literature is the diversity of areas of scientific activity which is reflected in the great variety of journals included in this listing. I have always been opposed to the formation of a journal devoted solely to bile and bile acids, but sometimes I think if such a journal were to be formed, its availability would make our lives easier.

Comments and criticisms are invited, and if the bibliography helps you, please let me know. Incidentally, there are undoubtedly a few errors in the subject index. If the article listed is incorrect, please check the article above or below the citation. If you find a major error, please write me.

In compiling the index, it is encouraging to see new areas develop a substantial body of data. For example, new areas include nucleation in bile, mesophase formation in bile, and an increased concern about gallstone calcification. In compiling the author index, one sees the entry of new personalities who literally explode like rockets with multiple articles in a short time period. Each such event signals the entry of a new energy force into cholanology. At the same time, some of the senior figures publish less, perhaps distracted by meetings, administrative obligations, or non-creatic writing tasks such as the compilation of a bibliography. Thus, a steady state obtains.

It is now 15 years since the first bulk shipment of chenodeoxycholic acid arrived in Rochester, and only this year will chenodeoxycholic acid be marketed in the USA. We have learned much about gallstone formation and dissolution, but there is still much, much more to learn.

Vicky Huebner, as editor and word processor, is responsible for the format of this version. Joseph Steinbach spent long hours in converting our word processor into a functioning computer. Kathy Kehr also assisted in the compilation. I acknowledge financial support from The Falk Foundation and the National Institutes of Health for the preparation of this bibliography.

The previous edition helped me in my own work, and I hope it has helped others. The reward for the tedious task of compiling these articles has been the pleasure at seeing our field prosper with an ever increasing volume of good science relevant to the diagnosis and treatment of biliary disease.

Bibliography

a Abaurre, R., Gordon, S.G., Mann, J.G., and Kern, F., Jr. The effects of ileal resection upon fasting bile salt pool size and composition. Gastroenterology 57:679-688, 1969.

b Abell, L.L., Levy, B.B., Brodie, B.B., and Kendall, F.E. Simplified method for estimation of total cholesterol in serum and demonstration of its specificity. J. Biol. Chem. 195:357-366, 1952.

c Abell, L.L., Mosbach, E.H., and Kendall, F.E. Cholesterol metabolism in the dog. J. Biol. Chem. 220:527-536, 1956.

d Accatino, L. and Simon, F.R. Identification and characterization of a bile acid receptor in isolated liver surface membrane. J. Clin. Invest. 57:496-508, 1976.

e Acosta, J.M. and Ledesma, C.L. Gallstone migration as a cause of acute pancreatitis. N. Engl. J. Med. 290:484-487, 1974 and 290:1201-1202, 1974 (Letter to Editor).

f Addleman, W. Cancer, cholesterol and cholestyramine. N. Engl. J. Med. 287:1047, 1972 (Letter to Editor).

g Adler, R.D., Metzger, A.L., and Grundy, S.M. Biliary lipid secretion before and after cholecystectomy in American Indians with cholesterol gallstones. Gastroenterology 66:1212-1217, 1974.

h Adler, R.D., Bennion, L.J., Duane, W.C., and Grundy, S.M. Effects of low dose chenodeoxycholic acid feeding on biliary lipid metabolism. Gastroenterology 68:326-334, 1975.

i Adler, M. Physiologie des sels biliaires et traitment medical de la lithiase biliaire par l'acide chenique. R. Med. Bruxelles 32:623-626, 1976.

j Admirand, W.H. and Small, D.M. The physicochemical basis of cholesterol gallstone formation in man. J. Clin. Invest. 47:1043-1052, 1968.

k Admirand, W.H. and Way, L.W. Medical treatment of retained gallstones. Trans. Assoc. Am. Phys. 85:382-387, 1972.

l Ahlberg, J., Angelin, B., Bjorkhem, I., and Einarsson, K. Individual bile acids in portal venous and systemic blood serum of fasting man. Gastroenterology 73:1377-1382, 1977.

m Ahlberg, J., Angelin, B., Einarsson, K., Hellstrom, K., and Leijd, B. Influence of deoxycholic acid on biliary lipids in man. Clin. Sci. & Mol. Med. 53:249-256, 1977.

n Ahlberg, J., Angelin, B., Einarsson, K., and Leijd, B. Biliary lipid composition and bile acid kinetics in patients with agenesis of the gallbladder with a note on the frequency of this anomaly. Acta Chir. Scand. 482(suppl.): 15-20, 1978.

a Ahlberg, J., Angelin, B., Bjorkhem, I., Einarsson, K., and Leijd, B. Hepatic cholesterol metabolism in normo- and hyperlipidemic patients with cholesterol gallstones. J. Lipid Res. 20:107-115, 1979.

b Ahlberg, J., Angelin, B., Einarsson, K., Hellstrom, K., and Leijd, B. Prevalence of gallbladder disease in hyperlipoproteinemia. Am. J. Dig. Dis. 24:459-464, 1979.

c Ahlberg, J., Angelin, B., Bjorkhem, I., Einarsson, K., Gustafsson, J.A., and Rafter, J. Effects of treatment with chenodeoxycholic acid on liver microsomal metabolism of steroids in man. J. Lab. Clin. Med. 95:188-194, 1980.

d Ahlberg, J., Angelin, B., Einarsson, K., Hellstrom, K., and Leijd, B. Biliary lipid composition in normo- and hyperlipoproteinemia. Gastroenterology 79:90-94, 1980.

e Ahlberg, J., Einarsson, K., and Westberg, G. Spontaneous dissolution of gallstones, a case report. Acta Chir. Scand. 500(suppl.):3-5, 1980.

f Ahlberg, J., Angelin, B., and Einarsson, K. Hepatic 3-hydroxy-3-methylglutaryl coenzyme A reductase activity and biliary lipid composition in man: Relation to cholesterol gallstone disease and effects of cholic acid and chenodeoxycholic acid treatment. J. Lipid Res. 22:410-422, 1981.

g Ahlberg, J., Curstedt, T., Einarsson, K., and Sjovall, J. Molecular species of biliary phosphatidylcholines in gallstone patients: The influence of treatment with cholic acid and chenodeoxycholic acid. J. Lipid Res. 22:404-409, 1981.

h Ahlsten, M., Hansson, R., Holmberg, I., Ljungdahl, I., and Wikvall, K. Reconstitution of cholesterol 7a-hydroxylase system from human liver microsomes. Biochem. Med. 26:307-313, 1981.

i Ahrens, E.H., Jr. and Craig, L.C. The extraction and separation of bile acids. J. Biol. Chem. 195:763, 1952.

j Ainsworth, C., Benslay, D.N., Davenport, J., Hudson, J.L., Kau, D., Lin, T.M., and Pfeiffer, R.R. Cholesterol-solubilizing agents related to the gallstone problem. J. Med. Chem. 10:158, 1967.

k Albers, J.J., Grundy, S.M., Cleary, P.A., Small, D.M., Lachin, J.M., and Schoenfield, L.J., for the National Cooperative Gallstone Study Group. NCGS: The effect of chenodeoxycholic acid on lipoproteins and apoproteins. Gastroenterology 82:638-646, 1982.

l Aldini, R., Barbara, L., Benelli, A., Borzatta, V., Geminiani, S., Mascellani, G., Morselli, A., Roda, A., and Roda, E. Effects of a salt of cholestyramine and 2-[4-(p-chlorobenzoyl)phenoxy]2-methyl propionic acid (a-1081) on biliary lipid secretion in rats. Br. J. Pharmac. 74:611-617, 1981.

a Aldini, R., Mazzella, G., Rossi, R.M., Cappelleri, G., Roda, E., and Barbara, L. Serum UDCA tolerance test in liver disease. 16th Meeting of the EASL, Lisbon, 1981 (abstract 98).

b Alegre, B., Garrido, G., Breto, M., Perez-Aguilar, F., et al. Efecto hipotrigliceridemiante del acido quenico en enfermos afectos de litasis biliar. Gastroenterol. y Hepatol. 2:173-177, 1979.

c Alessandrini, A., Ripoli, F., Boscaini, M., Archangeli, A., Gentilini, P., Blasi, A., Mangiameli, A., Fontana, G., Costa, L., Mazzacca, G., D'Arienzo, A., Okolicsanyi, L., et al. A multicentre clinical trial on ursodeoxycholic acid: effect of different dosages upon cholesterol gallstone dissolution. Ital. J. Gastroenterol. 12:185-188, 1980.

d Alfthan, O. and Kohler, R. Ether treatment of retained postoperative biliary tree stones. Acta Chir. Scand. 116:437-449, 1959.

e Ali, S.S., Kuksis, A., and Beveridge, J.M.R. Excretion of bile acids by three men on corn oil and butterfat diets. Can. J. Biochem. 44:1377-1388, 1966.

f Ali, S.S. and Javitt, N.B. Quantitative estimation of bile salts in serum. Canad. J. Biochem. 48:1054-1057, 1970.

g Ali, S.S. and Elliot, W.H. Bile Acids. XLVII. 12a-Hydroxylation of precursors of allo bile acids by rabbit liver microsomes. Biochim. Biophys. Acta 409:249-257, 1975.

h Allan, J.G., Gerskowitch, V.P., and Russell, R.I. Bile acids and post-vagotomy diarrhea. Brit. Med. J. 4:741, 1973 (Letter to Editor).

i Allan, R.N., Thistle, J.L., Hofmann, A.F., Carter, J.A., and Yu, P.Y.S. Lithocholate metabolism during chenotherapy for gallstone dissolution. I. Serum levels of sulphated and unsulphated lithocholates. Gut 17:405-412, 1976.

j Allan, R.N., Thistle, J.L., and Hofmann, A.F. Lithocholate metabolism during chenotherapy for gallstone dissolution. II. Absorption and sulphation. Gut 17:413-419, 1976.

k Allen, B.L., Deveney, C.W., and Way, L.W. Chemical dissolution of bile duct stones. World J. Surg. 2:429-437, 1978.

l Alling, C., Cahlin, E., and Schersten, T. Relationships between fatty acid patterns of serum, hepatic, and biliary lecithins in man. Effect of sucrose feeding. Biochim. Biophys. Acta 296:518-526, 1973.

m Almond, H.R., Vlahcevic, Z.R., Bell, C.C., Jr., Gregory, D.H., and Swell, L. Bile acid pools, kinetics and biliary lipid composition before and after cholecystecomy. N. Engl. J. Med. 289:1213-1216, 1973.

a Altomonte, L., Mingrone, G., Gattini, G., Pepe, M., and Greco, A.V. Molar percentages of bile acids: Cholesterol and phospholipids in bile of hyperlipemic subjects. Effect of a new hypolipemic drug: Etofibrate. Ital. J. Gastroenterol. 12:352, 1980 (abstract).

b Altomonte, L., Greco, A.V., Ghirlanda, G., Rebuzzi, A.G., and Manna, R. Concentration of bile acids and lipids in serum during normal menstrual cycle, after intake of oral contraceptive, and during normal pregnancy. Therapiewoche 31:8274, 8277-8278, 1981.

c Ammon, H.V. and Phillips, S.F. Inhibition of colonic water and electrolyte absorption by fatty acids in man. Gastroenterology, 65:744-749, 1973.

d Ammon, H.V. Conjugated bile acids in the canine gallbladder: Effect on water absorption in the absence and presence of lecithin. Gastroenterology 66:660, 1974 (abstract).

e Amos, B., Anderson, I.G., Haslewood, G.A.D., and Tokes, L. Bile salts of the lungfishes *Lepidosiren*, *Neoceratodus* and *Protopterus* and those of the Coelacanth *Latimeria chalumnae* Smith. Biochem. J. 161:201-204, 1977.

f Amuro, Y., Endo, T., Higashino, K., Uchida, K., and Yamamura, Y. Serum, fecal and urinary bile acids in patients with mild and advanced liver cirrhosis. Gastroenterol. Jpn. 16:506-513, 1981.

g Andersen, J.M. Chenodeoxycholic acid desaturates bile--but how? Gastroenterology 77:1146-1151, 1979.

h Anderson, E. and Hellstrom, K. Influence of fat-rich versus carbohydrate-rich diets on bile acid kinetics, biliary lipids, and net steroid balance in hyperlipidemic subjects. Metabolism 29:400-409, 1980.

i Anderson, I.G., Haslewood, G.A.D., Wiggins, H.S., and Wooten, I.D.P. Preparation of chenodeoxycholic acid from cholic acid. Nature 169:621, 1952.

j Anderson, K.E., Kok, E., and Javitt, N.B. Bile acid synthesis in man: Metabolism of 7-hydroxy-cholesterol-^{14}C- and 26-hydroxy-cholesterol-^{3}H. J. Clin. Invest. 51:112-117, 1972.

k Anfossi, A., Mortola, G.P., Cafiero, F., Parodi, E., Giusto, F., and Berti-Riboli, E. Choice between litholytic and surgical treatment in cholesterin cholecystic calculosis. Min. Med. 71:623-625, 1980.

l Angelico, M., Angelico, F., Amodeo, P., Attili, A.F., Puoti, C., Ricci, G., and Capocaccia, L. Individual bile acids in patients with primary hyperlipoproteinemias. Atherosclerosis 37:293-299, 1980.

m Angelin, B., Einarsson, K., and Hellstrom, K. Evidence for the absorption of bile acids in the proximal small intestine of normo- and hyperlipidaemic subjects. Gut 17:420-425, 1976.

a Angelin, B., Einarsson, K., Hellstrom, K., and Kallner, M. Elimination of cholesterol in hyperlipoproteinaemia. Clin. Sci. & Mol. Med. 51:393-397, 1976.

b Angelin, B. and Bjorkhem, I. Postprandial serum bile acids in healthy man. Evidence for differences in absorptive pattern between individual bile acids. Gut 18:606-609, 1977.

c Angelin, B., Bjorkhem, I., and Einarsson, K. Individual serum bile acid concentrations in normo- and hyperlipoproteinemia as determined by mass fragmentography: Relation to bile acid pool size. J. Lipid Res. 19:527-537, 1978.

d Angelin, B., Einarsson, K., and Hellstrom, K. Effect of cholestyramine on bile acid kinetics in patients with portal cirrhosis of the liver. Dig. Dis. & Sci. 23:1115-1120, 1978.

e Angelin, B., Einarsson, K., Hellstrom, K., and Leijd, B. Bile acid kinetics in relation to endogenous triglyceride metabolism in various types of hyperlipoproteinemia. J. Lipid Res. 19:1004-1016, 1978.

f Angelin, B., Einarsson, K., Hellstrom, K., and Leijd, B. Effects of cholestyramine and chenodeoxycholic acid on the metabolism of endogenous triglyceride in hyperlipoproteinemia. J. Lipid Res. 19:1017-1024, 1978.

g Angelin, B., Einarsson, K., and Leijd, B. Effect of chenodeoxycholic acid on serum and biliary lipids in patients with hyperlipoproteinemia. Clin. Sci. & Mol. Med. 54:451-455, 1978.

h Angelin, B., Ahlberg, J., Bjorkhem, I., Einarsson, K., and Ewerth, S. Serum levels of individual bile acids in portal venous and systemic circulation during treatment with chenodeoxycholic and cholic acid. In Biological Effects of Bile Acids, G Paumgartner, A Stiehl, W Gerok, eds. MTP Press, Lancaster, 1979, pp 107-108.

i Angelin, B., Einarsson, K., and Leijd, B. Biliary lipid composition during treatment with different hypolipidaemic drugs. Europ. J. Clin. Invest. 9:185-190, 1979.

j Angelin, B., Einarsson, K., Ewerth, S., and Leijd, B. Biliary lipid composition in patients with portal cirrhosis of the liver. Scand. J. Gastroenterol. 15:849-852, 1980.

k Angelin, B., Einarsson, K., Lindblad, L., Pettersson, H., and Schersten, T. Dissolution of gallstones with chenodeoxycholic acid. Lakartidningen 77:3872-2876, 1980.

l Angelin, B. and Leijd, B. Effects of cholic acid on the metabolism of endogenous plasma triglyceride and on biliary lipid composition in hyperlipoproteinemia. J. Lipid Res. 21:1-9, 1980.

m Angelin, B., Einarsson, K., Ewerth, S., and Leijd, B. Biliary lipid composition in obesity. Scand. J. Gastroent. 16:1015-1019, 1981.

a Angelin, B., Einarsson, K., and Leijd, B. Clofibrate treatment and bile cholesterol saturation: Short-term and long-term effects and influence of combination with chenodeoxycholic acid. Europ. J. Clin. Invest. 11:185-189, 1981.

b Antezana, C. and Csendes, A. In vitro dissolution of cholesterol gallstones with sodium cholate, heparin and monooctanoin. Med. Chile 109:601-605, 1981.

c Anver, M.R., Hunt, R.D.,and Califoux, L.V. Cholesterol gallstones in Aotus trivirgatus. J. Med. Primatol. 1:241-246, 1972.

d Anwer, M.S., Gronwall, R.R., Engelking, L.R., and Klentz, R.D. Bile acid kinetics and bile secretion in the pony. Am. J. Physiol. 229:592-597, 1975.

e Anwer, M.S., Kroker, R., and Hegner, D. Bile acid secretion and synthesis by isolated rat hepatocytes. Biochim. Biophys. Res. Commun. 64:603-609, 1975.

f Anwer, M.S., Engelking, L.R., Gronwall, R., and Klentz, R.D. Plasma bile acid elevation following CCl_4 induced liver damage in dogs, sheep, calves and ponies. Res. Vet. Sci. 20:127-130, 1976.

g Anwer, M.S., Kroker, R., and Hegner, D. Cholic acid uptake into isolated rat hepatocytes. Hoppe-Seyler's Z. Physiol. Chem. 357:1477-1486, 1976.

h Anwer, M.S., Kroker, R., and Hegner, D. Effect of albumin on bile acid uptake by isolated rat hepatocytes. Is there a common bile acid carrier? Biochem. Biophys. Res. Commun. 73:63-71, 1976.

i Anwer, M.S., Kroker, R., Hegner, D., and Petter, A. Cholic acid binding to isolated rat liver plasma membranes. Hoppe-Seyler's Z. Physiol. Chem. 358:543-553, 1977.

j Anwer, M.S. and Hegner, D. Effect of organic anions on bile acid uptake by isolated rat hepatocytes. Hoppe-Seyler's Z. Physiol. Chem. 359:1027-1030, 1978.

k Anwer, M.S. and Hegner, D. Effect of Na^+ on bile acid uptake by isolated rat hepatocytes. Evidence for a heterogeneous system. Hoppe-Seyler's Z. Physiol. Chem. 359:181-192, 1978.

l Anwer, M.S. and Hegner, D. Interaction of fusidates with bile acid uptake by isolated rat hepatocytes. Naunyn-Schmiedeberg's Arch. Pharmacol. 302: 329-332, 1978.

m Anwer, M.S., Kroker, R., and Hegner, D. Inhibition of hepatic uptake of bile acids by rifamycins. Naunyn-Schmiedeberg's Arch. Pharmacol. 302: 19-24, 1978.

n Anwer, M.S. and Hegner, D. An enzymatic method for the quantitative determination of 3-keto bile acids. Anal. Biochem. 99:408-414, 1979.

a Anwer, M.S. and Hegner, D. Study of cholic acid conjugation by isolated rat hepatocytes. Hoppe-Seyler's Z. Physiol. Chem. 360:515-522, 1979.

b Anwer, M.S. Effect of cations on bile acid choleresis in isolated perfused rat liver. Ital. J. Gastroenterol. 12:128-131, 1980.

c Arcangeli, A., Chirantini, E., Caramelli, L. and Buzzelli, G. Prove dinamiche con BSF in pazienti colelitiasici prima e dopo trattamento a lungo termine con acido chenodesossicolico. Minerva Med. 71:2405-2407, 1980.

d Areias, M.E., Menzes, M.L., Pinto Correia, J., and Tiago, M.E. Secrecao dos sais biliares. I. Metodos de estudo e valores normais; II. Resultados na cirrose hepatica. O. Medico 73:283-292, 1974 (Portugese).

e Aries, V., Crowther, J.S., Drasar, B.S., and Hill, M.J. Degradation of bile salts by human intestinal bacteria. Gut 10:575-576, 1969.

f Aries, V., Crowther, J.S., Drasar, B.S., Hill, M.J., and Williams, R.E.O. Bacteria and the aetiology of cancer of the large bowel. Gut 10:334-335, 1969.

g Aries, V.C. and Hill, M.J. Degradation of steroids by intestinal bacteria. I. Deconjunction of bile salts. Biochim. Biophys. Acta 202:526-534, 1970.

h Aries, V.C. and Hill, M.J. Degradation of steroids by intestinal bacteria. II. Enzymes catalysing the oxido-reduction of the 3a-,7a- and 12a-hydroxyl groups in cholic acid and the dehydroxylation of the 7-hydroxyl group. Biochim. Biophys. Acta 202:535-543, 1970.

i Aries, V.C. and Hill, M.J. The formation of unsaturated bile acids by intestinal bacteria. Biochem. J. 119:37P-38P, 1970.

j Arnesjo, B., Nilsson, A., Barrowman, J., and Borgstrom, B. Intestinal digestion and absorption of cholesterol and lecithin in the human. Scand. J. Gastroenterol. 4:653-665, 1969.

k Arnesjo, B. and Stahl, E. Taurocholate metabolism in patients with cholesterol gallstones. Scand. J. Gastroenterol. 8:369-375, 1973.

l Arnesjo, B., Bodvall, B., and Stahl, E. Bile acid patterns of gallbladder and hepatic bile in patients with and without cholesterol gallstones. Acta Chir. Scand. 141:135-138, 1975.

m Ashizawa, S., Ishi, N., and Ishihara, H., et al. Clinical study of gallstone dissolution with ursodeoxycholic acid. Igaku no ayumi (Progress in Medicine) 101:922-936, 1977.

n Ashkin, J., Hercker, E.S., and Ostrow, J.D. Regulation of the excretion of unconjugated bilirubin in bile. Gastroenterology 70:977, 1976 (abstract).

a Atsuta, Y. and Okuda, K. d-Hydroxylase for 5b-cholestane-3a,7a-diol in the biosynthesis of chenodeoxycholic acid. Arch. Biochem. & Biophys. 189: 137-143, 1978.

b Attias, J.L. Tratamiento. In Litiasis Biliar. JM Fregoso and J Cohen, eds. Editorial Diana, Mexico, 1978, pp 109-129.

c Attili, A.F., Angelico, M., Cantafora, A., Di Biase, A., Capocaccia, P., Gualdi, G.F., and Capocaccia, L. Effect of low doses of ursodeoxycholic acid on biliary lipid composition in non obese gallstone patients. Ital. J. Gastroenterol. 10:119-120, 1978.

d Attili, A.F., Angelico, M., Capocaccia, P., Gualdi, G., Cantafora, A., DiBiase, A., Capocaccia, L., and Giunchi, G. Effect of ursodeoxycholic acid on biliary lipid compostition. A double-blind study. Ital. J. Gastroenterol. 12:177-180, 1980.

e Aumiller, J. Krank und steinreich. Der Kosmos (7) 76-84, 1981.

f Austad, W.I., Lack, L., and Tyor, M.P. The importance of bile acids and of an intact distal small intestine for fat absorption. Gastroenterology 52:638-646, 1967.

g Ayaki, Y. and Yamasaki, K. In vitro conversion of 7a-hydroxycholesterol to come natural C_{24}-bile acids with special reference to chenodeoxycholic acid biogenesis. J. Biochem. 68:341-346, 1970 (Tokyo).

h Ayaki, Y., Tsuma-Date, T., Endo, S., and Ogura, M. Role of endogenous and exogenous cholesterol in liver as the precursor for bile acids in rats. Steroids 38:495-509, 1981.

i Ayengar, N.K.N., Singhal, A.K., McSherry, C.K., and Mosbach, E.H. The preparation of bile acid amides and oxazolines. Steroids 38:333-345, 1981.

j Baba, S., Uenoyama, R., Suminoe, K., Takeda, F., Hasegawa, S., and Kameno, Y. A measurement of individual bile acids in serum by high-performance liquid chromatography for clinical diagnostic information of hepatobiliary diseases. Kobe J. Med. Sci. 26:89-99, 1980.

k Baba, S., Suminoe, K., Uenoyama, R., Hasegawa, S., Takeda, F., and Kameno, Y. Studies on oral ursodeoxycholic acid tolerance test in hepatobiliary diseases with special reference to dynamic changes in individual serum bile acids. J. Clin. Chem. & Clin. Biochem. 19:605, 1981 (abstract).

l Back, P., Hamprecht, B., and Lynen, F. Regulation of cholesterol biosynthesis in rat liver: Diurnal changes of activity and influence of bile acids. Arch. Biochem. Biophys. 133:11, 1969.

m Back, P. Ausscheidung von Monohydroxy-Gallensauren im Urin bei Verschlussikterus und akuter Hepatitis. Z. Gastroenterologie 11:477, 1973.

n Back, P. Die Primare hepatische Synthese von Mono-Hydroxy-Gallensauren bei extrahepatischer Gallengangsatresie. Klin. Wschr. 51:926, 1973.

a Back, P. Synthesis and excretion of bile acids in a case of extrahepatic biliary atresia. Helv. Med. Acta 37:193-200, 1973.

b Back, P. and Ross, K. Identification of 3b-hydroxy-5-cholenic acid in human meconium. Z. Physiol. Chem. 354:83-89, 1973.

c Back, P. Differences in renal excretion of subgroups of bile acids depending on the introduction of polar groups. Digestion 10:322-323, 1974. (abstract).

d Back, P., Sjovall, J., and Sjovall, K. Monohydroxy bile acids in plasma in intrahepatic cholestasis of pregnancy. Identification by computerized gas chromatography-mass spectrometry. Med. Biol. 52:31, 1974.

e Back, P., Spaczynski, K., and Gerok, W. Bile salt glucuronides in urine. 3. Physiol. Chem. 355:749-752, 1974.

f Back, P. Bile acid glucuronides. II. Isolation and identification of a chenodeoxycholic acid glucuronide from human plasma in intrahepatic cholestasis. Hoppe-Seyler's Z. Physiol. Chem. Bd. 357:213-217, 1976.

g Back, P. and Walter, K. Developmental pattern of bile acid metabolism as revealed by bile acid analysis of meconium. Gastroenterology 78:671-676, 1980.

h Back, P. and Populoh, C. Induktion atypischer Gallensaurenhydroxylierungen. Z. Gastroenterol. XIX (9), 1981 (abstract 8).

i Bagheri, S.A., Bolt, M.G., Palmer, R.H., and Boyer, J.L. Lithocholic acid induced peliosis hepatis. Influence of microsomal enzyme metabolism on hepatic toxicity. In Advances in Bile Acid Research. ed S Matern, J Hackenschmidt, P Back, W Gerok. FK Schattauer Verlag, Stuttgart-New York, 1975, pp 249-254.

j Bagheri, S.A., Bolt, M.G., Boyer, J.L., and Palmer, R.H. Stimulation of thymidine incorporation in mouse liver and biliary tract epithelium by lithocholate and deoxycholate. Gastroenterology 74:188-192, 1978.

k Baillet-Guffroy, A., Baylocq, D., Rafidison, P., and Pellerin, F. Detection and determination of bile acids and their conjugated derivatives by liquid chromatography. Talanta 28:675-680, 1981.

l Baily, N.A., Keller, R.A., and Lasser, E.C. A computerized system for the measurement of gallstone volume in vivo. Med. Phys. 6(2) March/April, 1979.

m Baker, R.D. and Searle, G.W. Bile salt absorption at various levels of rat small intestine. Proc. Soc. Exptl. Biol. Med. 105:521-523, 1960.

n Balabaud, C., Noel, M., Beraud, C., and Dangoumau, J. The circadian rhythm of bile secretion in the rat. Digestion 10:325, 1974 (abstract).

a Balasubramaniam, S., Mitropoulos, K.A., and Myant, N.B. Rhythmic changes in the activity of cholesterol 7a-hydroxylase in the liver of fed and fasted rats. In Bile Acids in Human Disease. P Back and W Gerok, eds. FK Schattauer Verlag, Stuttgart-New York, 1972, pp 97-102.

b Balasubramaniam, S., Mitropoulos, K.A., and Myant, N.B. Evidence for the compartmentation of cholesterol in rat-liver microsomes. Europ. J. Biochem. 34:77-83, 1973.

c Balasubramaniam, S. and Mitropoulos, K.A. The role of cytochrome P-450 in the 7a-hydroxylation of cholesterol. Biochem. Soc. Trans. 3:964-967, 1975.

d Balasubramaniam, S., Mitropoulos, K.A., and Myant, N.B. Hormonal control of the acitivities of cholesterol 7a-hydroxylase and hydroxymethyl-glutaryl-CoA reductase in rats. In Advances in Bile Acid Research. S Matern, J Hacken-schmidt, P Back, W Gerok, eds. FK Schattauer Verlag, Stuttgart-New York, 1975, pp 61-70.

e Balasubramaniam, S., Mitropoulos, K.A., and Myant, N.B. The substrate for cholesterol 7a-hydroxylase. Biochim. Biophys. Acta 398:172-177, 1975.

f Balasubramaniam, S., Press, C.M., Mitropoulos, K.A., Magide, A.A., and Myant, N.B. Effect of portacaval anastomosis on the activities of hepatic enzymes related to cholesterol and bile acid metabolism in rats. Biochim. Biophys. Acta 441:308-315, 1976.

g Balint, J.A., Kyriakides, E.C., Spitzer, H.L., and Morrison, E.S. Lecithin fatty acid composition in bile and plasma of dog, man, rats, and oxen. J. Lipid Res. 6:96, 1965.

h Balint, J.A., Beeler, D.A., Treble, D.H., and Spitzer, H.L. Studies on the biosynthesis of hepatic and biliary lecithins. J. Lipid Res. 8:486-493, 1967.

i Balint, J.A., Beeler, D.A., Kyriakides, E.C., and Treble, D.H. The effect of bile salts upon lecithin synthesis. J. Lab. Clin. Med. 77:122-133, 1971.

j Balint, J.A., Kyriakides, E.C., Ainspan, J., and Beeler, D.A. Effect of dietary lipids on bile composition in rats. Gastroenterology 66:878, 1974 (abstract).

k Balistreri, W.F., Cowen, A.E., Hofmann, A.F., Szczepanik, P.A., and Klein, P.D. Validation of use of 11,12-^{2}H-labeled chenodeoxycholic acid in isotope dilution measurements of bile acid kinetics in man. Pediat. Res. 9:757-760, 1975.

l Balistreri, W.F., Korman, M.G., Cowen, A.E., and Hofmann, A.F. Sulfated lithocholic acid in Reye's Syndrome. In Reye's Syndrome. JD Pollack, ed. Grune and Stratton, New York, 1975, pp 269-271.

m Balistreri, W.F., Korman, M.G., Turcotte, J., and Hofmann, A.F. Radioimmunoasay of serum conjugates of cholic acid in infants and children. Pediat. Res. 9:301, 1975 (abstract).

a Balistreri, W.F., Partin, J.C., and Schubert, W.K. Bile acid malabsorption. A consequence of terminal ileal dysfunction in protracted diarrhea of infancy. J. Pediat. 90:21-28, 1977.

b Balistreri, W.F., Suchy, F.J., Farrell, M.K., and Heubi, J.E. Pathologic versus physiologic cholestasis: elevated serum concentration of a secondary bile acid in the presence of hepatobiliary disease. J. Pediatr. 98:399-402, 1981.

c Balistreri, W.F., Suchy, F.J., and Heubi, J.E. Serum bile acid response to a test meal stimulus: Sensitive test of ileal function. J. Pediat. (in press).

d Bandomer, G., Begemann, F., Kruger, W., and Schumpelick, V. Local cholesterol-lithogenicity in acute cholecystitis. 16th Meeting of the EASL, Lisbon, 1981 (abstract 104).

e Baqir, Y.A., Murison, J., Ross, P.E., and Bouchier, I.A.D. Radioimmunoassay of primary bile salts in serum. J. Clin. Path. 32:560-564, 1979.

f Baqir, Y.A., Ross, P.E., and Bouchier, I.A.D. Homogenous enzyme immunoassay of chenodeoxycholate conjugates in serum. Anal. Biochim. 93:361-365, 1979.

g Barbara, L., Roda, E., Roda, A., Festi, D., Sama, C., Mazzella, G., Aldini, R., and Labo, G. Results with chenodeoxycholic acid in the management of cholesterol lithiasis. Min. Med. 66:562-569, 1975.

h Barbara, L., Roda, A., Roda, E., Aldini, R., Mazzella, G., Festi, D., and Sama, C. Diurnal variations of serum primary bile acids in healthy subjects and hepatobiliary disease patients. Rendic. Gastroenterol. 8:194-198, 1976.

i Barbara, L. Roda, E., Roda, A., Sama, C., Festi, D., Mazzella, G., and Aldini, R. The medical treatment of cholesterol gallstones: Experience with chenodeoxycholic acid. Digestion 14:209-219, 1976.

j Barbara, L. Modificazioni dell'assetto lipidico biliare ed ematico dopo terapia con acido chenodesossicolico. Min. Med. 68:3023-3026, 1977.

k Barbara, L., Roda, E., Roda, A., Casanova, S., Festi, D., Sama, C., Mazzella, G. and Aldini, R. Progressi in terapia: Il trattamento medico della calcolosi biliare colesterolica nell'uomo con acido chenodesossicolico. Min. Med. 68:3355-3382, 1977.

l Barbara, L., Roda, E., Sassi, P., Festi, D., Sama, C., Aldini, R., Mazzella, G., and Roda, A. Chenodeoxycholic acid therapy of choledochal lithiasis. Min. Dietol. Gastroenterol. 24:13-23, 1978.

m Barbara, L., Roda, A., Mazzella, G., Festi, D., Aldini, R., Sama, C., Bazzoli, F., Morselli, A.M., and Roda, E. Efficacy of UDCA versus CDCA in cholesterol gallstones patients: A double blind trial. In: Drugs Affecting Lipid Metabolism. R Fumagalli, D Kritchevsky, R Paoletti, eds. Elsevier/North-Holland Biomedical Press, Amsterdam, New York, Oxford, 1980, pp 109-114.

a Bargeton, D., Salesse, J., Barber, J., and De Lavierre, C. Influence du nombre et de la position des functions hydoxylees et cetoniques sur l'activite choleretique et la toxicite de quelques acids biliares. Arch. Int. Pharmacodynam. 90:18-32, 1952.

b Barker, D.J.P., Gardner, M.J., Power, C., and Hutt, M.S.R. Prevalence of gall stones at necropsy in nine British towns: a collaborative study. Br. Med. J. 2:1389-1392, 1979.

c Barlattani, M., Carignola, W., Guglielmi, G., and Mammarella, A. Medical treatment to dissolve biliary cholesterol calculi. Biochemical and histological aspects of liver parenchyma in animals submitted to short- and long-term treatment with chenodeoxycholic acid. Influence of chenotherapy. Clin. Ter. 71:437-457, 1974.

d Barnes, S., Gollan, J.L., and Billing, B.H. Renal tubular reabsorption of bile acids by the isolated rat kidney. Clin. Sci. & Mol. Med. 51:14-15p, 1976 (abstract).

e Barnes, S., Gollan, J.L., and Billing, B.H. Role of renal tubular reabsorption of bile acids in cholestasis. Digestion 14:474, 1976 (abstract).

f Barnes, S., Thjodliefsson, B., Billing, B.H., and Sherlock, S. Plasma elimination of a tracer dose of cholyl-1-^{14}C-glycine in liver disease. Clin. Sci. & Mol. Med. 51:51p, 1976 (abstract).

g Barnes, S., Burhol, P.G., Zander, R., Haggstrom, G., Settine, R.L., and Hirschowitz, B.I. Enzymatic sulfation of glycochenodeoxycholic acid by tissue fractions from adult hamsters. J. Lipid Res. 20:952-959, 1979.

h Barnes, S., Burhol, P.G., Zander, R., and Hirschowitz, B.I. The effect of bile duct ligation on hepatic bile acid sulfotransferase activity in the hamster. Biochem. Med. 22:165-174, 1979.

i Barnes, S. Preparation and characterization of permethylated derivatives of bile acid and their application to gas chromatographic analysis. J. Chromatog. 183:269-276, 1980.

j Barnes, S., Waldrop, R., and Spenney, J.G. Diminished enzymatic bile salt sulfation in rhesus monkeys. Gastroenterology 80:1326, 1981 (abstract).

k Barnes, S., and J.M. Geckle. High resolution nuclear magnetic resonance spectroscopy of bile salts: individual proton assignments for sodium cholate in aqueous solution at 400 MHz. J. Lipid Res. 23:161-170, 1982.

l Barry, E.J. The effect of a deficiency of methionine and cystine on the conjugation of bile acids in the rat. Dissertation Abstracts, Ann Arbor, Michigan, Section B, 27:9100, 1966.

m Barth, C. and Hilmar, I. Taurocholate inhibits the glucocorticoid-induced rise of 3-hydroxy-3-methylglutaryl-CoA reductase in primary culture of hepatocytes. Europ. J. Biochem. 110:237-240, 1980.

a Barth, C., et al. Morphology and metabolism of adult rat hepatocytes in primary culture. Hoppe-Seyler's Physiol. Chem. 361:1017-1027, 1980.

b Bartrum, R.J., Crow, H.C., and Foote, S.R. Ultrasonic and radiographic cholecystography. N. Engl. Med. 296:538-541, 1977.

c Bashour, J.T. and Bauman, L. The solubility of cholesterol in bile salt solutions. J. Biol. Chem. 121:1-3, 1937.

d Bateson, M.C. and Bouchier, I.A.D. Prevalence of gallstones in Dundee: A necroscopy report. Brit. Med. J. 4:427-430, 1975.

e Bateson, M.C., Hopwood, D., and Bouchier, I.A.D. Effect of gallstone dissolution therapy on human liver structure. Am. J. Dig. Dis. 22:293-299, 1977.

f Bateson, M.C., Ross, P.E., Murison, J., and Bouchier, I.A.D. Effect of prolonged feeding with chenodeoxycholic acid on bile in patients with and without gallstones. Gut 18:599-605, 1977.

g Bateson, M.C., MacLean, D., Evans, J.R., and Bouchier, I.A.D. Chenodeoxycholic acid therapy for hypertriglyceridemia in men. Br. J. Clin. Pharm. 5:249-254, 1978.

h Bateson, M.D., MacLean, D., Ross, P.E., and Bouchier, I.A.D. Clofibrate therapy and gallstone induction. Dig. Dis. & Sci. 23:623-628, 1978.

i Bateson, M.C., Murison, J., Ross, P.E., and Bouchier, I.A.D. Comparison of fixed doses of chenodeoxycholic acid for gallstone dissolution. Lancet 1:1111-1114, 1978.

j Bateson, M.C., Ross, P.E., Murison, J.C., and Bouchier, I.A.D. Reversal of clofibrate-induced cholesterol oversaturation of bile with chenodeoxycholic acid. Brit. Med. J. 1:1171-1173, 1978.

k Bateson, M.C. and Iqbal, J. Ursodeoxycholic acid and serum-lipids. Lancet 2:151, 1979.

l Bateson, M.C. and Bouchier, I.A.D. Therapy with chenodeoxycholic acid (CDCA) and ursodeoxycholic acid (UDCA) in hyperlipidaemia. VII International Symposium on Drugs Affecting Lipid Metabolism, 1980.

m Bateson, M.C., Hill, A., and Bouchier, I.A.D. Analysis of response to ursodeoxycholic acid for gallstone dissolution. Digestion 20:358-364, 1980.

n Bateson, M.C., Ross, P.E., Murison, J.C., Saunders, J.H.B., and Bouchier, I.A.D. Ursodeoxycholic acid therapy and biliary lipids: A dose-response study. Gut 21:305-310, 1980.

o Bateson, M.C., Trash, D.B., and Bouchier, I.A.D. Can a six-month cholecystogram predict eventual response to gallstone dissolution therapy? Gut 21:A443, 1980 (abstract).

a Bateson, M.C., Bouchier, I.A.D., Trash, D.B., Maudgal, D.P., and Northfield, T.C. Calcification of radiolucent gall stones during treatment with ursodeoxycholic acid. Br. Med. J. 283:645-646, 1981.

b Bateson, M.C., Maudgal, D.P., Trash, D.B., Northfield, T.C., and Bouchier, I.A.D. Gallstone calcification caused by ursodeoxycholic acid (UDCA). Gut 22:A432, 1981 (abstract).

c Bateson, M.C. Dissolving gall stones. Brit. Med. J. 284:1-3, 1982 (editorial).

d Bateson, M.C. Ursodeoxycholic acid and gallstone calcification. (Letter) Lancet 1:47, 1982.

e Batey, R.G. Chenodeoxycholic acid in the management of gallstones. Drugs 14:116-119, 1977.

f Batta, A.K. and Salen, G. Taurine increases the effectiveness of urso deoxycholic acid as a gallstone dissolving agent. Hepatology 1:494, 1981 (abstract).

g Batta, A.K., Salen, G., and Shefer, S. The effect of feeding tauroursodeoxycholic acid on biliary bile acid composition. Gastroenterology 80:1106, 1981 (Abstract).

h Batta, A.K., Shefer, S., and Salen, G. Thin-layer chromatographic separation of conjugates of ursodeoxycholic acid from those of litho-, chenodeoxy-, deoxy-, and cholic acids. J. Lipid Res. 22:712-714, 1981.

i Bazzoli, F., Geminiani, S., Roda, A., Mazzella, G., Sama, C., Aldini, R., Morselli, A.M., Festi, D., Roda, E., and Barbara, L. Ursodeoxycholic acid in the dissolution of cholesterol gallstones: A blind-controlled trial. Ital. J. Gastroenterol. (Suppl 11) 115, 1979 (abstract).

j Bazzoli, F., Fromm, H., Roda, A., Sarva, R., and Roda, E. Bile acid metabolism in relation to hepatotoxicity after treatment with chenodeoxycholic and ursodeoxycholic acids in the rhesus monkey. Gastroenterology 78:1301, 1980 (abstract).

l Bazzoli, F., Sarva, R.P., Fromm, H., and Ceryak, S. Comparative formation of lithocholic acid (LC) from ursodeoxycholic acid (UDC) and chenodeoxycholic acids (CDC) in the human colon. Gastroenterology 79:1004, 1980 (abstract).

m Bazzoli, F., Sarva, R.P., Fromm, H., Ceryak, S., and Sembrat, R.F. Lithocholic acid is formed from chenodeoxycholic and ursodeoxycholic acids at a similar rate. Gastroenterology 80:1107, 1981 (Abstract).

n Bazzoli, F., Roda, A., Fromm, H., Sarva, R.P., Roda, E., and Barbara, L. Relation between serum and biliary bile acids as indicator of chenodeoxycholic and ursodeoxycholic acid-induced hepatotoxicity in the rhesus monkey. Dig. Dis. & Sci. (in press).

a Beaudoin, M., Carey, M.C., and Small, D.M. Effects of taurodihydrofusidate, a bile salt analogue, on bile formation and biliary lipid secretion in the Rhesus monkey. J. Clin. Invest. 56:1431-1441, 1975.

b Beckett, G.J., Douglas, J.G., Finlayson, N.D.C., and Percy-Robb, I.W. Differential timing of maximal postprandial concentrations of plasma chenodeoxycholate and cholate: its variability and implications. Digestion 22:248-254, 1981.

c Been, J.M., Bills, P.M., and Lewis, D. Electron probe microanalysis in the study of gallstones. Gut 18:836-842, 1977.

d Beesley, R. and Faust, R. Bile-salt inhibition of sodium ion-coupled d-glucose and L-alanine accumulation by brush-border-membrane vesicles from hamster jejunum. Biochem. J. 190:731-736, 1980.

e Begemann, F. Ein einfaches Verfahren zur Isolierung freier und konjugierter Gallensauren im Serum. Z. Klin. Chem. Klin. Biochem. 10:29-32, 1972.

f Begemann, F. Kinetik des Triglyzeridstoffwechsels unter Chenodesoxycholsauretherapie. Z. Gastroenterol. 13:314-317, 1975.

g Begemann, F. Zur Ursache der verminderten Triglyceridsynthese unter Chenodesoxycholsaure. 82. Tagung der Dtsch. Gesellsch. Inn. Med., Weisbaden, April, 1976.

h Begemann, F., Bandomer, G., and Herget, H.J. Die Beeinflussung der biliaren Lithogenitat durch Chenodesoxycholsaure und durch b-Sitosterin. 86. Tagung der I. Medizinischen Universitatsklinik, Hamburg, 22:27-28, 1976 (abstract).

i Begemann, F., Brunner, H., Caspary, W., Erb, W., Fromm, H., Leuschner, U., Mockel, G., Paumgartner, G., Stiehl, A., Weis, H., and Wolpers, C. Hinweise fur die Auflosung von Cholesteringallensteinen mit Chenodesoxycholsaure. Internist 18:114-115, 1977.

j Begemann, F. and Bandomer, G. Combination therapy with beta-sitosterin and chenic acid for the dissolution of biliary calculi. Verh. Dtsch. Ges. Inn. Med. 84:1103-1105, 1978.

k Begemann, F., Bandomer, G., and Herget, H.J. The influence of b-sitosterol on biliary cholesterol saturation and bile acid kinetics in man. Scand. J. Gastroenterol. 13:57-63, 1978.

l Begemann, F., Bandomer, G., Kruger, W., Schumpelick, V. Lokale Gallensaurenruckresorption als Lithogenitatsfaktor bei Cholecystitis. Z. Gastroenterol. XIX (9), 1981 (abstract 9).

m Beher, W.T. and Baker, G.D. Effect of dietary bile acids on in vivo cholesterol metabolism in the rat. Proc. Soc. Exptl. Biol. Med. 98:892-894, 1958.

a Beher, W.T., Beher, M.E., and Rao, B. Turnover of cholic and chenodeoxycholic acids in normal and hypophysectomised rats. Life Sciences 6:863-866, 1967.

b Beher, W.T., Rao, B., Beher, M.E., and Bertiasius, J. Bile acid synthesis in normal and hypophysectomised rats: A rate study using cholestyramine. Proc. Soc. Exptl. Biol. Med. 124:1193-1197, 1967.

c Beher, W.T., Filus, A.M., Rao, B., and Beher, M.E. A comparative study of bile acid metabolism in the rat, mouse, hamster, and gerbil. Proc. Soc. Exptl. Biol. Med. 130:1067-1074, 1969.

d Beher, W.T., Casazza, K.K., Beher, M.E., Filus, A.M., and Bertiasius, J. Effects of cholesterol on bile acid metabolism in the rat. Proc. Soc. Exptl. Biol. Med. 134:595-602, 1970.

e Beher, W.T., Lin, G.J., Casazza, K.K., and Bertiasius, J. Effects on anion-exchange polymers on bile acid metabolism in the rat. Atherosclerosis 16:169-174, 1972.

f Beke, R., DeWeerdt, G.A., Parijs, J., Huybrechts, W., and Barbier, F. Separation of conjugated and unconjugated bile acids by thin-layer chromatography. Clin. Chim. Acta 70:197-199, 1976.

g Beker, S. Treatment of cholesterol gallstones with chenic acid. A follow-up study of 25 patients. Am. J. Gastroenterol. 68:455-460, 1977.

h Bell, C.C., Jr., Vlahcevic, Z.R., and Swell, L. Alterations in the lipids of human hepatic bile after the oral administration of bile salts. Surg. Gyn. & Obst. 132:36-42, 1971.

i Bell, C.C., Jr., McCormick, W.C., III, Gregory, D.H., Law, D.H., Vlahcevic, Z.R., and Swell, L. Relationship of bile acid pool size to the formation of lithogenous bile in male Indians of the Southwest. Surg. Gyn. & Obst. 134:473-478, 1972.

j Bell, C.C., Jr., Almond, H.R., Vlahcevic, Z.R., Gregory, D.H., and Swell, L. The effect of cholecystectomy on bile acid pool size, kinetics, and biliary lipid composition in patients with cholesterol gallstones. Gastroenterology 64:879, 1973 (abstract).

k Bell, C.C., Jr., Vlahcevic, Z.R., Prazich, J., and Swell, L. Evidence that a diminished bile acid pool precedes the formation of cholesterol gallstones in man. Surg. Gyn. & Obst. 136:961-965, 1973.

l Bell, G.D., Sutor, D.J., Whitney, B., and Dowling, R.H. Factors influencing human gallstone dissolution in monkey, dog, and human bile. Gut 13:836, 1972 (abstract).

m Bell, G.D., Whitney, B., and Dowling, R.H. Gallstone dissolution in man using chenodeoxycholic acid. Lancet 2:1213-1216, 1972.

a Bell, G.D. and Dowling, R.H. The effects of chenodeoxycholic acid on bile composition in the Rhesus monkey and in man. Biol. Gastroenterol. 6:171-172, 1973.

b Bell, G.D., Lewis, B., Petrie, A., and Dowling, R.H. Serum lipids in cholelithiasis: Effect of chenodeoxycholic acid therapy. Brit. Med. J. 3:520-523, 1973.

c Bell, G.D., Mok, H.Y.I., Thwe, M., Murphy, G.M., Henry, K., and Dowling, R.H. Liver structure and function in cholelithiasis: Effect of chenodeoxycholic acid. Gut 15:165-172, 1974.

d Bell, G.D., Dowling, R.H., Whitney, B., and Sutor, D.J. The value of radiology in predicting gallstone type when selecting patients for medical treatment. Gut 16:359-364, 1975.

e Bell, G.D. The common gallstone: Take a closer look. Mod. Med. Asia 13:10-13, 1977.

f Bell, G.D. Medical treatment of gallstones. J. Royal Coll. Phys. London 13:47-52, 1979.

g Bell, G.D. and Doran, J. Gall stone dissolution in man using an essential oil preparation - Rowachol. Brit. Med. J. 1:24, 1979.

h Bell, G.D. Drugs used in the management of gallstones. In Side Effects of Drugs Annual, MNG Dukes, and J Elis, eds. Excerpta Medica Press, Amesterdam, Oxford, Princeton, 1981, pp 340-345.

i de Belle, R.C., Blacklow, N.R., Baylan, M., Little, J.M., and Lester, R. Bile acid conjugation in fetal hepatic organ culture. Gastroenterology 69:815, 1975 (abstract).

j Belobaba, D.T.E., Carlson, G.L., and LaRusso, N.F. A simple method for simultaneous specific activity measurements in a mixture of radiolabeled bile acids. J. Chromatogr. 172:410-416, 1979.

k Bennion, L.J. and Grundy, S.M. Effects of obesity and caloric intake on biliary lipid metabolism in man. J. Clin. Invest. 56:996-1011, 1975.

l Bennion, L.J., Ginsberg, R.L., Garnick, M.B., and Bennett, P.H. Effects of oral contraceptives on the gallbladder bile of normal women. N. Engl. J. Med. 294:189-192, 1976.

m Bennion, L.J. and Grundy, S.M. Effects of Diabetes Mellitus on cholesterol metabolism in man. N. Engl. J. Med. 296:1365-1371, 1977.

n Bennion, L.J., Drobny, E., Knowler, W.C., Ginsberg, R.L., Garnick, M.B., Adler, R.D., and Duane, W.C. Sex differences in the size of bile acid pools. Metabolism 27:961-969, 1978.

a Bennion, L.J. and Grundy, S.M. Risk factors for the development of cholelithiasis in man. N. Engl. J. Med. 299:1161-1167, 1978 (part I), 299:1221-1227, 1978 (part II).

b Bennion, L.J., Knowler, W.C., Mott, D.M., Spagnoia, A.M., and Bennett, P.H. Development of lithogenic bile during puberty in Pima Indians. N. Engl. J. Med. 300:873-876, 1979.

c Benoit, G., and Larrieu, H. Apport de la Radiokinesimetrie dans l' interpretation du reflux wirsungien dans les pancreatities aigues associees a une lithiase biliaire. Gastroenterol. Clin. Biol. 3:329-335, 1979.

d Beppu, T., Seyama, Y., Kasama, T., and Yamakawa, T. Quantitative determination of individual non-sulfated bile acids and sulfated lithocholic acid in serum by mass fragmentography. J. Biochem. 89:1963-1973, 1981.

e Beppu, T., Seyama, Y., Kasama, T., Serizawa, S., and Yamakawa, T. Serum bile acid profiles in cerebrotendinous xanthomatosis. Clin. Chim. Acta 118:167-175, 1982.

f van den Berg, G.W.O., van Blankenstein, M., Bosman-Jacobs, E.P., Frenkel, M., Horchner, P., Oost-Harwig, O.I., and Wilson, J.H.P. Solid phase radioimmunoassay for determination of conjugated cholic acid in serum. Clin. Chim. Acta. 73:277-283, 1976.

g van Berge Henegouwen, G.P., Ruben, A., and Brandt, K-H. Quantitative analysis of bile acids in serum and bile, using gas-liquid chromatography. Clin. Chim. Acta 54:249-261, 1974.

h van Berge Henegouwen, G.P., Brandt, K-H., Eyssen, H., and Parmentier, G. Sulfated and unsulfated bile acids in serum bile and urine of patients with cholestasis. Gut 17:861-869, 1976.

i van Berge Henegouwen, G.P. and Hofmann, A.F. A simple batch adsorption procedure for the isolation of sulfated and non-sulfated bile acids from serum. Clin. Chim. Acta 73:469-474, 1976.

j van Berge Henegouwen, G.P., Allan, R.N., Yu, P.Y.S., and Hofmann, A.F. A facile hydrolysis-solvolysis procedure for conjugated bile acid sulfates. J. Lipid Res. 18:118-122, 1977.

k van Berge Henegouwen, G.P., Hofmann, A.F., and Gaginella, T.S. Pharmacology of chenodeoxycholic acid. I. Pharmaceutical properties. Gastroenterology 73:291-299, 1977.

l van Berge Henegouwen, G.P., and Hofmann, A.F. Pharmacology of chenodeoxycholic acid. II. Absorption and metabolism. Gastroenterology 73:300-309, 1977.

m van Berge Henegouwen, G.P., Brandt, K-H., Ruben, A.Th., Schalm, S.W., and Taal, B. High frequency of lithogenic bile in primary biliary cirrhosis. Neth. J. Med. 25:89-93, 1982.

a Bergman, F. and van der Linden, W. Diet-induced cholesterol gallstones in hamsters: Prevention and dissolution by cholestyramine. Gastroenterology 53:418-421, 1967.

b Bergman, F., van der Linden, W., and Sjovall, J. Biliary bile acids and hepatic ultra-structure in hamsters fed gallstone-inducing and -dissolving diets. Acta Physiol. Scand. 74:480-491, 1968.

c Bergman, F., Juul, A.H., and van der Linden, W. Development and regression of morphological and biochemical changes in hamsters and mice fed a cholesterol-cholic acid containing diet. Acta Path. Microbiol. Scand. 78:179-191, 1970.

d Bergman, F. and van der Linden, W. Reaction of the Mongolian gerbil to a cholesterol-, cholic acid-containing gallstone-inducing diet. Acta Path. Microbiol. Scand. 79:476-486, 1971.

e Bergman, F. and van der Linden, W. Importance of diet for reaction of bile acid pattern to altered thyroid function. Z. Ernahr. 11:40-46, 1972.

f Bergman, F. and van der Linden, W. Effect of chenodeoxycholic acid on gallstone formation and liver morphology in hamsters and mice. Biol. Gastroent. 6:173, 1973.

g Bergman, F. and van der Linden, W. Liver morphology and gallstone formation in hamsters and mice treated with chenodeoxycholic acid. Acta Path. Microbiol. Scand. 81:213-221, 1973.

h Bergman, F. and van der Linden, W. Bile acid pool size in hamsters during gallstone formation and after cholecystectomy. Scand. J. Gastroenterol. 10:35, 1975.

i Bergman, F. and van der Linden, W. Effect of dietary fiber on gallstone formation in hamsters. Z. Ernahrungswiss, 14:218-224, 1975.

j von Bergmann, J., von Bergmann, K., Hadorn, B., and Paumgartner, G. Biliary lipid composition in early childhood. Clin. Chim. Acta 64:241, 1975.

k von Bergmann, K., Paumgartner, G., and Preisig, R. Increased cholesterol saturation in dog bile induced by chenodeoxycholic acid. Digestion 8:440, 1973 (abstract).

l von Bergmann, K., Schultheiss, H.R., and Paumgartner, G. Contrasting effects of different types of enzyme inducers on cholesterol saturation of rat bile. Digestion 10:317, 1974 (abstract).

m von Bergmann, K., Mok, H.Y.I., and Grundy, S.M. Regulation of bile acid pool size in man. Gastroenterology 69:877, 1975 (abstract).

n von Bergmann, K., Schultheiss, H.R., Paumgartner, G., and Preisig, R. Die Konjugation von Chenodesoxycholsaure und Cholsaure wahrend einer Leberpassage. Schweiz. med. Wschr. 105:413-415, 1975.

a von Bergmann, K., Mok, H.Y.I., and Grundy, S.M. Distribution of the bile acid pool in the fasting state in man. Gastroenterology 71:934, 1976 (abstract).

b von Bergmann, K., Gutsfeld, M., Schulz-Hagen, K., and von Unruh, G. Comparison of urso versus chenodeoxycholic acid on biliary lipid secretion in man. Gastroenterology 75:955, 1978 (abstract).

c von Bergmann, K., Mok, H.Y.I., Hardison, W.G.M., and Grundy, S.M. Cholesterol and bile acid metabolism in moderately advanced, stable cirrhosis of the liver. Gastroenterology 77:1183-1192, 1979.

d von Bergmann, K., Gutsfeld, M., Schulze-Hagen, K., and von Unruh, G. Effects of ursodeoxycholic acid on biliary lipid secretion in patients with radiolucent gallstones. In Biological Effects of Bile Acids. G Paumgartner, A Stiehl, and W Gerok, eds. MTP Press, Lancaster, 1979, pp 61-66.

e von Bergmann, K., Strottkoter, H., and Leiss, O. Decreased cholesterol absorption during ursodeoxycholic acid administration. Hepatology 1:670, 1981 (abstract).

f Bergmann, M. Ueber die peristaltische Wirksamikeit der Gallensauren und ihre klinische Anwendung. Wien. Klin. Wschr. 64:704-707, 1952.

g Bergstrom, S., Rottenberg, M., and Voltz, J. The preparation of some carboxyl-labelled bile acids. Acta Chem. Scand. 7:481-484, 1953.

h Bergstrom, S., Sjovall, J., and Voltz, J. Metabolism of lithocholic acid in the rat. Acta Physiol. Scand. 30:22, 1953.

i Bergstrom, S. and Sjovall, J. Occurrence and metabolism of chenodeoxycholic acid in the rat. Acta Chem. Scand. 8:611, 1954.

j Bergstrom, S. and Borgstrom, B. The intestinal absorption of fats. In Prog. Chem. Fats Other Lipids. RT Holman, WO Lundberg, T Malkin, eds. Pergammon Press, Ltd., New York, 1955, pp 351-393.

k Bergstrom, S. and Paabo, K. Preparation of 3a-hydroxychol-5-enic acid from hyodesoxycholic acid and corresponding 24-^{14}C-labelled acids. Acta Chem. Scand. 9:699, 1955.

l Bergstrom, S. and Danielsson, H. On the regulation of bile acid formation in the rat liver. Acta Physiol. Scand. 43:1, 1958.

m Bergstrom, S., Danielsson, H., and Goransson, A. On the bile acid metabolism in the pig. Acta Chem. Scand. 13:776, 1959.

n Bergstrom, S., Lindstedt, S., and Samuelsson, B. Bile Acids and Steroids 82: On the mechanism of deoxycholic acid formation in the rabbit. J. Biol. Chem. 234:2022-2025, 1959.

o Bergstrom, S. Metabolism of bile acids. Fed. Proc. 21:28-32, 1962.

p Bergstrom, S. and Danielsson, H. Formation and metabolism of bile acids. In Handbook of Physiology. Section 6: Alimentary Canal. CF Code, W Heidel eds. American Physiology Society, Washington, 5:2391, 1968.

a Berk, R.N. and Lasser, E.C. Altered concepts of the mechanism of nonvisualization of the gallbladder. Radiology 82:296-302, 1964.

b Berk, R.N. and Wheeler, H.O. The role of water reabsorption by the gallbladder in the mechanism of nonvisualization at cholecystography. Radiology 103:37-40, 1972.

c Berk, R.N., Loeb, P.M., Goldberger, L.E., and Sokoloff, J. Oral cholecystography with iopanoic acid. N. Eng. J. Med. 290:204-210, 1974.

d Berman, A.L., Snapp, E., Ivy, A.C., and Atkinson, A.J. On the regulation or homeostasis of the cholic acid output in biliary duodenal fistula dogs. Am. J. Physiol. 131:776-782, 1941.

e Berman, A.L., Snapp, E., Ivy, A.C., Hough, V.H., and Atkinson, A.J. The effect of dessicated hog bile and hog bile acid preparations on the volume and constituents of bile. Am. J. Physiol. 131:752-759, 1941.

f Bermann, C., Berourne, C., Brette, R., Chaput, J.C., Debray, C., Etienne, J.P., Gerolami, A., Paraf, A., Petite, J.P., Rautureau, J., and Sarles, H. Medical treatment of biliary cholesterol lithiasis by chenodeoxycholic acid (chenic acid). French multicenter controlled test. Nouv. Presse Med. 6:41-43, 1977.

g Bermann, C., Brette, R., Chaput, J.C., Debray, C., Etienne, J.P., Gerolami, A., Paraf, A., Petite, J.P., Rautureau, J., and Sarles, H. Multicenter study of the effect of different doses of chenodeoxycholic acid in cholesterol biliary lithiasis. Therapie 32:403, 1977.

h Bernades, P., Bertrand, L., Bouvry, M., Colin, R., Geffroy, Y., Hecht, Y., Klepping, C., Lambert, R., Levy, V.G., Michel, H., Paliard, P., Paris, J., and Quinton, A. Traitement de la lithiase biliaire cholesterolique par l'acide ursodesoxycholique. Resultats d'une etude multicentrique en double insu. Nouv. Presse Med. 11:587-589, 1982.

i Bernstein, L.H., Gutstein, S., and Weiner, S. Folic acid conjugate: Inhibition by unconjugated dihydroxy bile acids. Proc. Soc. Exptl. Biol. Med. 132:1167-1169, 1969.

j Berretta, S. Perfusione del coledoco con acido ursacolico nel trattamento della calcolosi residua. Min. Diet. Gastroenterol. 27:11-16, 1981.

k Berseus, O. Conversion of cholesterol to bile acids in rat: Purification and properties of a d^4-3-ketosteroid-5b-reductase and a 3a-hydroxysteroid dehydrogenase. Bile Acids and Steroids 187. Europ. J. Biochem. 2:493-502, 1967.

l Berthelot, P., Erlinger, S., Dhumeaux, D., and Preaux, A-M. Mechanism of phenobarbital-induced choleresis in the rat. Am. J. Physiol. 219:809-813, 1970.

a Besancon, F. and Marche, C. Lithase de cause medicamenteuse chez la souris: Comparison entre le dehydrocholate et d'autres choleretiques. Therapie 25:487-501, 1970.

b Besancon, F., Marche, C., Barret, C., et al. Pharmachologie de la lithiase vesiculare. Effets preventif et curatif de diverses medications chez la souris. Therapie 25:463-485, 1970.

c Besancon, F., Marche, C., Barret, C., et al. Therapeutique experimentale de la lithiase vesiculaire. Effet preventif et curatif de diverses medications chez la souris. Arch. Fran. Mal. App. Dig. 59:353-376, 1970.

d Besancon, F., Marche, C., and Parrot, J. Lithiase experimentale par exces d'acide cholique chez la souris. Bio. Gastroenterol. 2:147-160, 1970.

e Besancon, F., Marche, C., and Parrot, J. Pathologie experimentale de la lithiase vesiculaire. Relations entre la lithiase et les lesions. Arch. Fran. Mal. App. Dig. 59:429-452, 1970.

f Besancon, F. and Marche, C. Similitudes pathologiques et therapeutiques entre l'atherosclerose et al cholecystite lithiasique. Ann. Med. Interne 122:1037-1044, 1971.

g Besancon, F. Les lithiases biliaires et cholecystites lithiasiques experimentales. M.C.D. 4(Suppl. 1):39-44, 1975.

h Besancon, F. La formation des calculs biliaires. Mat. Med. Polona, 1, 1976.

i Best, R., Rasmussen, J., and Wilson, C. An evaluation of solutions for fragmentation and dissolution of gallstones and their effect on liver and ductal tissue. Ann. Surg. 138:570-581, 1953.

j Betteridge, D., Krone, W., Middleton, C., and Galton, D. Regulation of sterol synthesis in human intestinal mucosa. Eur. J. Clin. Invest. 10:227-230, 1980.

k Bevan, G., Engert, R., Klipstein, F.A., Maldonado, N., Rubulis, A., and Turner, M.D. Bile salt metabolism in tropical sprue. Gut 15:254-259, 1974.

l Bevans, M. and Mosbach, E.H. Biological studies of dihydrocholesterol: Production of biliary concrements and inflammatory lesions of the biliary tract in rabbits. Arch. Path. 62:112-117, 1956.

m Bhattacharyya, A.K., Connor, W.E., and Spector, A.A. Abnormalities of cholesterol turnover in hypercholesterolemic (type II) patients. J. Lab. Clin. Med. 88:202-214, 1976.

n Biffl, H., Pristautz, H., Parsche, P., Passath, A., and Leb, G. Clinical evaluation of serum bile acids as a new liver function test. Acta Med. Austriaca 7:52-55, 1981.

a Bikhazi, A.B. and Higuchi, W.I. An interfacial barrier limited transport of cholesterol across an aqueous polysorbate 80-hexadecane interface. J. Pharm Sci. 59:744, 1970.

b Bikhazi, A.B. and Higuchi, W.I. Interfacial barriers to the transport of sterols and other organic solutes at the oil/water interface. Biochem. Biophys. Acta 233:676, 1971.

c Bilton, R.F., Mason, A.N., and Smith, D.V. The localization and induction of bile acid dehydrogenases in Pseudomonas N.C.I.B. 10590. Biochem. Soc. Trans. 5:1717-1719, 1977.

d Binder, H.J. and Rawlins, C.L. Effect of conjugated dihydroxy bile salts on electrolyte transport in rat colon. J. Clin. Invest. 52:1460-1466, 1973.

e Binder, H.J., Filburn, B., and Floch, M. Bile acid inhibition of intestinal anaerobic organisms. Am. J. Clin. Nutr. 28:119-125, 1975.

f Binder, H.J., Filburn, C., and Volpe, B.T. Bile salt alteration of colonic electrolyte transport: Role of cyclic adenosine monophosphate. Gastroenterology 68:503-508, 1975.

g Binet, S., Delage, Y., and Erlinger, S. Influence of taurocholate, taurochenodeoxycholate, and taurodehydrocholate on sulfobromophthalein transport into bile. Am. J. Physiol. 236:E10-E14, 1979.

h Birkett, D. and Silen, W. The pH-dependent effect of sodium taurocholate on increasing gastric mucosal permeability. Gut 15:336, 1974 (abstract).

i Birkner, H.J. and Kern, F., Jr. In vitro adsorption of bile salts to food residues, salicylazosulfapyridine, and hemicellulose. Gastroenterology 67:237-244, 1974.

j Bjorkhem, I., Danielsson, H., Issidorides, C., and Kallner, A. On the synthesis and metabolism of cholest-4-en-7a-ol-3-one. Acta Chem. Scand. 19:2151, 1965.

k Bjorkhem, I., Danielsson, H., Einarsson, K., and Johansson, G. Formation of bile acids in man: Conversion of cholesterol into 5b-cholestane-3a,7a,12a-triol in liver homogenates. J. Clin. Invest. 47:1573-1582, 1968.

l Bjorkhem, I., Einarsson, K., and Johansson, G. Formation and metabolism of 3b-hydroxycholest-5-en-7-one and cholest-5-one-3b,7b-diol. Acta Chem. Scand. 22:1595, 1968.

m Bjorkhem, I. and Gustafsson, J. On the conversion of cholestanol into allocholic acid in rat liver. Europ J. Biochem. 18:207-213, 1971.

n Bjorkhem, I., Danielsson, H., and Wikvall, K. 7a-Hydroxylation of taurodeoxycholic acid by a reconstituted system from rat liver microsomes. Biochem. Biophys. Res. Comm. 53:609-616, 1973.

a Bjorkhem, I., Einarsson, K., and Hellers, G. Metabolism of mono- and dihydroxylated bile acids in preparations of human liver. Europ. J. Clin. Invest. 3:459-465, 1973.

b Bjorkhem, I. and Gustafsson, J. Omega-hydroxylation of steroid side-chain in biosynthesis of bile acids. Europ. J. Biochem. 36:201-212, 1973.

c Bjorkhem, I. and Danielsson, H. Assay of liver microsomal cholesterol 7a-hydroxylase using deuterated carrier and gas chromatography-mass spectrometry. Anal. Biochem. 59:508, 1974.

d Bjorkhem, I., Danielsson, H., and Wikvall, K. Hydroxylations of bile acids by reconstituted systems from rat liver microsomes. J. Biol. Chem. 249:6439-6445, 1974.

e Bjorkhem, I., Danielsson, H., and Wikvall, K. Cytochrome P-450 - Dependent hydroxylations in biosynthesis and metabolism of bile acids. Biochem. Soc. Transact. 3:825-828, 1975.

f Bjorkhem, I., Gustafsson, J., Johansson, G., and Persson, B. Biosynthesis of bile acids in man: Hydroxylation of the C27-steroid side chain. J. Clin. Invest. 55:478-486, 1975.

g Bjorkhem, I. and Angelin, B. Evidence for differences in absorptive pattern between individual bile acids in man. Gut 17:420-426, 1976.

h Black, R.B., Hole, D., and Rhodes, J. Bile damage to the gastric mucosal barrier: The influence of pH and bile acid concentration. Gastroenterology 61:178-184, 1971.

i Blaskiewicz, R.J., O'Neil, G.J., Jr., and Elliot, W.H. Bile acids. XLI. Hepatic microsomal 12a-hydroxylation of allochenodeoxycholate to allocholate. Proc. Soc. Exptl. Biol. Med. 146:92-95, 1974.

j Bloch, C.A. and Watkins, J.B. Determination of conjugated bile acids in human bile and duodenal fluid by reverse-phase high-performance liquid chromatography. J. Lipid Res. 19:510-513, 1978.

k Bloch, H.M., Thornton, J.R., and Heaton, K.W. Effects of fasting on the composition of gallbladder bile. Gut 21:1087-1089, 1980.

l Bloch, K., Berg, B.N., and Rittenberg, D. The biological conversion of cholesterol to cholic acid. J. Biol. Chem. 149:511, 1943.

m Bloomfield, D.K. Dynamics of cholesterol metabolism. I. Factors regulating total sterol biosynthesis and accumulation in the rat. Proc. Natl. Acad. Sci. U.S. 50:117-124, 1963.

n Blow, D.M. and Rich, A. Studies on the formation of helical deoxycholate complexes. J. Am. Chem. Soc. 82:3566-3571, 1960.

o Blum, L. and Spritz, N. The metabolism of intravenously injected isotopic cholic acid in Laennec's cirrhosis. J. Clin. Invest. 45:187-193, 1966.

a Bode, J.C., Zelder, O., and Neuberger, H.O. Effect of taurocholate, dehydrocholate and secretin on biliary output alkaline phosphatase. Helv. Med. Acta 37:143-151, 1973.

b Bode, J.C., Zelder, O., and Bode, C. Qualitative and quantitative altera tions of hepatic bile flow during recovery from extrahepatic cholestasis. In Problems in Intrahepatic Cholestasis. P Gentilini, H Popper, S Sherlock, and U Teodori, eds., Karger, Basel, 1979, pp 83-87.

c Bogren, A. and Larsson, K. Crystalline components of biliary calculi. Scand J. Clin. Lab. Invest. 15:457-462, 1963.

d Bojanowicz, K. and Witkowska, A. Possibility of gallstone dissolution of biliary calculi with chenodeoxycholic acid. Pol. Tyg. Lek. 32:1299-1302, 1977.

e Bokkenheuser, V., Hoshita, T., and Mosbach, E.H. Bacterial 7-dehydroxylation of cholic acid and allocholic acid. J. Lipid Res. 10:421-426, 1969.

f Bolton, C., Nicholls, J., and Heaton, K. Estimation of cholesterol in bile: Assessment of an enzymatic method. Clin. Chim. Acta 105:225-230, 1980.

g Bongfiglio, M., Casamichiela, M., and Garagnani, A. Preliminary experience with the use of ursodeoxycholic acid in the treatment of biliary calculosis. Clin. Ter. 88:491-497, 1979.

h Bonorris, G.G., Coyne, M., Chung, A., and Schoenfield, L.J. Mechanism of estrogen-induced saturated bile in the hamster. J. Lab. Clin. Med. 90:963-970, 1977.

i Booyapisit, S.T., Trotman, B.W., Ostrow, J.D., Olivieri, P.J., and Gallo, D. Measurement of conjugated and unconjugated bilirubin in bile. A new thin-layer chromatographic method. J. Lab. Clin. Med. 88:857-863, 1976.

j Booyapisit, S.T., Trotman, B.W., and Ostrow, J.D. Unconjugated bilirubin and the hydrolysis of conjugated bilirubin in gallbladder bile of patients with cholelithiasis. Gastroentrology 74:70-74, 1978.

k Borel, G.A. Lithogenese biliaire. Physiopathologie et applications theraputiques. Schweiz. med. Wschr. 103:161-163, 1973.

l Borel, G.A., Lemp, R., Diallo, T.H., and Magnenat, P. Cholic acid clearance in normal subjects and in patients with liver disease. Helv. med. Acta 37:201-207, 1973.

m Borel, G.A. and Magnenat, P. The clearance of a tracer dose of cholic acid in liver cirrhosis. Helv. med. Acta 37:129-135, 1973.

n Borgman, R.F. and Haselden, F.H. Cholelithiasis in rabbits: Effects of several treatments on formation and dissolution of gallstones. Am. J. Vet. Res. 30:1979-1984, 1969.

a Borgman, R.F. and Haselden, F.H. Cholelithiasis in rabbits: Effects of cod liver oil on dissolution of gallstones. Am. J. Vet. Res. 32:427-432, 1971.

b Borgman, R.F. and Haselden, F.H. Cholelithiasis in rabbits: Influence of dietary roughage on gallstone formation. Am. J. Vet. Res. 32:433, 1971.

c Borgman, R.F. and Haselden, F.H. Cholelithiasis in rabbits: Effects of steroids on dissolution of gallstones. Am. J. Vet. Res. 33:847-851, 1972.

d Borgstrom, B., Dahlqvist, A., Lundh, G., and Sjovall, J. Studies of intestinal digestion and absorption in the human. J. Clin. Invest. 36:1521-1536, 1957.

e Borgstrom, B. Studies of intestinal cholesterol absorption in the human. J. Clin. Invest. 39:809-815, 1960.

f Borgstrom, B., Lundh, G., and Hofmann, A.F. The site of absorption of conjugated bile salts in man. Gastroenterology 45:299-308, 1963.

g Borgstrom, B. The behavior of micellar solution during gel filtration. Surface Chemistry 225-230, 1965.

h Borgstrom, B. The dimension of the bile salt micelle: Measurements by gel filtration. Biochim. Biophys. Acta 106:171-183, 1965.

i Borgstrom, B. Partition of lipids between emulsified oil and micellar phases of glyceride-bile salt dispersions. J. Lipid Res. 8:598-608, 1967.

j Borgstrom, B. and Erlanson, C. Pancreatic lipase and co-lipase. Interactions and effects of bile salts and other detergents. Europ. J. Biochem. 37:60-68, 1973.

k Borgstrom, B. Bile salts - their physiological functions in the gastrointestinal tract. Acta Med. Scand. 196:1-10, 1974.

l Borgstrom, B. and Donner, J. Binding of bile salts to pancreatic colipase and lipase. J. Lipid Res. 16:287-292, 1975.

m Borgstrom, B. Interactions of pancreatic lipase with bile salts and dodecyl sulfate. J. Lipid Res. 17:491-496, 1976.

n Borgstrom, B. Phospholipid absorption. In Lipid Absorption: Biochemical and Clinical Aspects. K Rommel, H Goebell, eds. MTP Press, Lancaster, 1976, pp 65-70.

o Borowsky, S.A., Bonorris, G.G., Goldstein, L.I., and Schoenfield, L.J. Effects of chenodeoxycholic and lithocholic acids on hamster liver ultrastructure. Gastroenterology 66:668, 1974 (abstract).

p Bortz, W.M. and Steele, L.A. Synchronization of hepatic cholesterol synthesis, cholesterol and bile acid content, fatty acid synthesis and plasma free fatty acid levels in the fed and fasted rat. Biochim. Biophys. Acta 306:85, 1973.

a Bortz, W.M., Steele, L.A., Arkens, L., and Grundhofer, B. Studies on the alteration of hepatic cholesterol synthesis in the rat. Biochim. Biophys. Acta 316:366-377, 1973.

b Bose, A.K., Pramanik, B.N., and Fujiwara, H. Identification and quantitation of bile acids using stable isotope labels. In Proc. II Intl. Conf. Stable Isotopes. ed. ER Klein and PD Klein, Conf. 751027. National Technical Information Service, Springfield, VA, 1975, pp 711-715.

c Boston Collaborative Drug Surveillance Programme. Oral contraceptives and venous thromboembolic disease, surgically confirmed gallbladder disease and breast tumors. Lancet 1:1399-1404, 1973.

d Boston Collaborative Drug Surveillance Programme. Surgically confirmed gallbladder disease, venous thromboembolism, and breast tumors in relation to postmenopausal estrogen therapy. N. Eng. J. Med. 290:15-19, 1974.

e Botham, K.M., Lawson, M.E., Beckett, G.J., Percy-Robb, I.W., and Boyd, G.S. The effect of portal blood bile salt concentrations on bile salt synthesis in rat liver. Biochim. Biophys. Acta 666:238-245, 1981.

f Botham, K.M., Lawson, M.E., Beckett, G.J., Percy-Robb, I.W., and Boyd, G.S. Portal blood concentrations of conjugated cholic and chenodeoxycholic acids. Relationships to bile salt synthesis in liver cells. Biochim. Biophys. Acta 665:81-87, 1981.

g Bouchier, I.A.D., Cooperband, S.R., and Ei Kodsi, B.M. Mucous substances and viscosity of normal and pathological human bile. Gastroenterology 49:343-353, 1965.

h Bouchier, I.A.D. Macromolecular material in bile and its relationship to gallstone formation. S. Afr. Med. J. 40:735-738, 1966.

i Bouchier, I.A.D. and Cooperband, S.R. Isolation and characterization of a macromolecular aggregate associated with bilirubin. Clin. Chim. Acta 15:291-302, 1967.

j Bouchier, I.A.D. and Cooperband, S.R. Sephadex filtration of a macromolecular aggregate associated with bilirubin. Clin. Chim. Acta 15:303-313, 1967.

k Bouchier, I.A.D. and Freston, J.W. The aetiology of gallstones. Lancet 1:340-344, 1968.

l Bouchier, I.A.D. Recent concepts of gallstone formation. Tijdschr. Gastroenterol. 13:301-308, 1970.

m Bouchier, I.A.D. The vagus, the bile and gallstones. Gut 11:799-803, 1970.

n Bouchier, I.A.D. Experimental cholelithiasis. Sci. Basis Med. Ann. Rev. 232-243, 1971.

o Bouchier, I.A.D. Gallstone formation. Lancet 1:711-715, 1971.

a Bouchier, I.A.D. The biochemistry of gallstone formation. Clin. Gastroenterol. 2:49-66, 1973.

b Bouchier, I.A.D. Gallstones. In Modern Trends in Gastroenterology. AE Read, ed. Butterworths, 1975, pp 203-223.

c Bouchier, I.A.D. Gallstones. Brit. Med. J. 2:870-872, 1976.

d Bouchier, I.A.D. Gallstones. Proc. R. Soc. Med. 70:597-599, 1977.

e Bouchier, I.A.D. Medical treatment of gallstones. Ann. Rev. Med. 31:59-77, 1980.

f Bouma, M., Levy, V., and Infante, R. Liver ultrastructure in cholesterolic gallstone patients before and after treatment with chenodeoxycholic acid. Gastroenterol. Clin. Biol. 4:569-576, 1980.

g Bourges, M., Small, D.M., and Dervichian, D.G. Biophysics of lipidic association. II. The ternary systems: Cholesterol-lecithin-water. Biochim. Biophys. Acta 137:157-167, 1967.

h Bourges, M., Small, D.M., and Dervichian, D.G. Biophysics of lipidic associations. III. The quaternary systems lecithin-bile salt-cholesterol-water. Biochim. Biophys. Acta 144:189-201, 1967.

i Boyd, G.S. and Percy-Robb, I.W. Enzymatic regulation of bile acid synthesis. Am. J. Med. 51:580-587, 1971.

j Boyer, J.L. and Klatskin, G. Canalicular bile flow and bile secretory pressure - evidence of a non-bile salt dependent fraction in the isolated perfused rat liver. Gastroenterology 59:853-859, 1970.

k Boyer, J.L., Scheig, R.L., and Klatskin, G. The effect of sodium taurocholate on the hepatic metabolism of sulfobromophthalein sodium (BSP): The role of bile flow. J. Clin. Invest. 49:206-215, 1970.

l Boyer, J.L. Canalicular bile formation in the isolated perfused rat liver. Am. J. Physiol. 221:1156-1163, 1971.

m Boyer, J.L. Effect of chronic ethanol feeding on bile formation and secretion of lipids in the rat. Gastroenterology 62:294-301, 1972.

n Boyer, J.L. and Bloomer, J.R. Canalicular bile secretion in man. Studies utilizing the biliary clearance of ^{14}C-mannitol. J. Clin. Invest. 54:773-781, 1974.

o Boyer, J.L., Bloomer, J.R., Maddrey, W.C., and Tilson, D. Variation in hepatic bile composition following cholecystectomy in patients with previous gallstones. Yale J. Biol. Med. 47:211-217, 1974.

p Boyer, J.L. and Reno, D. Properties of (Na^+ + K^+)-activated ATPase in rat liver plasma membranes enriched with bile canaliculi. Biochem. Biophys. Acta 401:59-72, 1975.

a Brandau, K. and Keup, U. Studies on the determination and induction of cholesterol 7a-hydroxylase. Arzneimittel-Forschung 26:1837-1842, 1976.

b Brandli, H.H., Hefti M.L., and Blum, A.L. Dissolution of gallstones by chenodoxycholic acid. Schweiz. med. Wschr. 107:1770-1773, 1977.

c Brandt, L.J. and Bernstein, L.H. Bile salts: Their role in cholesterol synthesis, secretion and lithogenesis. Am. J. Gastroenterol. 65:17-30, 1976.

d Brandt, P. and Ungeheuer, E. Gallensteine - eine Zivilisationskrankheit. Frankfurter Allgemeine Zeitung, 26, 1980.

e Brandt, P., Ungeheuer, E., and Schroder, D. Gallensteinleiden. Operation oder Steinauflosung? Der Informierte Arzt 9:4-11, 1981.

f Braverman, D.Z., Johnson, M.L., and Kern, F., Jr. Effects of pregnancy and contraceptive steroids on gallbladder function. N. Engl. J. Med. 302:362-364, 1980.

g Bray, G.A. and Gallagher, T.F., Jr. Suppression of appetite by bile acids. Lancet 1:1066-1067, 1968.

h Bray, G.A. and Gallagher, T.F., Jr. Weight gain and intestinal histology in rats fed cholic, lithocholic, hyodeoxycholic, chenodeoxycholic, and deoxycholic acid. Proc. Soc. Exptl. Biol. Med. 130:175-177, 1969.

i Bremer, J. Species differences in the conjugation of free bile acids with taurine and glycine. Biochem. J. 63:507, 1956.

j Bremmelgaard, A. and Pedersen, L. Bile acids in bile during long-term chenodeoxycholic acid treatment. Scand. J. Gastroenterol. 4:161-165, 1975.

k Bremmelgaard, A. and Sjovall, J. Hydroxylation of cholic, chenodeoxycholic and deoxycholic acids in patients with intrahepatic cholestasis. J. Lipid Res. 21:1072-1081, 1980.

l Brenneman, D.E., Connor, W.E., Forker, E.L., and DenBesten, L. The formation of abnormal bile and cholesterol gallstones from dietary cholesterol in the prarie dog. J. Clin. Invest. 51:1495-1503, 1972.

m Brodersen, R. Dimerisation of bilirubin anion in aqueous solution. Acta Chem. Scand. 20:2895, 1966.

n Brown, B.D. and Ammon, H.V. Effect of glucose on jejunal water and solute absorption in the presence of glycodeoxycholate and oleate in man. Dig. Dis. & Sci. 26:710-717, 1981.

o Brown, M.S., Dana, S., Dietschy, J.M., and Siperstein, M.D. 3-Hydroxy-3-methylglutaryl coenzyme A reductase: Solubilization and purification of a cold sensitive enzyme. J. Biol. Chem. 248:4731-4738, 1973.

a Brown, M.S., Dana, S.E., and Goldstein, J.L. Regulation of 3-hydroxy-3-methylglutaryl coenzyme A reductase activity in cultured human fibroblasts. J. Biol. Chem. 249:789-796, 1974.

b Brown, M.S. and Goldstein, J.L. Familial hypercholesterolemia: Defective binding of lipoproteins to cultured fibroblasts associated with impaired regulation of 3-hydroxy-3-methyl-glutaryl coenzyme A reductase activity. Proc. Nat. Acad. Sci. 71:788-792, 1974.

c Brucke, H. Galle und Gallensauren, Ihre Therapeutische Anwendung. Wiener Med. Woch. 100:581-584, 1950.

d Bruhl, W. Ursachen der Gallensteinbildung (Cholesterinsteine). Schweiz. med. Wschr. 102:1766-1768, 1972.

e Bruhl, W. and Zepke, D. Gallensauren im Leberparenchym bei Gallensteintragern und Normalpersonen. Schw. med. Wschr. 103:870-873, 1973.

f Bruhl, W. Der Einfluss der abfuhrenden Gallenwege auf die Zusammensetzung der Gallensauren. Z. Gastroenterol. 13:3-7, 1975.

g Bruhl, W. Der Einfluss der abfuhrenden Gallenwege auf die Zusammensetzung der Gallensauren. Untersuchungen bei Cholesterinsteintragern und einer steinfreien Vergleichsgruppe. Z. Gastroenterol. Bd. 13:690-694, 1975.

h Bruhl, W. Der Einfluss der Cholezystektomie auf die Lipidzusammensetzung der Lebergalle. Schw. med. Wschr. 105:494-496, 1975.

i Brunner, H., Northfield, T.C., Hofmann, A.F., Go, V.L.W., and Summerskill, W.H.J. Daily secretion of biliary lipids and pancreatic enzymes in relation to food intake and gastric emptying in man. Mayo Clin. Proc. 49:851-860, 1974.

j Bruusgaard, A. Quantitative determination of the thin-layer chromatographic separation. Clin. Chim. Acta 28:495, 1970.

k Bruusgaard, A., Sorensen, T.I.A., Justesen, T., and Krag, E. Changes in bile acid metabolism after intestinal by-pass operation for extreme obesity. Scand. J. Gastroenterol. 10:33, 1975.

l Bruusgaard, A. and Andersen, R.B. Chenodeoxycholic acid treatment of rheumatoid arthritis. Lancet 1:700, 1976 (Letter to Editor).

m Bruusgaard, A., Malver, E., Pedersen, L.R., Schlichting, P., and Sylvest, J. Criteria for selection of patients for medical treatment (chenodeoxycholic acid therapy) of gallstones. Scand. J. Gastroenterol. 7:97-102, 1976.

n Bruusgaard, A., Sorensen, T.I.A., Justesen, T., and Krag, E. Bile acid metabolism after jejunoileal bypass operation for obesity. Scand. J. Gastroenterol. 11:833-838, 1976.

o Brydon, W.G., Borup-Christensen, S., van der Linden, W., and Eastwood, M. The effect of dietary psyllium hydrocolloid and lignin on bile. Z. Ernahrungswiss 18:77-80, 1979.

a Brydon, W., Tadesse, K., and Eastwood, M. The effect of dietary fibre on bile acid metabolism in rats. Br. J. Nutr. 43:101, 1980.

b Buchwald, H. and Varco, R.L. Partial ileal bypass for hypercholesterolemia and atherosclerosis. Surg. Gyn. & Obst. 124:1231-1238, 1967.

c Budai, K. and Javitt, N.B. Lithocholic acid: Notes on purification. J. Lipid Res. 21:1136-1137, 1980.

d Budillon, G., D'Arienzo, A., Mazzacca, G., Parrilli, G., Capuano, G. D-glucaric acid excretion during chenodeoxycholic therapy for gallstones. Lancet 1:206, 1978.

e Burhenne, H.J. Complications of nonoperative extraction of retained common duct stones. Am. J. Surg. 131:260-262, 1976.

f Burke, C.W., Lewis, B., Panveliwalla, D., and Tabaqchali, S. The binding of cholic acid and its taurine conjugate to serum proteins. Clin. Chim. Acta 32:207-214, 1971.

g Burke, V. and Anderson, C.M. Bile and bacteria. II. Bacterial flora of the upper gastrointestinal tract. In Paediatric Gastroenterology. CM Anderson, V Burke, eds. Blackwell Scientific Publications, Oxford, 1975, pp 397-410.

h Burnett, W. The composition of gall stones. Tijdschr. Gastroenterol. 14:34-45, 1971.

i Burnett, W., Dwyer, K.R., Kennard, C.H., and Roberts, G. In vitro studies of gallstone dissolution using the scanning electron microscope. Aust. N.Z. J. Surg. 49:131-133, 1979.

j Burns, M.J. and Self, K.S. Effects of cystine, niacin and taurine on cholesterol and bile acid metabolism in rabbits. Metabolism 18:427-432, 1969.

k Burstein, S. and Lieberman, S. Hydrolysis of keto steroid hydrogen sulfates by solvolysis procedures. J. Biol. Chem. 233:331-335, 1958.

l Buscher, H-P., Gerok, W., Schneider, S., and Kurz, G. Untersuchung des Gallensauretransports mit fluoreszierenden Derivaten. Z. Gastroenterol. 19:3739, 1981.

m Butt, J. and Hanson, K. Effect of frequency of feeding upon human biliary lipid output. Gastroenterology 66:670, 1974 (abstract).

n Cahlin, E., Gottfries, A., Jonsson, J., and Schersten, T. The origin of lysolecithin in hepatic bile in acute cholecystitis. An experimental study on rabbits. Acta Chir. Scand. 139:372-376, 1973.

o Cahlin, E., Jonsson, J., Nilsson, S. and Schersten, T. Biliary lipid composition in normolipidemic and prebeta hyperlipoproteinemic gallstone patients. Influence of sucrose feeding of the patients on the biliary lipid composition. Scand. J. Gastroenterol. 8:449-456, 1973.

a Calandra, S., Tarugi, P., Battistini, N., Crovetti, F. Cholesterol synthesis in isolated rat hepatocytes in vitro. Effect of sterol and bile acids. Exptl. & Mol. Path. 30:434-448, 1979.

b Calcraft, B., LaRusso, N.F., Hofmann, A.F., and Belobaba, D.T.E. Development of a simple, safe, bile acid clearance test: The radio-cholate clearance test. Gastroenterology 69:812, 1975 (abstract).

c Caldwell, F.T., Jr., Levitsky, K., and Rosenberg, B. Dietary production and dissolution of cholesterol gallstones in the mouse. Am. J. Physiol. 209:473-478, 1965.

d Camarri, E., Fici, F., and Marcolongo, R. Influence of chenodeoxychoic acid on serum triglycerides in patients with primary hypertriglyceridemia. Int. J. Clin. Pharmacol. 16:523-526, 1978.

e Camarri, E., Marcolongo, R., and Fici, F. Hypotriglyceridemic effect of chenodeoxycholic acid after a short time of administration. Int. J. Clin. Pharmacol. 16:527-528, 1978.

f Camarri, E., Marcolongo, R., Zaccherotti, L., and Marini, G. The hypotriglyceridemic effect of chenodeoxycholic acid in type IV hyperlipemia. Biomed. 29:193-198, 1978.

g Cameron, A. Advertising chenodeoxycholic acid. Br. Med. J. 15:1586-1587, 1979 (Letter to Editor).

h Camilleri, M., Murphy, R., and Chadwick, V.S. Dose-related effects of chenodeoxycholic acid in the rabbit colon. Dig. Dis. Sci. 25:433-438, 1980.

i Camilleri, M., Murphy, R., and Chadwick, V.S. Inhibition of chenodeoxycholic acid induced secretion in the rabbit colon. Europ. J. Clin. Invest. 11:34, 1981 (abstract).

j Campa, P.P., Marcellini, G., and Tomassini, P. Effetto dell'associazione di acido chenodesossicolico e di fentonio sulla dinamica della via biliare principale in colecistect-omizzati. Min. Diet. Gastr. 24:43-47, 1978.

k Campa, P.P. Chenodeoxycholic acid versus ursodeoxycholic acid in biliary tract dynamics in cholecystectomised patients. Ital. J. Gastroenterol. 12:348-349, 1980.

l Campbell, C.B., Spencer, J., and Dowling, R.H. Bile salt secretion and pool size in rhesus monkeys with controlled interruption of the enterohepatic circulation. Gut 10:1050, 1969 (abstract).

m Campbell, C.B., Burgess, P., Roberts, S.A., Dowling, R.H., and White, J. The use of rhesus monkeys to study biliary secretion with an intact enterohepatic circulation. Aust. N. Z. J. Med. 2:49-56, 1971.

n Campbell, C.B., Cowley, D.J., and Dowling, R.H. Dietary factors affecting biliary lipid secretion in the rhesus monkey. A mechanism for the hypocholesterolaemic action of polyunsaturated fat? Europ. J. Clin. Invest. 2:332-341, 1972.

a Campbell, C.B., McGuffie, C., and Powell, L.W. The measurement of sulfated and non-sulfated bile acids in serum using gas liquid chromatography. Clin. Chim. Acta 63:249-262, 1975.

b Campbell, C.B. and Cowen, A.E. Bile salt metabolism. II. Bile salts and disease. Aust. N.Z. J. Med. 7:587-595, 1977.

c Canepa, A., Volpi, C., Ciravegna, C., Dodero, M., and Celle, G. Clinical experiences concerning gallstone dissolution with ursodeoxycholic acid. Acta Gastroenterol. Belg. 43:502-507, 1980.

d Capocaccia, L., Attili, A.F., Cantafora, A., Bracci, F., Paciscopi, L., Puoti, C., Pieche, U., and Angelico, M. Sulfated bile acids in serum, bile, and urine of cirrhotic patients before and after portacaval anastomosis. Dig. Dis. Sci. 26:513-517, 1981.

e Caprini, J.A., Crampton, A.R., and Swan, V.M. Nonoperative extraction of retained common duct stones. Arch. Surg. 111:445-451, 1976.

f Capron, J.P. Essais therapeutiques de la lithiase biliaire en dehous de l'acide chenodesoxycholique. Therapie 32:409-416, 1977.

g Capron, J.P., Dupas, J.L., Capron-Chivrac, D., Aubin, J.P., and Delamarre, J. Unconjugated hyperbilirubinemia during treatment with chenodeoxycholic acid. Gastroenterology 77:121-122, 1979.

h Capron, J.P. Effets indesirables de l'acide chenodesoxycholique et l'acide ursodesoxycholique: Ce que l'oie et l'ours n'ont pas en commun. Gastroenterol. Clin. Biol. 4:526-530, 1980.

i Carella, M., Einarsson, K., and Hellstrom, K. The formation of deoxycholic acid in patients with Type II and IV hyperlipoproteinemia. Atherosclerosis 24:293-299, 1976.

j Carey, J.B., Jr. Chenodeoxycholic acid in human blood. Science 123:892, 1956.

k Carey, J.B., Jr. The serum trihydroxy-dihydroxy bile acid ratio in liver and biliary tract disease. J. Clin. Invest. 37:1494-1503, 1958.

l Carey, J.B., Jr. Bile acids in the serum of jaundiced patients. Gastroenterology 41:285-287, 1961.

m Carey, J.B., Jr. and Williams, G. Relief in the pruritis of jaundice with a bile acid sequestering resin. J. Am. Med. Assn. 176:432-435, 1961.

n Carey, J.B., Jr. and Williams, G. Metabolism of lithocholic acid in bile fistula patients. J. Clin. Invest. 42:450-455, 1963.

o Carey, J.B., Jr. Bile acids, cirrhosis, and human evolution. Gastroenterolgy 46:490-493, 1964 (Editorial).

a Carey, J.B., Jr. and Williams, G. Lithocholic acid in human-blood serum. Science 150:620-622, 1965.

b Carey, J.B., Jr., Wilson, I.D., Zaki, F.G., and Hanson, R.F. The metabolism of bile acids with special reference to liver injury. Medicine 45:461-470, 1966.

c Carey, J.B., Jr., Wilson, I.D., Zaki, F.G., and Williams, G. Predominance of the dihydroxy primary bile acid pathway in cholesterol catabolism in liver cirrhosis: A potential source of liver injury. J. Lab. Clin. Med. 68:862, 1966 (abstract).

d Carey, J.B., Jr. Bile salts and hepatobiliary disease. In Diseases of the Liver, L Schiff, ed. JB Lippincott Co., Philadelphia, 1969, pp 103-146.

e Carey, M.C. and Small, D.M. Micellar properties of dihydroxy and trihydroxy bile salts: Effects of counterion and temperature. J. Coll. Inter. Sci. 31:382-396, 1969.

f Carey, M.C. and Small, D.M. The characteristics of mixed micellar solutions with particular reference to bile. Am. J. Med. 49:590-608, 1970.

g Carey, M.C. and Small, D.M. Micellar properties of sodium fusidate, a steroid antibiotic structurally resembling the bile salts. J. Lipid Res. 12:604-613, 1971.

h Carey, M.C. and Small, D.M. Micelle formation by bile salts. Physical-chemical and thermodynamic considerations. Arch. Intern. Med. 130:506-527, 1972.

i Carey, M.C. and Small, D.M. Solution properties of taurine and glycine conjugates of fusidic acid and its derivatives. Biochim. Biophys. Acta 306:51-57, 1973.

j Carey, M.C., Hirom, P.C. and Small, D.M. Precipitation of bile salts by chlorpromazine (CPZ): The protective effect of lecithin (LEC). Gastroenterology 66:671, 1974 (abstract).

k Carey, M.C. Cheno and urso: What the goose and the bear have in common. N. Engl. J. Med. 293:1255-1257, 1975.

l Carey, M.C., Montet, J.C., and Small, D.M. Surface and solution properties of steroid antibiotics, 3-acetoxyl fusidic acid, cephalosporin P1 and helvolic acid. Biochemistry 14:4896-4905, 1975.

m Carey, M.C., Hirom, P.C., and Small, D.M. A study of the physical-chemical interactions between biliary lipids and chlorpromazine hydrocholoride. Bile salt precipitation as a mechanism for phenothiazine-induced bile secretory failure. Biochem. J. 153:519-531, 1976.

a Carey, M.C. Critical tables for calculating the cholesterol saturation of native bile. J. Lipid Res. 19:945-955, 1978.

b Carey, M.C. and Small, D.M. The physical chemistry of cholesterol solubility in bile. J. Clin. Invest. 61:998-1026, 1978.

c Carey, M.C. and Ko, G. The importance of total lipid concentration in determining cholesterol solubility in bile and the development of critical tables for calculating "% cholesterol saturation" with a correction factor for ursodeoxycholate-rich bile. In Biological Effects of Bile Acids, G Paumgartner, A Steihl, and W Gerok, eds. MTP Press, Lancaster, 1979, pp 299-308.

d Carey, M.C., Mazer, N.A. and Benedek, G.B. Novel physical-chemical properties of ursodeoxycholic acid (UDCA) and its conjugates: Relevance to gallstone dissolution in man. Gastroenterology 72:1036, 1979 (abstract).

e Carey, M.C., Montet, J., Igimi, H., Mazer, N. and Phillips, M. Chenodeoxycholic acid (CDC) ursodeoxycholic acid (UDC) and their glycine and taurine conjugates: Comparison of bulk and surface properties in dilute solution. Gastroenterology 77:A6, 1979 (abstract).

f Carey, M.C.. Wu, S.F., and Watkins, J.B. Solution properties of sulfated monohydroxy bile salts. Relative insolubility of the disodium salt of glycolithocholate sulfate. Biochim. Biophys. Acta 575:16-26, 1979.

g Carey, M.C. Differential detergent effects of taurochenodeoxycholate (TCDC) and tauroursodeoxycholate (TUDC) on lecithin and cholesterol secretion from model membranes: Description of a novel in vitro perfusion system. IVth Internat'l Gstaad Symposium, 1981 (abstract).

h Carey, M.C., Montet, J.C., Phillips, M.C., Armstrong, M.J., and Mazer, N.A. Thermodynamic and molecular basis for dissimilar cholesterol-solubilizing capacities by micellar solutions of bile salts: cases of sodium chenodeoxycholate and sodium ursodeoxycholate and their glycine and taurine conjugates. Biochemistry 20:3637-3648, 1981.

i Carlisle, V.F. and Tasman-Jones, C. Prevention of gallstone formation in rabbits by the oral administration of Kanamycin. Surg. Gyn. & Obst. 144:195-198, 1977.

j Carlstrom, K., Kirk, D.N., and Sjovall, J. Microbial synthesis of 1b- and 15b-hydroxylated bile acids. J. Lipid Res. 22:1225-1234, 1981.

k Carulli, N., Ponz de Leon, M., Manenti, F., Zeneroli, M.L. Drug metabolism in jaundice: Effects of bilirubin and bile acids in man. Digestion 8:470-471, 1973 (abstract).

l Carulli, N., and Ponz de Leon, M. Terapia medica della colelitiasi colesterinica con acido chenodesossicolico. Il Fegato 24:3-7, 1977.

a Carulli, N., Zironi, F., Ponz de Leon, M., Pinetti, A., and Ferrari, P. Comparative effects of short-term feeding of chenodeoxycholic and ursodeoxycholic acid on hepatic metabolism in man. Gut 19:A994, 1978 (abstract).

b Carulli, N., Ponz de Leon, M., Zironi, F., Iori, R., and Loria, P. Bile acid feeding and hepatic sterol metabolism: Effect of deoxycholic acid. Gastroenterology 79:637-641, 1980.

c Carulli, N., Ponz de Leon, M., Zironi, F., Pinetti, A., Smerieri, A., Iori, R., and Loria, P. Hepatic cholesterol and bile acid metabolism in subjects with gallstones: Comparative effects of short-term feeding of chenodeoxycholic acid and ursodeoxycholic acid. J. Lipid Res. 21:35-43, 1980.

d Carulli, N., Zironi, F., Ponz de Leon, M., Iori, R., and Loria, P. Bile acid pool composition and hepatic cholesterol metabolism in man. The effect of deoxycholic acid administration. Ital. J. Gastroenterol. 12:233, 1980.

e Carulli, N., Ponz de Leon, M., Loria, P., Iori, R., Rosi, A., and Romani, M. Effect of the selective expansion of cholic acid pool on bile lipid composition: Possible mechanism of bile acid induced biliary cholesterol desaturation. Gastroenterology 81:539-546, 1981.

f Carulli, N., Ponz de Leon, M., Podda, M., Zuin, M., Strata, A., Frigerio, G., and DiGrisolo, A. Chenodeoxycholic acid and ursodeoxycholic acid effects in endogenous hypertriglyceridemias. A controlled double-blind trial. J. Clin. Pharmacol. 21:436-442, 1981.

g Casanova, S., Roda, A., Festi, D., Mazzella, G., Aldini, R., Bazzoli, F., Sama, C., Morselli, A.M., Barbara, L., and Roda, E. Effect of chenodiol on the small intestine. Unimpaired structure and function during therapy for gallstone dissolution. JAMA 246:2597-2601, 1981.

h Caspary, W.F. Inhibition of active hexose and amino acid transport by conjugated bile salts in rat ileum. Europ. J. Clin. Invest. 4:17-24, 1974.

i Caspary, W.F. and Katterman, R. Einfluss der konservativen cholelitholytischen Therapie mit Chenodesoxycholsaure auf Cholesterin und Triglyzeride im Serum von Gallensteintragern. Z. Gastroenterol. Bd. 13:644-647, 1975.

j Caspary, W.F. and Gunther, G. Effect of bile acids and antacids on transmural gastric potential difference in humans. 10th Intl. Cong. Gastroenterol., Budapest, June, 1976.

k Caspary, W.F. and Graf, S. Binding von Gallensauren an Antacida. Dtsch. med. Wschr. 103:825-827, 1978.

l Caspary, W.F. and Meyne, K. Comparative effects of urso- and chenodeoxycholic acid on colonic and small intestinal function in rats. _In_ Biological Effects of Bile Acids. G Paumgartner, A Stiehl, and W Gerok, eds. MTP Press, Lancaster, 1979, pp 233-240.

a Caspary, W.F. and Meyne, K. Effects of chenodeoxy- and ursodeoxycholic acid on absorption, secretion, and permeability in rat colon and small intestine. Digestion 20:168-174, 1980.

b Cass, O.W., Cowen, A.E., Hofmann, A.F., and Coffin, S.B. Thin-layer chromatographic separation of sulfated and unsulfated lithocholic acid and its glycine and taurine conjugates. J. Lipid. Res. 16:159-160, 1975.

c Celle, G. and Dodero, M. Pathophysiology of cholesterol lithiasis. Pathologica 69:431-440, 1977.

d Celle, G., Ciravegna, G., Deconca, V., Mansi, C., Picciotto, A., Savarino, V., and Dodero, M. Dissolution of cholesterol biliary calculi with chenodeoxycholic acid. Med. Chir. Dig. 7:321-324, 1978.

e Celle, G., Cavanna, M., Bocchini, R., Robbiano, L., Dodero, M., Volpi, C., Dellepiane, F., Cuneo-Crovari, P., Scarvaglieri-Giuliano, R., and Sigari-Canu, G. Chenodeoxycholic acid (CDCA) versus ursodeoxycholic acid (UDCA): a comparison of their effects in pregnant rats. Arch. Int. Pharmacodyn. Ther. 246:149-158, 1980.

f Chadwick, V.S., Modha, K., and Dowling, R.H. Mechanism for hyperoxaluria in patients with ileal dysfunction. N. Engl. J. Med. 289:172-176, 1973.

g Chadwick, V.S., Phillips, S.F., and Hofmann, A.F. Measurements of intestinal permeability using low molecular weight polyethylene glycols (PEG 400). II. Application to studies of normal and abnormal permeability states in man and animals. Gastroenterology 73:247-251, 1977.

h Chadwick, V.S., Gaginella, T., Carlson, G., Debongnie, J-C, Phillips, S.F., and Hofmann, A.F. Effect of molecular structure on bile acid induced alterations in absorptive function, permeability, and morphology in the perfused rabbit colon. J. Lab. Clin. Med. 94:661-674, 1979.

i Chang, F.C. Potential bile acid metabolites. 2. 3,7,12-trisubstituted 5b-cholanic acids. J. Org. Chem. 44:4567-4572, 1979.

j Chapple, M.J., Nolan, D., Low-Beer, T.S., et al. Gallbladder emptying measured by a radioisotope method. Brit. J. Radiol. 48:19-22, 1975.

k Charles, M., Sari, H., Entressangles, B., and Desnuelle, P. Interaction of pancreatic colipase with a bile salt micelle. Biochim. Biophys. Res. Comm. 65:744-745, 1975.

l Chenderovitch, J., Raizman, A., and Infante, R. Effect of phenobarbital and carbon tetrachloride on dehydrocholate induced choleresis in the guinea-pig. Biol. Gastroenterol. 7:171-178, 1974.

m Chen, E-J., Imperato, T.J., and Bolt, R.J. Enzymatic sulfation of bile salts. II. Studies on bile salt sulfotransferase from rat kidney. Biochim. Biophys. Acta 522:443-451, 1978.

a Cherayil, G.D., Hsia, S.L., Matschiner, J.T., Soidy, E.A., Elliot, W.H., and Thayer, S.A. Bile acids. XVII. Metabolism of a a-muricholic acid-24-^{14}C in the rat. J. Biol. Chem. 238:1973-1978, 1963.

b Cheung, L.Y., Englert, E., Moody, R.G., et al. Dissolution of gallstones with bile salts, lecithin, and heparin. Surgery 76:500-503, 1974.

c Chevrel, B. Chenodeoxycholic acid. Indications in biliary pathology and hyperlipoproteinemias. Med. Chir. Dig. 9:31-34, 1980.

d Chirantini, E., Arcangeli, A., Romagnoli, P., Buzzelli, G., Salvadori, G., and Gentilini, P. Functional and ultrastructural changes in the liver during CDCA treatment. Ital. J. Gastroenterol. 12:224-227, 1980.

e Chitranukroh, A., Billing, B.H., and Barnes, S. Protein binding of bile salts in blood in cholestasis. Hepatology 1:503, 1981 (abstract).

f Cho, M. Study on dissolution of human cholesterol gallstones by using scanning electron microscope. Jpn. J. Gastroenterol. 76:1979-1992, 1979.

g Ciravegna, G., Volpi, C., Canepa, A., Michetti, P., Dodero, M., and Celle, G. Ursodeoxycholic acid and cholesterol lithiasis. Clinical observations. Ital. J. Gastroenterol. 12:346, 1980.

h Clain, J., Malagelada, J-R, Chadwick, V.S., and Hofmann, A.F. Binding properties in vitro of antacids for conjugated bile acids. Gastroenterlogy 73:556-559, 1977.

i Clark, M.L., Lanz, H.C., and Senior, J.R. Bile salt regulation of fatty acid absorption and esterification in rat everted jejunal sacs in vitro and into thoractic duct lymph in vivo. J. Clin. Invest. 48:1587-1599, 1969.

j Classen, M. and Ossenberg, J.W. Non-surgical removal of common bile duct stones. Gut 18:760-769, 1977.

k Clausen, J., Kruse, I., and Dam, H. Fractionation and characterization of proteins and lipids in bile. Scand. J. Clin. Lab. Invest. 17:325-335, 1965.

l Clearfield, H.R. Drug dissolution of gallstones. Am. Fam. Physician 25:202-204, 1982.

m Cleave, T.L. and Castleden, W.M. Diseases of Western civilization. Brit. Med. J. 1:678-679, 1973.

n Cleave, T.L. Effect of bran on blood lipids and calcium. Lancet 1:137, 1974 (Letter to Editor).

o Cobb, M., Turkki, P., Linscheer, W., and Raheja, K. Lecithin supplementation in healthy volunteers: Effect on cholesterol esterification and plasma and bile lipids. Nutr. Metab. 24:228-237, 1980.

a Cochran, K.M., Mackenzie, J.F., and Russell, R.I. Role of taurocholic acid in production of gastric mucosal damage after ingestion of aspirin. Brit. Med. J. 1:183-185, 1975.

b Cohen, B.I., Raicht, R.F., and Mosbach, E.H. Effect of dietary bile acids, cholesterol, and b-sitosterol upon formation of coprostanol and 7-dehydroxylation of bile acids by rat. Lipids 9:1024-1029, 1974.

c Cohen, B.I., Raicht, R.F., and Mosbach, E.H. Effects of dietary plant sterols and bile acids on sterol metabolism. Biochim. Biophys. Acta 487:287-296, 1977.

d Cohen, B.I., Raicht, R.F., and Mosbach, E.H. Sterol metabolism studies in the rat. Effects of primary bile acids (sodium taurochenodeoxycholate and sodium taurocholate) on sterol metabolism. J. Lipid Res. 18:223-231, 1977.

e Cohen, B.I., Budai, K., and Javitt, N.B. Solvolysis of chenodeoxycholic acid sulfates. Steroids 37:621-626, 1981.

f Cohen, B.I. and Raicht, R.F. Effects of bile acids on colon carcinogenesis in rats treated with carcinogens. Cancer Res. 2:3759-3760, 1981.

g Cohen, H., Bonorris, G.G., Marks, J.W., and Schoenfield, L.J. Effect of Zanchol and chenic acid on bile acid pool size and gallstones in hamsters. Am. J. Med. Sci. 283:23-31, 1982.

h Cohen, S., Kaplan, M., Gottleib, J., and Patterson, J. Liver disease and gallstones in regional enteritis. Gastroenterology 60:237-245, 1971.

i Collins, D.M., Bates, J.H.T., Maslowski, A.H., McKinnon, A.E., and Campbell, C.B. The extent of reflux of unconjugated ^{14}C-cholic acid from the liver in subjects with normal liver function. Aust. J. Exp. Biol. Med. Sci. 59: 779-790, 1981.

j Comess, L.J., Bennett, P.H., and Burch, T.A. Clinical gallbladder disease in Pima Indians. N. Engl. J. Med. 277:894-898, 1967.

k Comfort, M.W., Gray, H.K., and Wilson, J.M. The silent gallstone: A ten to twenty year follow-up study of 112 cases. Ann. Surg. 128:931-937, 1948.

l Conley, D.R. and Goldstein, L.I. Pathogenesis and therapy of cholesterol gallstones: With emphasis on the metabolic effects of chenodeoxycholic acid. Med. Clin. North Am., WB Saunders, Co., Philadelphia. 5,:1025-1034, 1975.

m Conley, D.R., Coyne, M.J., Bonorris, G.G. Chung, A., and Schoenfield, L.J. Bile acid stimulation of colonic adenylate cyclase and secretion in the rabbit. Am. J. Dig. Dis. 21:453-458, 1976.

n Conley, D.R., Coyne, M.J., Chung, A., Bonorris, G.G. and Schoenfield, L.J. Propranolol inhibits adenylate cyclase and secretion stimulated by deoxycholic acid in the rabbit colon. Gastroenterology 71:72-75, 1976.

a Connor, W.E., Witiak, D.T., Stone, D.B., and Armstrong, M.L. Cholesterol balance and fecal neutral steroid and bile acid excretion in normal men fed dietary fats of different fatty acid composition. J. Clin. Invest. 48:1363-1375, 1969.

b Connor, W.E. The effects of dietary lipid and sterols on the sterol balance. In Athersclerosis, Proc 2nd Int'l. Symp. RJ Jones, ed. Springer Verlag, New York, 1970, pp 253-261.

c Conte, D., Bozzani, A., Sironi, L., Rocca, F., Camassa, L., and Bianchi, P.A. Radiolucent gallstone dissolution with bedtime UDCA administration. Digestion 22:302-304, 1981.

d Cook, J.W., Kennaway, N.M., and Kennaway, E.L. Production of tumors in mice by deoxycholic acid. Nature 145:627-628, 1940.

e Cooper, R.A., Diloy-Paray, M., Lando, P., and Greenberg, M.S. An analysis of lipoproteins, bile acids and red cells in patients with liver disease. J. Clin. Invest. 51:3182-3192, 1972.

f Cooper, R.A., Garcia, F.A., and Trey, C. The effect of lithocholic acid on red cell membranes in vivo. J. Lab. Clin. Med. 79:7-18. 1972.

g Cooperberg, P.L. and Burhenne, H.J. Real-time ultrasonography. N. Engl. J. Med. 302:1277-1279, 1980.

h Corazza, G.R., Simeone, E., DiGiammarco, A.M., Ciccarelli, R., and Tenaglia, G. Positive effects of chenodeoxycholic acid (CDCA) on the biohumoral clinical aspect of cholesterin calculosis of the gallbladder. Minerva Med. 69:758-761, 1978.

i Corazza, G.R., Ciccarelli, R., Caciagli, F., and Gasbarrini, G. Cyclic AMP and cyclic GMP levels in human colonic mucosa before and during chenodeoxycholic acid therapy. Gut 20:489-492, 1979.

j Corazziari, E., Pozzessere, C., Cani, S., Piccinni-Leopardi, M., Anzini, F., and Alessandrini, A. Chenodeoxycholic acid and diarrhoea. Lancet 2:266-267, 1978.

k Corbett, C.L., Bartholomew, T.C., Billing, B.H., and Summerfield, J.A. Urinary excretion of bile acids in cholestasis: Evidence for renal tubular secretion in man. Clin. Sci. 61:773-780, 1981.

l Corrigan, O.I., Su, C., Higuchi, W., and Hofmann, A.F. Mesophase formation during cholesterol dissolution in ursodeoxycholate-lecithin solutions: New mechanism for gallstone dissolution in humans. J. Pharm. Sci. 69:869-871, 1980.

m Cotton, P.B., Vallon, A.G., and Mason, R. Intra-ductal infusion of monooctanoin for common duct stones. Lancet 1:436-437, 1981.

n Cousar, C.D. and Gadacz, T.R. Comparison of antacids on the binding of bile salts. Gastroenterology 80:1357, 1981 (abstract).

a Cowen, A.E., Korman, M.G., Hofmann, A.F., and Cass, O.W. Metabolism of lithocholate in healthy man. I. Biotransformation and biliary excretion of intravenously administered lithocholate, lithocholylglycine, and their sulfates. Gastroenterology 69:59-66, 1975.

b Cowen, A.E., Korman, M.G., Hofmann, A.F., Cass, O.W., and Coffin, S.B. Metabolism of lithocholate in healthy man. II. Enterohepatic circulation. Gastroenterology 69:67-76, 1975.

c Cowen, A.E., Korman, M.G., Hofmann, A.F., and Thomas, P.J. Metabolism of lithocholate in healthy man. III. Plasma disappearance of labeled lithocholate and its derivatives. Gastroenterology 69:77-82, 1975.

d Cowen, A.E., Korman, M.G., Hofmann, A.F., and Thomas, P.J. Plasma disappearance of radioactivity after intravenous injection of labelled bile acids in man. Gastroenterology 68:1567-1573, 1975.

e Cowen, A.E., Hofmann, A.F., Hachey, D.L., Thomas, P.J., Belobaba, D.T.E., Klein, P.D., and Tokes, L. Synthesis of 11,12-$^3H_2$- and 11,12-$^3H_2$-labeled chenodeoxycholic and lithocholic acids. J. Lipid Res. 17:231-238, 1976.

f Cowen, A.E. and Campbell, C.B. Bile salt metabolism. I. The physiology of bile salts. Aust. N. Z. J. Med. 7:579-586, 1977.

g Cowen, A.E., Korman, M.G., Hofmann, A.F., Turcotte, J., and Carter, J. Radioimmunoassay of unsulfated lithocholates. J. Lipid Res. 18:692-697, 1977.

h Cowen A.E., Korman, M.G., Hofmann, A.F., Turcotte, J., and Carter, J. Radioimmunoassay of sulfated lithocholates. J. Lipid Res. 18:698-703, 1977.

i Cowie, A.G. and Clark, C.G. Bile composition in dogs with and without gallbladders, and the effect of vagotomy. Brit. J. Surg. 58:867, 1971.

j Cowie, A.G. and Clark, C.G. The lithogenic effect of vagotomy. Bull. Soc. Int. Chir. 31:7-10, 1972.

k Cowie, A.G. and Clark, C.G. The lithogenic effect of vagotomy. Brit. J. Surg. 59:365-367, 1972.

l Cowie, A.G., Sutor, D.J., Wooley, S.E., et al. The calcium palmitate gall-stone. Brit. J. Surg. 60:16-18, 1973.

m Coyne, M.J., Bonorris, G.G., Chung, A., Goldstein, L.I., Lahana, D., and Schoenfield, L.J. Treatment of gallstones with chenodeoxycholic acid and phenobarbital. N. Engl. J. Med. 292:604-607, 1975.

n Coyne, M.J. and Schoenfield, L.J. Gallstone disease. Post Grad. Med. 57:153-158, 1975.

a Coyne, M.J., Bonorris, G.G., Goldstein, L.I., and Schoenfield, L.J. Effect of chenodeoxycholic acid and phenobarbital on the rate-limiting enzymes of hepatic cholesterol and bile acid synthesis in patients with gallstones. J. Lab. Clin. Med. 87:281-291, 1976.

b Coyne, M.J. and Schoenfield, L.J. Gallstone formulation and dissolution. In Progress in Liver Disease. Popper and Schaffner, eds. Grune & Stratton, New York, 1976, pp 622-635.

c Coyne, M.J., Bonorris, G.G., Chung, A., Conley, D., and Schoenfield, L.J. Propanolol inhibits bile acid and fatty acid stimulation of cyclic AMP in human colon. Gastroenterology 73:971-974, 1977.

d Coyne, M.J., Bonorris, G.G., Chung, A., Cove, H., and Schoenfield, L.J. Dietary cholesterol affects chenodeoxycholic acid action on biliary lipids. Gastroenterology 72:927-931, 1977.

e Coyne, M.J., Marks, J.W., and Schoenfield, L.J. Mechanism of cholesterol gallstone formation. Clin. Gastroenterol. 6:129-139, 1977.

f Coyne, M.J., Bonorris, G., Chung, A., Winchester, R., and Schoenfield, L.J. Estrogen enhances dietary cholesterol induction of saturated bile in the hamster. Gastroenterology 75:76-79, 1978.

g Crawford, N. A study on human bile and some of its constituents. II. Concerning the physical-chemical characteristics of the bile salts and cholesterol solubilization. J. Med. Lab. Tech. 13:351-359, 1956.

h Cronholm, T., Burlingame, A.L., and Sjovall, J. Utilization of the carbon and hydrogen atoms of ethanol in the biosynthesis of steroids and bile acids. Europ. J. Biochem. 49:497-510, 1974.

i Cronholm, T., Einarsson, K., and Gustafsson, J.A. Changes in vivo metabolism of bile acids in rat after treatment with phenobarbital. Lipids 9:844-849, 1974.

j Crouse, J.R. and Grundy, S.M. Effects of sucrose polyester on cholesterol metabolism in man. Metabolism 28:994-1000, 1979.

k Crowell, M.J. and Macdonald, I.A. Enzymic determination of 3a-, 7a-, and 12a-hydroxyl groups of fecal bile salts. Clin. Chem. 26:1298-1300, 1980.

l Crowther, J.S., Drasar, B.S., Goddard, P., Hill, M.J., and Johnson, K. The effect of a chemically defined diet on the faecal flora and faecal steroid concentration. Gut 14:790-793, 1973.

m Crummy, A.B. and Mack, E. Infusion therapy of choledocholithiasis: Technique for catheter placement. Am. J. Roentgen. 136:622-623, 1981.

n Cuchet, P., Morrier, C., Cand, F., and Keriel, C. Effects of clofibrate and tiadenol on the elimination of lipids and bile acids in rat bile. Lipids 16:732-738, 1981.

a Cussler, E.L., Evans, D.F., and DePalma, R.G. A model for gallbladder function. Proc. Nat'l. Acad. Sci. 67:400, 1970.

b Czygan, P., Greim, H., Trulzsch, D., Rudick, J., Hutterer, F., Schaffner,F., Rosenthal, O., Popper, H., and Cooper, D.Y. Hydroxylation of taurolithocholate by isolated human microsomes. II. Cytochrome P-450 dependency. Biochim. Biophys. Acta 354:168-171, 1974.

c Czygan, P. and Stiehl, A. Untersuchungen zur Toxizitat sulfatierter und nicht sulfatierter Gallensauren. Z. Gastroenterol. 13:468-473, 1975.

d Czygan, P., Stiehl, A., and Kommerell, B. Behandlung der Hepato-Choledocholithiasis mit Chenodesoxycholsaure bei intrahepatischen Gallengangszysten (M. Caroli). Verh. Dtsch. Ges. Inn. Med. 81:1305-1307, 1975.

e Czygan, P., Stiehl, A., Frohling, W., Kommerell, B., and Encke, A. Therapie intrahepatischer Cholesterinsteine durch Chenodesoxycholsaure. Dtsch. med. Wschr. 102:518-520, 1977.

f Czygan, P., Stiehl, A., Gotz, R., Raedsch, R., and Kommerell, B. Serumelimination und renale clearance glukuronidierter, sulfatierter und freier ^{14}C-chenodesoxycholsaure bei patienten mit leberzirrhose und cholestase. Z. Gastroenterol. 17:643, 1979 (abstract).

g Czygan, P., Seitz, H., Waldherr, R., Stiehl, A., and Kommerell, B. Untersuchungen zur kokarzinogenen Wirkung von Ursodeoxycholsaure und Chenodeoxycholsaure beim Dimethylhydrazine-induzierten Kolonkarzinom der Ratte. Z. Gastroenterol. XIX (9), 1981 (abstract 87).

h Czygan, P., Seitz, H.K., Weber, E., and Kommerell, B. Effect of chenodeoxycholic acid and ursodeoxycholic acid on cell regeneration in the colon. Internat'l Symp on IBD, Jerusalem, 1981 (abstract).

i Czygan, P., Seitz, H., Weber, E., Stiehl, A., and Kommerell, B. DNA synthesis in the rat colon: Influence of chenodeoxycholic acid and ursodeoxycholic acid. Gastroenterology 80:1131, 1981 (abstract).

j Czygan, P., Stiehl, A., Raedsch, R., Manner, Ch., and Kommerell, B. Cholesterol gallstone dissolution rate with urso and combined urso-cheno treatment. 16th Meeting of the EASL, Lisbon, 1981 (abstract 152).

k Dahl Iverson, E., and Westgaard, E. La cholecystendese dans la lithiase vesiculaire. Lyon Chir. 58:695, 1962.

l Dam, H., Kruse, I., Kallehauge, H.E., Hartkopp, O.E., and Krogh Jensen, M. Studies on human bile. I. Composition of bladder bile from cholelithiasis patients and surgical patients with normal bile compared with data for bladder bile of hamsters on different diets. Scand. J. Clin. Lab. Invest. 18:385-404, 1966.

m Dam, H., Kruse, I., Krogh Jensen, M., Kallehauge, H.E., and Hartkopp, O.E. The influence of two different fats on the composition of human bile. Proc. 7th Int'l. Cong. Nutr. 1:2-7, 1966.

a Dam, H., Christensen, F., and Prange, I. The relationship between diet and composition of bladder bile in mice. Z. Ernahrungswiss. 9:200-208, 1969.

b Dam, H. Nutritional aspects of gallstone formation with particular reference to alimentary production of gallstones in laboratory animals. World Rev. Nutr. Diet 11:199-239, 1969.

c Dam, H. Determinants of cholesterol cholelithiasis in man and animals. Am. J. Med. 51:596-613, 1971.

d Dam, H. and Hegardt, F.G. The relation between formation of gallstones rich in cholesterol and the solubility of cholesterol in aqueous solutions of bile salts and lecithin. Z. Ernahrungswiss. 10:239-252, 1971.

e Dam, H., Kruse, I, Prange, I., Kallehauge, H.E., Fenger, H.J., Krogh Jensen, M. Studies on human bile. III. Composition of duodenal bile from healthy young volunteers compared with composition of bladder bile from surgical patients with and without uncomplicated gallstone disease. Z. Ernahrungswiss. 10:160-177, 1971.

f Dam, H., Prange, I., Krogh Jensen, M., Kallehauge, H.E., and Fenger, H.J. Studies on human bile. IV. Influence of ingestion of cholesterol in the form of eggs on the composition of bile in healthy subjects. Z. Ernahrungswiss. 10:178-187, 1971.

g Dam, H., Prange, I., Krogh Jensen, M., Kallehauge, H.E., and Fenger, H.J. Studies on human bile. V. Influence of cholestyramine treatment on the composition of bile in healthy subjects. Z. Ernahrungswiss. 10:188-197, 1971.

h Dam, H., Prange, I., and Sondergaard, E. Alimentary production of gallstones in hamsters. XXIV. Influence of orally ingested chenodeoxycholic acid and hyodeoxycholic acid on formation of gallstones. Z. Ernahrungswiss. 11:80-94, 1972.

i Dam, H., Prange, I., and Sondergaard, E. Alimentary production of gallstones in hamsters. XXV. Inhibition of production of cholesterol gallstones by 2-(p-chlorophenoxy)-isobutyric acid ethyl ester (clofibrate). Z. Ernahrungswiss. 11:95-104, 1972.

j Dam, H., Prange, I., Krogh Jensen, M., Stilling, B., and Bremmelgaard, A. Studies of human bile. VI. Influence of diets low in fat on the composition of bile in healthy subjects. Z. Ernahrungswiss. 14:1-17, 1975.

k Dancygier, H., Schneider, M., Leuschner, U., and Hubner, K. Effect of chenodeoxycholic acid and ursodeoxycholic acid on liver cell proliferation in the rat--a morphometric and histoautoradiographic study. Ital. J. Gastroenterol. 12:44-48, 1980.

l Danielsson, H. and Kazuno, T. On the metabolism of bile acids in the guinea pig. Acta Chem. Scand. 13:1137, 1959.

a Danielsson, H., Eneroth, P., Hellstrom, K., and Sjovall, J. Synthesis of some 3b-hydroxylated bile acids and the isolation of 3b,12a-hydrocholanic acid from feces. J. Biol. Chem. 237:3657, 1962.

b Danielsson, H. Present status of research on catabolism and excretion of cholesterol. In Advances in Lipid Research. R Paoletti and D Kritchevsky, eds. Academic Press, New York, vol. I, 1963, pp 335-385.

c Danielsson, H., Eneroth, P., Hellstrom, K., Lindstedt, S., and Sjovall, J. On the turnover and excretory products of cholic acid and chenodeoxycholic acid in man. J. Biol. Chem. 238:2299-2304, 1963.

d Danielsson, H., Kallner, A., and Sjovall, J. On the composition of the bile acid fraction of rabbit feces and the isolation of a new bile acid: 3a, 12a-dihydroxy-5a-cholanic acid. J. Biol. Chem. 238:3846, 1963.

e Danielsson, H. and Einarsson, K. Further studies on the formation of bile acids in the guinea pig. Acta Chem. Scand. 18:732-738, 1964.

f Danielsson, H., Einarsson, K., and Johansson, G. Effect of biliary drainage on individual reactions in the conversion of cholesterol to taurocholic acid. Europ. J. Biochem. 2:44, 1967.

g Danielsson, H. and Tchen, T.T. Steroid Metabolism in Metabolic Pathways, Edition 3, Volume 2. DM Greenberg, ed. Academic Press, New York, 1968.

h Danielsson, H. Formation and metabolism of bile acids. In The Biological Basis of Medicine. Bittar & Bittar, eds. Chapter 8, 1969.

i Danielsson, H. Effect of biliary obstruction on formation and metabolism of bile acids in rat. Steroids 22:567-579, 1973.

j Danielsson, H. Influence of dietary bile acids in formation of bile acids in the rat. Steroids 22:667-676, 1973.

k Danielsson, H. and Johansson, G. Effects of long term feeding of chenodeoxycholic acid on biosynthesis and metabolism of bile acids in the rat. Gastroenterology 67:126-134, 1974.

l Danielsson, H. Bile acid metabolism and its control. Second NATO Advanced Study Institute on the Biliary System. August 24-30, 1975, Aalborg, Denmark, p 80 (abstract).

m Danielsson, H. and Sjovall, J. Bile acid metabolism. In Annual Review of Biochemistry, 44:233, 1975.

n Danzinger, R.G., Hofmann, A.F., Schoenfield, L.J., and Thistle, J.L. Altered bile acid metabolism in patients with cholesterol cholelithiasis. J. Clin. Invest. 50:24a, 1971 (abstract).

o Danzinger, R.G.,, Gordon, H., Schoenfield, L.J., and Thistle, J.L. Lithogenic bile in siblings of young women with cholelithiasis. Mayo Clin. Proc. 47:762-766, 1972.

a Danzinger, R.G.,, Hofmann, A.F., Schoenfield, L.J., and Thistle, J.L. Dissolution of cholesterol gallstones by chenodeoxycholic acid. N. Engl. J. Med. 286:1-8, 1972.

b Danzinger, R.G.,, Hofmann, A.F., Schoenfield, L.J., and Thistle, J.L. Expansion of decreased bile acid pool and dissolution of gallstones by chenodeoxycholic acid. Gastroenterology 62:178, 1972 (abstract).

c Danzinger, R.G., Hofmann, A.F., Schoenfield, L.J., and Thistle, J.L. Surgeons react to medical gallstone treatment. N. Engl. J. Med. 286:792-793, 1972 (Letter to editor).

d Danzinger, R.G., Hofmann, A.F., Schoenfield, L.J., and Thistle, J.L. Effect of oral chenodeoxycholic acid on bile acid kinetics and biliary lipid composition in women with cholelithiasis. J. Clin. Invest. 52:2809-2821, 1973.

e Danzinger, R.G., Kurtas, T.K., and Torchia, M.G. Low-dose chenodeoxycholic acid for gallstone dissolution: A randomized trial in poor operative risk patients. Dig. Dis. & Sci. 25:785-789, 1980.

f Danzinger, R.G., Hofmann, A.F., DiPietro, R.A., Ljungwe, E.B., and Barnhart, J.L. Metabolism and physiological properties of two 7-keto bile acids in the dog. Hepatology 1:505, 1981 (abstract).

g Danzinger, R.G., Hofmann, A.F., DiPietro, R.A., Lorenzo, D., and Nazareno, G. Metabolism and physiological properties of 7a- and 7b-monohydroxy bile acids. Hepatology 1:505, 1981 (abstract).

h Darnis, F. and Poupon, R. Dietary fats and cholesterol biliary calculi. Med. Chir. Dig. 8:221-224, 1979.

i D'Ascenzo, G. and Marino, A. Effect of chenodeoxycholic acid on cholesterol calculi. Farmaco Ed. Prat. 30:328-339, 1975.

j Davenport, H.W. Absorption of taurocholate-24-^{14}C through the canine gastric mucosa. Proc. Soc. Exptl. Biol. Med. 125:670-673, 1967.

k Davenport, H.W. Destruction of the gastric mucosal barrier by detergents and urea. Gastroenterology 54:175-181, 1968.

l Davidson, N.O., Samuel, P., Lieberman, S., Shane, S.P., Crouse, J.R., and Ahrens, E.H., Jr. Measurement of bile acid production in hyperlipidemic man: Does phenotype or methodology make the difference? J. Lipid Res. 22:620-631, 1981.

m Davis, J.W. and Elliot, W.H. Bile acids. LVIII. Bile acids and colorectal cancer. Lipids 13:976-981, 1978.

n Davis, R.A. and Kern, F., Jr. Effects of ethinyl estradiol and phenobarbital on bile acid synthesis and biliary bile acid and cholesterol excretion. Gastroenterology 70:1130-1135, 1976.

a Davis, R.A., Showalter, J.P., and Kern, F., Jr. Reversal of ethinyl estradiol induced hypocholesterolemia and cholestasis by Triton WR-1339. In Bile Acid Metabolism in Health and Disease, G Paumgartner and A Stiehl, eds. MTP Press, Lancaster, 1977, pp 25-31.

b Dawson, A.M., Isselbacher, K.J., and Bell, V.M. Studies on lipid metabolism in the small intestine with observations on the role of bile salts. J. Clin. Invest. 39:730-740, 1960.

c DeBarros, S.G., Balistreri, W.F., Soloway, R.D., Weiss, S.G., Miller, P.C., and Soper, K. Response of total and individual serum bile acids to endogenous and exogenous bile acid input to the enterohepatic circulation. Gastroenterology 82:647-652, 1982.

d Debongnie, J-C and Phillips, S.F. Colonic function and diarrhea. Gastroenterology 72:1046, 1977 (abstract).

e Dehesa, M. and Landa, L. Tratamiento de la litiasis vesicular con acido quenodesoxicolico (AQD). Informe de 50 casos. Rev. Gastroent. Mex. 46: 163-166, 1981.

f Deitrick, J.E., McSherry, C.K., Thorbjarnarson, B., and Glenn, F. The study of bile salt kinetics in the experimental animal using a new technique. J. Surg. Res. 16:559-563, 1974.

g Deleze, G., von Bergmann, J., von Bergmann, K., Hadorn, B., and Paumgartner, G. Composition en acides biliaires et saturation en cholesterol de la bile du jeune enfant. Schw. med. Wschr. 106:322, 1976.

h Deleze, G., Paumgartner, G., Karlaganis, G., Giger, W., Reinhard, M., and Sidiropoulos, D. Bile acid pattern in human amniotic fluid. Europ. J. Clin. Invest. 8:41-45, 1978.

i Delmont, J., Rampal, P., Math, M, Faure, X., and Renson, M. Treatment of biliary lithiasis with ursodeoxycholic acid. Sem. Hop Paris 56:1613-1616, 1980.

j DeMark, B.R., Everson, G.T., Klein, P.D., Showalter, R.B., and Kern, F., Jr. A method for the accurate measurement of isotope ratios of chenodeoxycholic and cholic acids in serum. J. Lipid Res. 23:204-210, 1982.

k Demers, L.M. and Hepner, G.W. Levels of immunoreactive glycine conjugated bile acids in health and hepatobiliary disease. Am. J. Clin. Path. 66:831-839, 1976.

l Demers, L.M. and Hepner, G.W. Radioimmunoassay of serum bile acids. Clin. Chem. 22:602-606, 1976.

m Demers, L.M. and Jones, D.E. Serum concentration of bile acids in maternal blood and cord blood at parturition. Am. J. Obstet. Gynecol. 137:146-147, 1980.

n Demeulenaere, L. and van Waes, L. Lithiase biliaire et acide chenique. Faits acquis et perspectives. Acta Gastro-Ent. Belg. 38:7-12, 1975 (Editorial).

a DenBesten, L., Connor, W.E., and Bell, S. The effect of dietary cholesterol on the composition of human bile. Surgery 73:266-273, 1973.

b DenBesten, L., Reyna, R.H., Connor, W.E., and Stegink, L.D. The different effects on the serum lipids and fecal steroids of high carbohydrate diets given orally or intravenously. J. Clin. Invest. 52:1384-1393, 1973.

c DenBesten, L., Safaie-Shirazi, A., Connor, W.E., and Bell, S. Early changes in bile induced by a high cholesterol diet in prairie dogs. Gastroenterology 66:1036-1045, 1974.

d Denk, H., Schenkman, J.B., Bacchin, P.G., Hutterer, F., Schaffner, F., and Popper, H. Mechanism of cholestasis. III. Interaction of synthetic detergents with the microsomal cytochrome P-450 dependent biotransformation system in vitro. A comparison between the effects of detergents, the effects of bile acids, and the findings in bile duct ligated rats. Exp. Molec. Path. 14:263-276, 1971.

e Devers, T.J., Gallo, D., and Ostrow, J.D. Effects of bile lipids and pH on the solubility of unconjugated bilirubin. Gastroenterology 68:1082, 1975 (abstract).

f Devers, T.J., Gallo, D., and Ostrow, J.D. Mechanism of solubilization of unconjugated bilirubin by taurocholate. Gastroenterology 69:816, 1975 (abstract).

g Dew, M.J., van Berge Henegouwen, G.P., Huijbregts, A.W.M., and Allan, R.N. Hepatotoxic effect of bile acids in inflammatory bowel disease. Gastroenterology 78:1393-1401, 1980.

h Dew, M.J., Hawker, P., Nutter, S., Allan, R. Human intestinal sulphation of lithocholate. A new site for bile acid metabolism. Life Sci. 27:317-323, 1980.

i Dew, M.J., Hawker, P., Nutter, S., van Berge Henegouwen, G., Huijbregts, A., and Allan, R. Lithocholate metabolism in colonic carcinoma. Gut (in press).

j DeWitt, E.H. and Lack, L. Effects of sulfation patterns on intestinal transport of bile salt sulfate esters. Am. J. Physiol. 238:G34-G39, 1980.

k Diamond, J.M. and Wright, E.M. Biological membranes: The physical basis of ion and non-electrolyte selectivity. Ann. Rev. Physiol. 31:581-646, 1969.

l DiCicco, M., Ferraris, R., Spampinato, L., and De La Pierre, M. Evaluation of the treatment of cholelithiasis using chenodeoxycholic acid. Min. Dietol. Gastroenterol. 25:41-46, 1979.

m Dietschy, J.M. and Wilson, J.D. Cholesterol synthesis in the gastrointestinal tract: Localization and mechanisms of control. J. Clin. Invest. 44:1311-1327, 1965.

a Dietschy, J.M. Recent developments in solute and water transport across the gall bladder epithelium. Gastroenterology 50:692-707, 1966.

b Dietschy, J.M., Salomon, H.S., and Siperstein, M.D. Bile acid metabolism. I. Studies on the mechanisms of intestinal transport. J. Clin. Invest. 45:832-846, 1966.

c Dietschy, J.M. Effects of bile salts on intermediate metabolism of the intestinal mucosa. Fed. Proc. 26:1589, 1967.

d Dietschy, J.M. and Siperstein, M.D. Effect of cholesterol feeding and fasting on sterol synthesis in seventeen tissues of the rat. J. Lipid Res. 8:97-104, 1967.

e Dietschy, J.M. Mechanism for the intestinal absorption of bile acids. J. Lipid Res. 9:297-309, 1968.

f Dietschy, J.M. The role of bile salts in controlling the rate of intestinal cholesterogenesis. J. Clin. Invest. 47:286-300, 1968.

g Dietschy, J.M. and Wilson, J.D. Cholesterol synthesis in the squirrel monkey: Relative rates of synthesis in various tissues and mechanism of control. J. Clin. Invest. 47:166-174, 1968.

h Dietschy, J.M. and Wilson, J.D. Regulation of cholesterol metabolism. N. Engl. J. Med. 282:1128-1138, 1970.

i Dietschy, J.M. and Gamel, W.G. Cholesterol synthesis in the intestine in man: Regional differences and control mechanisms. J. Clin. Invest. 50:872-880, 1971.

j Dietschy, J.M. and Weis, H.J. Cholesterol synthesis in the gastrointestinal tract. Am. J. Clin. Nutr. 24:70-76, 1971.

k Dietschy, J.M. The biology of bile acids. Arch. Intern. Med. 130:473-474, 1972.

l Dietschy, J.M. The uptake of lipids into the intestinal mucosa. In Physiology of Membrane Disorders. TE Andreoli, JF Hoffman, and DD Fanestil, eds. Plenum Pub. Corp., New York, 1978, pp 577-592.

m DiFilippo, N.M. and Blumenthal, H.J. Experimental cholelithiasis in the golden hamster: Effect of glucuronolactone. Am. J. Osteopath. Assn. 72:288-293, 1972.

n DiPadova, C., Tritapepe, R., Marabini, L., DiPadova, F., Rovagnati, P., and Mazzocchi, M. Ursodeoxycholic acid and liver microsomal mixed function oxidase system in man. Methods Find. Exp. Clin. Pharmacol. 3:209-211, 1981.

o DiPietro, R., Danzinger, R., Hofmann, A.F., Schmack, B., Jones, C., Gupta, S., and Flynn, B. New, potent cholesterol dissolving agents for dissolution of retained duct stones. Gastroenterology 80:1330, 1981 (abstract).

a DiTullio, N.W. and Stack, E.J. Alterations in biliary lipids of mice during dehydrocholic acid feeding. J. Lipid Res. 14:552-556, 1973.

b Dolgrin, S.M., Schwartz, J.S., Kressel, H.Y., Soloway, R.D., Wallace, T.M., Trotman, B.W., Soloway, A.S., and Good, L.I. Identification of patients with cholesterol or pigment gallstones by discriminant analysis of radiographic features. N. Engl. J. Med. 304:808-811, 1981.

c Dolkart, R.E., Lorenz, M., Jones, K.K., and Brown, D.F.G. Relation of fatty acids and bile salts to the formation of gallstones. Arch. Int. Med. 66:1087-1094, 1940.

d Doman, D.B. and Ginsberg, A.L. Glucagon infusion therapy for biliary tree stones. Gastroenterology 80:1137, 1981 (abstract).

e Domellof, L., Eriksson, S., Mori, H., Weisburger, J.H., and Williams, G.M. Effect of bile acid gavage or vagotomy and pyloroplasty on gastrointestinal carcinogenesis. Am. J. Surg. 142:551-554, 1981.

f Doous, T.W. Gallstones and carcinoma of the large bowel. N. Z. Med. J. 77:162, 1973.

g Doran, J., Keighley, M.R.B., and Bell, G.D. Rowachol--A possible treatment for cholesterol gallstones? Gut 20:312-317, 1979.

h Doty, J.E., DenBesten, L., Roslyn, J.J., Pitt, H.A., Kuchenbecker, S.L., and Porter-Fink, V. Interaction of chenodeoxycholic acid and dietary cholesterol in the treatment of cholesterol gallstones. Am. J. Surg. 143: 48-54, 1982.

i Douglas, J.G., Beckett, G.J., Nimmo, I.A., Finlayson, N.D.C., and Percy-Robb, I.W. Bile salt measurements in Gilbert's syndrome. Europ. J. Clin. Invest. 11:421-423, 1981.

j Dowling, R.H., Mack, E., Picott, J., Berger, J., and Small, D.M. Experimental model for the study of the enterohepatic circulation of bile in the Rhesus monkey. J. Lab. Clin. Med. 72:169-176, 1968.

k Dowling, R.H., Mack, E., and Small, D.M. Effects of controlled interruption of the enterohepatic circulation of bile salts by biliary diversion and by ileal resection on bile salt secretion, synthesis, and pool size in the Rhesus monkey. J. Clin. Invest. 49:232-242, 1970.

l Dowling, R.H., Mack, E., and Small, D.M. Primate biliary physiology. IV. Biliary lipid secretion and bile composition after acute and chronic interruption of the enterohepatic circulation in the Rhesus monkey. J. Clin. Invest. 50:1917-1926, 1971.

m Dowling, R.H. The enterohepatic circulation. Gastroenterology 62:122-140, 1972.

n Dowling, R.H., Bell, G.D., White, J. Lithogenic bile in patients with ileal dysfunction. Gut 13:415-420, 1972.

a Dowling, R.H. Chenodeoxycholic acid: The British experience. Hosp. Prac. 9:85-93, 1974.

b Dowling, R.H. The goose that laid the golden bile: Gall-stone dissolution in man with chenodeoxycholic acid. Irish J. Med. Sci. (supplement) 115-127, 1974.

c Dowling, R.H., Mok, H.Y.I., and Bell, G.D. Chenodeoxycholic acid and the liver. Lancet 2:875-876, 1974.

d Dowling, R.H. Chenodeoxycholic acid therapy of gallstones. Clin. Gastroenterol. 6:141-163, 1977.

e Dowling, R.H. Physiopathologie de la lithiase biliaire et son traitement par l'acide chenodesoxycholique. Med. Chir. Dig. 6:6-9, 1977.

f Dowling, R.H., Iser, J.H., Murphy, G.M., Ponz de Leon, M., and Isaacs, P. The Guys experience with chenotherapy for gallstone dissolution. In Liver and Bile, L Bianchi, ed. Baltimore Univ. Park Press, Baltimore, 1977, pp 281-295.

g Dowling, R. The gallstone dissolution story. Hosp. Update 2:1081-1103, 1979.

h Dowling, R.H., Hofmann, A.F., and Barbara, L. Workshop on Ursodeoxycholic Acid. University Park Press, Baltimore, 1979.

i Dowling, R. A personal view of gallstone dissolution. Hepatology 111:ix-xii, 1980 (Editorial).

j Dowling, R.H. Medical treatment of gallstones with CDCA and UDCA. In Bile Acids and Lipids. G Paumgartner, A Stiehl, and W Gerok, eds. MTP Press, Lancaster, 1981, pp 329-339.

k Dreher, K.D., Schulman, J.H., and Hofmann, A.F. Surface chemistry of the monoglyceride-bile salt system: Its relationship to the function of bile salts in fat absorption. J. Colloid Interface Sci. 25:71-83, 1967.

l Druke, T., Ganeval, D., and Marche, C. Chenodeoxycholic acid: Possible intestinal injury? N. Engl. J. Med. 290:405-406, 1974 (Letter to Editor).

m Duane, W.C. The intermicellar bile salt concentration in equilibrium with the mixed micelles of human bile. Biochim. Biophys. Acta 398:275, 1975.

n Duane, W.C., Adler, R.D., Bennion, L.J., and Ginsberg, R.L. Determination of bile acid pool size in man: A simplified method with advantages of increased precision, shortened analysis and decreased isotope. J. Lipid Res. 16:155-158, 1975.

o Duane, W.C., Ginsberg, R.L., and Bennion, L.J. Effects of fasting on bile acid metabolism and biliary lipid composition in man. J. Lipid Res. 17:211-219, 1976.

a Duane, W.C. Taurocholate- and taurochenodeoxycholate-lecithin micelles. BBRC 74:223, 1977.

b Duane, W.C. Simulation of the defect of bile acid metabolism associated with cholesterol cholelithiasis by sorbitol ingestion in man. J. Lab. Clin. Med. 91:969-978, 1978.

c Duane, W. and Hanson, K. Role of gallbladder emptying and small bowel transit in regulation of bile acid pool size in man. J. Lab. Clin. Med. 92:859-872, 1978.

d Duane, W.C., Gilberstadt, M.L., and Wiegand, D.M. Diurnal rhythms of bile acid production in the rat. Am. J. Physiol. 236:R175-R179, 1979.

e Duane, W.C. and Bond, J.H., Jr. Prolongation of intestinal transit and expansion of bile acid pools by propantheline bromide. Gastroenterology 78:226-230, 1980.

f Duane, W.C. and Wiegand, D.M. Mechanism by which bile salt disrupts the gastric mucosal barrier in the dog. J. Clin. Invest. 66:1044-1049, 1980.

g Duane, W.C., Wiegand, D.M., and Gilberstadt, M.L. Intragastric duodenal lipids in the absence of a pyloric sphincter: Quantitation, physical state, and injurious potential in the fasting and postprandial states. Gastroenterology 78:1480-1487, 1980.

h Dubin, M., Maurice, M., Feldmann, G., and Erlinger, S. Phalloidin induced cholestasis in the rat: Relation to changes in microfilaments. Gastroenterology 75:450-455, 1978.

i Dujovne, C.A. and Mardiat, J. Is the hepatotoxic potential of bile acids, chlorpromazine and erythromycin estolate related to their detergent potency? Gastroenterology 69:818, 1975 (abstract).

j Dumont, M., Berthelot, P., and Dhumeaux, D. Comparison of the choleretic effects of dehydrocholate and glycodeoxycholate in the rabbit. Digestion 4:144-145, 1971.

k Dumont, M., Erlinger, S., and Uchman, S. Hypercholeresis induced by ursodeoxycholic acid and 7-ketolithocholic acid in the rat. Possible role of bicarbonate transport. Gastroenterology 79:82-89, 1980.

l Dupont, T., Baylocq, D., Guffroy, A., Champault, G., Beaugrand, M., Hecht, Y., and Ferrier, J.P. Separation and dosage of bile acid by high performance liquid chromatography. Application to the study of normal and lithogenous bile. Gastroenterol. Clin. Biol. 3:349-354, 1979.

m Dusza, J.P., Jospeh, J.P., and Bernstein, S. Steroid conjugates. IV. The preparation of steroid sulfates with triethylamine-sulfur trioxide. Steroids 12:49, 1968.

a Dutt, M.K., Murray, B., Jazrawi, R., Kupfer, R., Northfield, T.C., and Thompson, R.P.H. Bilirubin-cholesterol saturation index (BrCSI): a new index to predict lithogenicity in cholesterol gall stone (CGS) disease. Gut 22:A887, 1981.

b Duvaldestin, P., Mahu, J.L., Metreau, J.M., Arcondel, J., Preaux, A.M., and Berthelot, P. Possible role of a defect in hepatic bilirubin glucuronidation in the initiation of cholesterol gallstones. Gut 21:650-655, 1980.

c Dyer, D.L. The effect of pH on solubilization of weak acids and bases. J. Colloid Interface Sci. 14:640-645, 1959.

d Dyfverman, A. and Sjovall, J. A novel liquid-gel chromatographic method for extraction of unconjugated steroids from aqueous solutions. Anal. Lett. B11:485-499, 1978.

e Dyrszka, H., Chen, T., Salen, G., and Mosbach, E.H. Toxicity of chenodeoxycholic acid in the Rhesus monkey. Gastroenterology 69:333-337, 1975.

f Dyrszka, H., Salen, G., Zaki, F.G., Chen, T., and Mosbach, E.H. Hepatic toxicity in the Rhesus monkey treated with chenodeoxycholic acid for 6 months: Biochemical and ultrastructural studies. Gastroenterology 70:93-104, 1976.

g Eastwood, M.A. The distribution of bile salts along the small intestine of rats. Biochim. Biophys. Acta 137:393, 1967.

h Eastwood, M.A., and Hamilton, D. A sensitive non-destructive method for the determination of bile acids on thin layer chromatography. Biochem. J. 105:370, 1967.

i Eastwood, M.A. and Hamilton, D. Studies on the adsorption of bile salts to non-absorbed components of diet. Biochim. Biophys. Acta 152:165-173, 1968.

j Eastwood, M.A. A method for the estimation of bile acid conjugates in biological fluids. J. Chromatog. 65:407-411, 1972.

k Eastwood, M.A. Physiology of bile acids in the ileum and colon. Scot. Med. J. 18:142-145, 1973.

l Eastwood, M.A., Findlay, J.M. and Mitchell, W.D. The physical state of bile acids in the diarrhea stool of ileal dysfunction. Gut 14:319-323, 1973.

m Eastwood, M. and Kay, R. An hypothesis for the action of dietary fiber along the gastrointestinal tract. Am. J. Clin. Nutr. 32:364-367, 1979.

n Eaton, D.L. and Klaassen, C.D. Effects of acute administration of taurocholic and taurochenodeoxycholic acid on biliary lipid excretion in the rat. Proc. Soc. Exptl. Biol. Med. 151:198-202, 1976.

o Edenharder, R. and Deser, H-J. The significance of the bacterial steroid degradation for the etiology of large bowel cancer. VIII. Transformation of cholic-, chenodeoxycholic-, and deoxycholic acid by lecithinase-lipase-negative clostridia. Zbl. Bakt. Hyg. 174:91-104, 1981.

a Edenharder, R. and Knaflic, T. Epimerization of chenodeoxycholic acid to ursodeoxycholic acid by human intestinal lecithinase-lipase-negative Clostridia. J. Lipid Res. 22:652-658, 1981.

b Editorial. Abnormal bile or faulty gall bladder? Brit Med. J. 4:571-572, 1970.

c Editorial. Cholesterol absorption versus cholesterol synthesis in man. Nutr. Rev. 28:11-15, 1970.

d Editorial. Gallstones: A new liver disease? N. Engl. J. Med. 283:96-97, 1970.

e Editorial. Carcinoma of the gallbladder: Can the outlook be improved? Lancet 2:967, 1971

f Editorial. Epidemiology of large bowel cancer. Lancet 2:120, 1971.

g Editorial. Atromid-S and cholecystitis. Brit. Med. J. 1:106, 1972.

h Editorial. The dissolution of gallstones. JAMA 221:600, 1972.

i Editorial. Dissolving gall stones. Brit. Med. J. 1:525, 1972.

j Editorial. Gallbladder disorders: An insurance experience. Statistical Bull. (Metropolitan LIfe) August, 1972.

k Editorial. Les calculs biliaires sont soluble. Medicine Mondiale No. 106, p 73, May, 1972.

l Editorial. Les fantasies de l'acide chenodeoxycholique. Medicine Mondiale No. 111, p 70, Sept., 1972.

m Editorial. Manipulating bile acids: Key to aborting cholelithiasis. Hosp. Prac. 7(9), 1972.

n Editorial. Medical treatment of gallstone disease. Lancet 1:360-361, 1972.

o Editorial. Stagnation of bile. Brit. Med. J. 3:779-781, 1972.

p Editorial. Bile acid breath test: Extremely simple, moderately useful. Ann. Intern. Med. 79:743-744, 1973.

q Editorial. Diet and cholesterol gallstones. Lancet 1:471-472, 1973.

r Editorial. Dissolution of gallstones. Nutr. Rev. 31:113-114, 1973.

s Editorial. More about chenodeoxycholic acid. Brit. Med. J. 4:629, 1973.

t Editorial. Steine erweicht. Der Speigel, No. 6, p 108, 1973.

a Editorial. Complications of anticholesterol treatment. Brit. Med. J. 1:324, 1974.

b Editorial. Determination of the cholesterol saturation of human bile and its relevance to gallstone formation. Am. J. Dig. Dis. 19:268-270, 1974.

c Editorial. Effects of cholecystectomy. Brit. Med. J. 2:72-73, 1974.

d Editorial. Oestrogens, lipids and gallstones. Brit. Med. J. 3:132-133, 1974.

e Editorial. Dangers of silent gallstones. Brit. Med. J. 3:415, 1975.

f Editorial. Progress in dissolving gallstones. Brit. Med. J. 1:699-700, 1975.

g Editorial. Choosing patients for chenodeoxycholic acid treatment. Brit. Med. J. 1:1119-1120, 1977.

h Editorial. Chenic acid for gall stones. Brit. Med. J. 2:847, 1978.

i Editorial. Chenodeoxycholic acid therapy of gallstones. S. Afr. Med. J. 54:724-725, 1978.

j Editorial. Chenodeoxycholic acid. Med. Chir. Dig. 7:343-344, 1978.

k Editorial. Chenotherapy: Questions--Answers. Med. Chir. Dig. 7:347-351, 1978.

l Editorial. Formation and dissolution of gallstones. J. Assoc. Physicians India 26:852-855, 1978.

m Editorial. Medical treatment of gallstones. Drug Ther. Bull. 16:69-71, 1978.

n Editorial. Dissolving gallstones. Med. J. Aust. 1:456-457, 1980.

o Editorial. Dissolution of bile duct stones. Lancet 1:336, 1981.

p Editorial. Dissolving hopes for gallstone disslution? Lancet 2:905-906, 1981.

q Egberts, E-H., Cain, H., Dolle, W., Fischer, R., Frommhold, W., Kohler, F., and Martini, G.A. Die angeborene Erweiterung der grossen intrahepatischen Gallenwege: Carolische Krankheit. Internist 17:149-159, 1976.

r Eggen, D.A. Cholesterol metabolism in Rhesus monkey, Squirrel monkey and baboon. J. Lipid Res. 15:139-144, 1974.

s Einarsson, K. On the formation of hyodeoxycholic acid in the rat. J. Biol. Chem. 241:534-539, 1966.

t Einarsson, K. On the properties of the 12a-hydroxylase in cholic acid biosynthesis. Europ. J. Biochem. 5:101-108, 1968.

a Einarsson, K. and Johansson, G. Effect of phenobarbital on the conversion of cholesterol to taurocholic acid. Europ. J. Biochem. 6:293, 1968.

b Einarsson, K. and Johansson, G. Effect of carbon monoxide and phenobarbital on hydroxylation of bile acids by rat liver microsomes. FEBS Letters 4:177, 1969.

c Einarsson, K., Gustafsson, J.A., and Goldman, A.S. Metabolism of steroid hormones, sterols, and bile acids in liver microsomes from male, female, and male-pseudohermophroditic rats. Eur. J. Biochem. 31:345-353, 1972.

d Einarsson, K. and Hellstrom, K. The formation of bile acids in patients with three types of hyperlipoproteinemia. Europ. J. Clin. Invest. 2:225-230, 1972.

e Einarsson, K., Hellstrom, K., and Kallner, M. The effect of clofibrate on the elimination of cholesterol as bile acid in patients with hyperlipoproteinemia type II and IV. Europ. J. Clin. Invest. 3:345-351, 1973.

f Einarsson, K., Hellstrom, K., and Kallner, M. Feedback and regulation of bile acid formation in man. Metabolism 22:1477-1483, 1973.

g Einarsson, K. and Gustafsson, J. Effect of 16a-cyanopregnenolone on the hydroxylation of lithocholic acid by rat liver microsomes. Biochem. Pharm. 23:9-12, 1974.

h Einarsson, K. and Hellstrom, K. The formation of deoxycholic and chenodeoxycholic acid in man. Clin. Sci. Mol. Med. 46:183-190, 1974.

i Einarsson, K., Hellstrom, K., and Kallner, M. Bile acid kinetics in relation to sex, serum lipids, body weights, and gallbladder disease in patients with various types of hyperlipoproteinemia. J. Clin. Invest. 54:1301-1311, 1974.

j Einarsson, K., Hellstrom, K., and Kallner, M. The effect of cholestyramine on the elimination of cholesterol as bile acids in patients with hyperlipoproteinemia types II and IV. Europ. J. Clin. Invest. 4:405-410, 1974.

k Einarsson, K., Hellstrom, K., and Kallner, M. Effect of cholic acid feeding on bile acid kinetics and neutral fecal steroid excretion in hyperlipoproteinemia (types II and IV). Metabolism 23:863-873, 1974.

l Einarsson, K., Hellstrom, K., and Kallner, M. Influence of deoxycholic acid feeding on the elimination of cholesterol in normolipidaemic subjects. Clin. Sci. Mol. Med. 47:425-433, 1974.

m Einarsson, K., Hellstrom, K., and Kallner, M. Randomly tritium-labelled chenodeoxycholic acid as tracer in the determination bile acid turnover in man. Clin. Chim. Acta 56:235-239, 1974.

n Einarsson, K., Hellstrom, K., and Kallner, M. Gallbladder disease in hyperlipoproteinemia. Lancet 1:484-494, 1975.

a Einarsson, K., Hellstrom, K., and Schersten, T. The formation of bile acids in patients with portal liver cirrhosis. Scand. J. Gastroenterol. 10:299-304, 1975.

b Einarsson, K., Hellstrom, K., and Leijd, B. Bile acid kinetics and steroid balance during nicotinic acid therapy in patients with hyperlipoproteinemia types II and IV. J. Lab. Clin. Med. 90:613-622, 1977.

c Einarsson, K., Ahlberg, J., Angelin, B., and Holmstrom, B. Evidence for the presence of different hepatic cholesterol precursor pools in man. In The Liver. R Preisig, J Bircher, eds. Editio Cantor, Aulendorf, 1978, pp 233-238.

d Einarsson, K., Grundy, S., and Hardison, W.G.M. Enterohepatic circulation rates of cholic acid and chenodeoxycholic acid in man. Gut 20:1078-1082, 1979.

e Einarsson, K. and Grundy, S. Effects of feeding cholic acid and chenodeoxycholic acid on cholesterol absorption and hepatic secretion of biliary lipids in man. J. Lipid Res. 21:23-34, 1980.

f Ekwall, P. and Sjoblom, L. On the solubilization of steroid hormones by association colloids. Acta Chem. Scand. 3:1179-1180, 1949.

g Ekwall, P. Micelle formation in sodium cholate solutions. Acta Acad. Aboensis Math. Phys. 17:3-10, 1951.

h Ekwall, P., Lindstrom, E.V., and Setala, K. The stability of the micelles in bile acid salt solutions of different acidities. Acta Chem. Scand. 5:990-994, 1951.

i Ekwall, P. The solubilization of lipophilic substances by bile acid salts. In Proc. of the 1st Int'l Conf on Biochem. Prob. of Lipids. R Ruyssen, ed. Brussels, 1953, pp 103-119.

j Ekwall, P. and Fontell, K. Small angle scattering of x-rays in aqueous solutions of bile acid salts. Acta Chem. Scand. 10:327-340, 1956.

k Ekwall, P. and Ekholm, R. Monolayers of bile acid. In Proc of the 2nd Int'l Cong. Surf. Act., Gas-Liquid and Liquid-Liquid Interface. JH Schulman, ed. Butterworths Scientific Pub., London, 1957, pp 22-30.

l Ekwall, P., Ekholm, R., and Norman, A. Surface balance studies of bile acid monolayers. I. Cholanic and glycocholanic acid monolayers. Acta Chem. Scand. 11:693-702, 1957.

m Ekwall, P., Ekholm, R., and Norman, A. Surface balance studies of bile acid monolayers. II. Monolayers of lithocholic and glycolithocholic acids. Acta Chem. Scand. 11:703-709, 1957.

n Ekwall, P., Fontell, K., and Norman, A. Small-angle scattering of x-rays in aqueous solutions of sodium salts of conjugated and unconjugated bile acids. Acta Chem. Scand. 11:190-192, 1957.

a Ekwall, P., Rosendahl, T., and Lofman, N. Studies on bile acid salt solutions. I. The dissociation constants of the cholic and deoxycholic acids. Acta Chem. Scand. 11:590-598, 1957.

b El Kodsi, B., Cooperband, S.R., and Bouchier, I.A.D. Variations in the ultracentrifugal characteristics of human gallbladder bile and hepatic bile with diseases of the biliary tree. J. Lab. Clin. Med. 72:592-601, 1968.

c Elliott, W.H., Walsh, L.B., Mui, M.M., Thorn, M.A., and Siegfried, C.M. Bile acids. XXVIII. Gas chromatography of new bile acids and their derivatives. J. Chromatog. 44:452, 1969.

d Elliott, W.H. and Hyde, P.M. Metabolic pathways of bile acid synthesis. Am. J. Med. 51:568-579, 1971.

e Ellis, W.R., Rose, D.H., Richmond, C.R., Nehru, A.Y., Middleton, A., and Bell, G.D. Radio-opaque gallstones--reduction in size and calcium content on treatment with Rowachol. Gut 21:A910, 1980 (abstract).

f Ellis, W.R., Bell, G.D., Clegg, R.J., Middleton, B., and White, D.A. Mechanisms for adjuvant cholelithiolytic properties of the monoterpene mixture Rowachol (R). Gastroenterology 80:1141, 1981 (abstract).

g Ellis, W.R., Bell, G., Middleton, B., and White, D. Adjunct to bile-acid treatment for gall-stone dissolution: Low-dose chenodeoxycholic acid combined with a terpene preparation. Brit. Med. J. 282:611-612, 1981.

h Ellis, W.R., Bell, G.D., Somerville, K., Clegg, R.J., Middleton, B., and White, D.A. Mechanisms for adjuvant cholelitholytic properties of the monoterpene mixture Rowachol (R). Clin. Sci. 61:38, 1981 (abstract).

i Emerman, S. and Javitt, N.B. Metabolism of taurolithocholic acid in the hamster. J. Biol. Chem. 242:661-664, 1967.

j Encrantz, J-C., and Sjovall, J. On the bile acids in duodenal contents of infants and children. Clin. Chim. Acta 4:793, 1959.

k Endo, T., Uchida, K., Amuro, Y., Higashino, K., and Yamamura, Y. Bile acid metabolism in benign recurrent intrahepatic cholestasis. Gastroenterology 76:1002-1006, 1979.

l Eneroth, P. Thin-layer chromatography of bile acids. J. Lipid Res. 4:11-16, 1963.

m Eneroth, P., Gordon, B., Ryhage, R., and Sjovall, J. Identification of mono- and dihydroxy bile acids in human feces by gas-liquid chromatography and mass spectrometry. J. Lipid Res. 7:511-523, 1966.

n Eneroth, P., Gordon, B., and Sjovall, J. Characterization of trisubstituted cholanic acids in human feces. J. Lipid Res. 7:425-430, 1966.

o Eneroth, P., Hellstrom, K., and Sjovall, J. Bile acids and steroids. CXCV. A method for quantitative determination of bile acids in human feces. Acta Chem. Scand. 22:1729, 1968.

a Eneroth, P. Thin-layer chromatography of bile alcohols and bile acids. In Lipid Chromatographic Analysis. GV Marinetti, ed. Marcel Dekker, Inc., New York, 1969, pp 149-183.

b Eneroth, P. and Sjovall, J. Methods of analysis in the biochemistry of bile acids. In Methods in Enzymology. RB Clayton, ed. Academic Press, New York, 1969, p 237.

c Eneroth, P., Ryhage, R., and Sjovall, J. Mass spectra of bile acids. In The Bile Acids: Chemistry, Physiology, and Metabolism. D Kritchevsky, PP Nair, eds. Plenum Press, New York, 1971, p 209.

d Eng, C. and Javitt, N.B. Chenodeoxycholic-3-sulfate: Metabolism and excretion in hamster and rat. Gastroenterology 80:1331, 1981 (abstract).

e Engelking, L.R., Gronwall, R., and Anwer, M.S. Effect of bile acid on hepatic excretion and storage of bilirubin in ponies. Am. J. Vet. Res. 37:47-50, 1976.

f Engelking, L.R., Barnes, S., Hirschowitz, B.I., Dasher, C.A., Spenney, J.G., and Naftel, D. Determination of the pool size and synthesis rate of bile acids by measurements in blood of patients with liver disease. Clin. Sci. 58:485-492, 1980.

g Engelking, L.R., Gronwall, R., and Anwer, M.S. Effect of dehydrocholic, chenodeoxycholic, and taurocholic acids on the excretion of bilirubin. Am. J. Vet. Res. 41:355-361, 1980.

h Englert, E., Jr., Harman, C.G., and Wales, E., Jr. Gallstones induced by normal foodstuffs in dogs. Nature 224:280-281, 1969.

i Englert, E., Jr., Harman, C.G., Freston, J.W., Straight, R.C., and Wales, E.E., Jr. Studies on the pathogenesis of diet-induced dog gallstones. Am. J. Dig. Dis. 22:305-314, 1977.

j Entenman, C., Holloway, R.J., Albright, M.L., and Leong, G.F. Bile acids and lipid metabolism. II. Essential role of bile acids in bile phospholipid excretion. Arch. Biochem. Biophys. 130:253-256, 1969.

k Erb, W., Schreiber, J., and Walczak, M. Gaschromatographische Untersuchungen der Serumgallensauren: Methodik sowie Ergebnisse bei Patienten mit akuter Hepatitis. Z. Gastroenterol. 10:349-358, 1972.

l Erb, W. and Leuschner, U. Die Entstehung von Gallensteinen. Med. Klin. 68:131-135, 1973.

m Erb, W., Schreiber, J., and Walczak, M. Untersuchungen der Gallensauren im Serum von Patienten mit extrahepatischer Cholostase und mit chonischen Lebererkrankungen. Z. Gastroenterol. 11:279-288, 1973.

a Erb, W. Die Auflosung von Cholesteringallensteinen. Ein aktuelles therapeutisches Problem. Med. Klin. 70:1199-1207, 1975.

b Erickson, S.K., Cooper, A.D., Matshui, S.M., and Gould, R.G. 7-ketocholesterol. Its effects on hepatic cholesterogenesis and its hepatic metabolism in vivo and in vitro. J. Biol. Chem. 252:5186-5193, 1977.

c Eriksson, S. Biliary excretion of bile acids and cholesterol in bile fistula rats. Proc. Soc. Exptl. Biol. Med. 94:578-583, 1957.

d Eriksson, S. Bile acid pool in the rat. Bile acids and steroids. Acta Physiol. Scand. 48:439, 1960.

e Erlinger, S. La dissolution medicale des calculs biliaires: Un vieux reve devenu relite. Le Monde 13-14, January 5, 1977.

f Erlinger, S. Treatment of biliary calculi: The place of chenodeoxycholic acid. Rev. Infirm. 27:683-685, 1977.

g Erlinger, S., Poupon, R., and Dumont, M. Hepatic uptake, storage and biliary transport maximum of bile acids in the dog. In Bile Acid Metabolism in Health and Disease. G Paumgartner and A Stiehl, eds. MTP Press, Lancaster, 1977, pp 107-112.

h Erlinger, S. Cholestasis: Pump failure, microvilli defect, or both? Lancet 1:533-534, 1978.

i Ertan, A., Brooks, F.P., Ostrow, J.D., Arvan, D.A., Williams, C.N., and Cerda, J.J. Effect of jejunal amino acid perfusion and exogenous cholecystokinin on the exocrine pancreatic and biliary secretions in man. Gastroenterology 61:686-692, 1971.

j Etienne, J.P. Conclusions: Current concepts in the treatment of biliary lithiasis by chenodeoxycholic acid. Therapie 32:417-421, 1977.

k Everson, G.T., Braverman, D.Z., Johnson, M.L., and Kern, F., Jr. A critical evaluation of real-time ultrasonography for the study of gallbladder volume and contraction. Gastroenterology 79:40-46, 1980.

l Evrard, E. and Janssen, G. Gas-liquid chromatographic determination of human fecal bile acids. J. Lipid Res. 9:226-236, 1968.

m Evrard, E. Some current trends in bile salt research. Digestion 5:108-115, 1972.

n Exner, T. and Koppel, J.L. The effect of bile salts on the esterase activities of plasmin and some other enzymes. Biochim. Biophys. Acta 321:303-318, 1973.

o Eyssen, H., Vandeputte, M., and Evrard, E. Effect of various dietary bile acids in nutrient absorption and on liver size in chicks. Arch. Int. Pharmacodyn. 158:292-306, 1965.

a Eyssen, H., Evrard, E., and Vanderhaeghe, H. Cholesterol-lowering effects of N-methylated neomycin and basic antibiotics. J. Lab. Clin. Med. 68:753-768, 1966.

b Eyssen, H., Parmentier, G., Compernolle, F., Boan, J., and Eggermont, E. Trihydroxycoprostanic acid in the duodenal fluid of two children with intrahepatic bile duct anomalies. Biochem. Biophys. Acta 272:212, 1972.

c Eyssen, H., Smets, L., Parmentier, G., and Janssen, G. Sex-linked differences in bile acid metabolism of germfree rats. Life sciences 21:707-712, 1977.

d Fairclough, P.D., Feest, T.G., Chadwick, V.S., and Clark, M.L. The effect of chenodeoxycholic acid on oxalate absorption from the excluded human colon. A mechanism for "enteric" hyperoxaluria. Gut 18:240-244, 1977.

e Falaiye, J.M. Bile salt patterns in Nigerians on a high fibre diet. Lancet 1:1002, 1974 (Letter to Editor).

f Falconer, J.D., Smith, A.N., and Eastwood, M.A. The effects of bile acids on colonic motility in the rabbit. Steroids 21:36, 1980 (abstract).

g Falk, H. Bile duct flushing solutions. CA Selects-Steroids 14:9, 1981 and 14:19, 1981.

h Fallon, H.J. and Woods, J.W. Cholestyramine treatment of hyperlipidemias. Clin. Res. 15:73, 1967 (abstract).

i Faloon, W.W. Gallstone prophylaxis and therapy. Am. J. Dig. Dis. 19:81-87, 1974.

j Faloon, W.W., Rubulis, A., Hussain, I., Randhawa, I., Flood, M.S. Bile acid pattern in gallstone and cholecystectomised patients receiving chenodeoxycholic acid, and in 'normal obese' patients. Gastroenterology 66:884, 1974 (abstract).

k Faloon, W.W., Rubulis, A., and Flood, M.S. Lithogenic and hepatotoxic potential in intestinal by-pass: Bile acid and sterol changes. Gastroenterology 68:1073, 1975 (abstract).

l Farivar, S., Fromm, H., Schindler, D., and Schmidt, F.W. Sensitivity of bile acid breath test in the diagnosis of bacterial overgrowth in the small intestine with and without the stagnant (blind) loop syndrome. Dig. Dis. & Sci. 24:33-40, 1979.

m Farivar, S., Fromm, H., Schindler, D., McJunkin, B., and Schmidt, F.W. Tests of bile-acid and vitamin B_{12} metabolism in ileal Crohn's disease. Am. J. Clin. Path. 72:69-74, 1980.

n Farrell, K.E., Smith, D.C., and Mackay, C. Gallstone dissolution in vitro. Brit. J. Surg. 60:900, 1973 (abstract).

o Fausa, O. Duodenal bile acids after a test meal. Scand. J. Gastroenterol. 9:567-570, 1974.

a Fausa, O. and Skalhegg, B.A. Quantitative determination of bile acids and their purified 3-hydroxysteroid dehydrogenase. Scand. J. Gastroenterol. 10:747-752, 1975.

b Fausa, O. Serum bile acid concentration after a test meal. Scand. J. Gastroenterol. 11:229-232, 1976.

c Fausa, O. and Gjone, E. Serum bile acid concentrations in patients with liver disease. Scand. J. Gastroenterol. 11:537-543, 1976.

d Fedorowski, T., Salen, G., Calallilo, A., Tint, G.S., Mosbach, E.H., and Hall, J.C. Metabolism of ursodeoxycholic acid in man. Gastroenterology 73:1131-1137, 1977.

e Fedorowski, T., Salen, G., Zaki, F.G., Shefer, S., and Mosbach, E.H. Comparative effects of ursodeoxycholic acid and chenodeoxycholic acid in the Rhesus monkey. Gastroenterology 74:75-81, 1978.

f Fedorowski,. T., Salen, G., Tint, G.S., and Mosbach, E. Transformation of chenodeoxycholic acid and ursodeoxycholic acid by human intestinal bacteria. Gastroenterology 77:1068-1073, 1979.

g Feher, T., Papp, J., and Kazik, M.H. Spectrofluorometric determination of individual bile acids in biological fluids: Duodenal content and bile. Z. Klin. Chem. Klin. Biochem. 11:376-380, 1973.

h Feher, T., Papp, J., and Kazik, M.H. Spectrofluorometric determination of individual bile acids in biological fluids: Peripheral plasma. Clin. Chim. Acta 44:409-418, 1973.

i Feld, K.M. and Higuchi, W.I. Dissolution rate behavior of solid cholesterol preparations in bile acid solutions. J. Pharm. Sci. 70:717-723, 1981.

j Feldman, S. and Gibaldi, M. Bile salt-induced permeability changes in the isolated rat intestine. Proc. Soc. Exptl. Biol. Med. 132:1031-1033, 1969.

k Fernholz, E. Die isolierung der 3-oxy-6-keto-allocholansaure aus schweinegalle. Z. Physiol. Chem. 232:202, 1935.

l Ferrari, A., Scholastico, C., and Beretta, L. On the mechanism of cholic acid 7a-dehydroxylation by a clostridium difermentans cell-free extract. FEBS Letters 75:166-167, 1977.

m Ferrari, V. Chenodeoxycholic acid. Lancet 1:1314, 1978 (Letter to Editor).

n Ferraris, R., Fiorentini, M.T., Falco, M., Deleide, G., and DeLaPierre, M. Direct radioimmunoassay for cholic and chenodeoxycholic conjugates using ^{125}I tracers. J. Nucl. Med. Allied Sci. 25:99-106, 1981.

o Festi, D., Sama, C., Malavolti, M., Messale, E., Morselli, A.M., Roda, A., and Roda, E. Assessment of liver disease by serum primary bile acids: Critical evaluation. Ital. J. Gastroenterol. 13:214-215, 1981 (abstract).

a Festi, D., Aldini, R., Rossi, R.M., Frabboni, R., Onorato, G., Roda, A., Fugazza, R., Ornati, S., and Barbara, L. Postprandial primary bile acid determination versus ursodeoxycholic acid oral load in liver disease. Gastroenterology 82:1227, 1982 (abstract).

b Fevery, J., van Hees, G.P., Leroy, P., Compernolle, F., and Heirwegh, K.P.M. Excretion in dog bile of glucose and xylose conjugates of bilirubin. Biochem. J. 125:803-810, 1971.

c Fevery, J. Pathogenesis of Gilbert's syndrome. Europ. J. Clin. Invest. 11:417-418, 1981.

d Fex, H., Lundvall, K.E., and Olsson, A. Hydrogen sulfates of natural estrogens. Acta Chem. Scand. 22:254-264, 1968.

e Fieser, L.F. Napthoquinone antimalarials. XVI. Water-soluble derivatives of alcoholic and unsaturated compounds. J. Am. Chem. Soc. 70:3232-3237, 1948.

f Fieser, L.F. and Rajagopolan, S. Selective oxidation with N-bromosuccinimide. I. Cholic acid. J. Am. Chem. Soc. 71:3935-3938, 1949.

g Fieser, L.F. and Rajagopolan, S. Oxidation of steroids. III. Selective oxidation and acylations in the bile acid series. J. Am. Chem. Soc. 72: 5530, 1950.

h Filho, G.G. Hepatotoxicidade do acido quenodesoxicolico: Estudo histopatologico e ultra-estrutural em coelhos. Arq Gastroent 14:76-82, 1977.

i Filly, R.A., Allen, B., Minton, M.J., Bernhoft, R., and Way, L.W. In vitro investigation of the origin of echoes within biliary sludge. J. Clin. Ultrasound 8:193-200, 1980.

j Findlay, J.M., Smith, A.N., Mitchell, W.D., Anderson, A.J.B., and Eastwood, M.A. Effects of unprocessed bran on colon function in normal and in diverticular disease. Lancet 1:146-149, 1974.

k Finni, K., Simila, S., Koivisto, M., Heikura, S., Maentausta, O., and Janne, O. Serum cholic acid and chenodeoxycholic acid concentrations in neonatal hyperbilirubinemia. Biol. Neonate 40:264-268, 1981.

l Fischer, C.D., Cooper, N.S., Rothschild, M.A., and Mosbach, E.H. Effect of dietary chenodeoxycholic acid and lithocholic acid in the rabbit. Am. J. Dig. Dis. 18:877-886, 1974.

m Fischmeister, I. Infrared spectra of bile acid and peptide conjugated bile acids. Arkiv. Kemi 16:151, 1960.

n Fisher, M.M. and Farber, E. Lithocholate induced choledocholithiasis. Gastroenterology 58:281, 1970 (abstract).

o Fisher, M.M., Magnusson, R., and Mivai, K. Bile acid metabolism in mammals. I. Bile acid-induced intrahepatic cholestasis. Lab. Invest. 21:88-91, 1971.

a Fisher, M.M., Magnusson, R., Phillips, M.J., and Miyai, K. Bile acid metabolism in mammals. IV. Sex differences in chenodeoxycholic acid metabolism in the rat. Lab. Invest. 27:254-262, 1972.

b Fisher, M.M. and Yousef, I.M. Sex differences in the bile acid composition of human bile: Studies in patients with and without gallstones. Canad. Med. Assn. J. 109:190-193, 1973.

c Fisher, M.M., Price, V.M., Magnusson, R.J., and Yousef, I.M. Bile acid metabolism in mammals. VII. Studies on the sex differences in deoxycholic acid metabolism in the isolated perfused rat liver. Lipids 9:786-794, 1974.

d Fisher, M.M., Bloxam, D.L., Oda, M., Phillips, M.J., and Yousef, I.M. Characterization of rat liver cell plasma membranes. Proc. Soc. Exptl. Biol. Med. 150:177-184, 1975.

e Fisher, M.M., Kakis, G., and Yousef, I.M. Bile acid pool in Wistar rats. Lipids 11:93-96, 1976.

f Fisher, M.M., Price, V.M., and Yousef, I.M. Biliary lipids in pregnancy. In The Hepatobiliary System. W Taylor, ed. Plenum Press, New York, 1976, pp 555-571.

g Fisher, M.M., Bloxam, D.L., Nagy, B.R., and Yousef, I.M. Rate-limiting steps in the biliary secretion of chenodeoxycholic acid (CDCA) and its metabolites. Gastroenterology 72:79, 1977 (abstract).

h Fisher, R.L. and Binder, H.J. Cholesterol cholelithiasis. Conn. Med. 41:467-469, 1977.

i Fisher, R.L. Progress in the medical management of gallstones. Med. Times 107:30-35, 1979.

j Fisher, R.L., Anderson, D.W., Boyer, J.L., Ishak, K., Klatskin, G., Lachin, J.M., Phillips, M.J., and the Steering Committee of the National Cooperative Gallstone Study Group. A prospective morphologic evaluation of hepatic toxicity of chenodeoxycholic acid in patients with cholelithiasis: the National Cooperative Gallstone Study. Hepatology 2:187-201, 1982.

k Fiske, C.H. and Subbarow, Y. The colorometric determination of phosphorous. J. Biol. Chem. 66:375-400, 1925.

l Fitzpatrick, G., Neutra, R., and Gilbert, J.P. Cost-effectiveness of cholecystectomy for silent gallstones. In Costs, Risks, and Benefits of Surgery. JP Bunker, BA Barnes, F Mosteller, eds. Oxford University Press, New York, 1977, pp 246-261.

m Floch, M.H., Gershengoren, W., Elliot, S., and Spiro, H.M. Bile acid inhibition of the intestinal microflora. A function for simple bile acids? Gastroenterology 61:228-233, 1971.

n Floch, M.H., Binder, H.J., Filburn, B., and Gershengoren, W. The effect of bile acids on intestinal microflora. Am. J. Clin. Nutr. 25:1418-1426, 1972.

a Flugel, H. Auflosung von Gallensteinen mit Chenodesoxycholsaure. Fortschr. Med. 92:272-274, 1974.

b Flugel, H. Cholelithlysis. Fortschr. Med. 96:1139-1142, 1978.

c Flynn, M., Darby, C., Hyland, J., Hammond, P., and Taylor, I. The effect of bile acids on colonic myoelectrical activity. Brit. J. Surg. 66:776-779, 1979.

d Fon, G.T., Goldin, A.R., and Thomson, K.R. Non-operative removal of retained gall stones experience in Flinders Medical Centre. Aust. Radiol. 23:248-251, 1979.

e Fontell, K. Micellar behavior in solutions of bile-acid salts. I. Vapor pressure of the aqueous solutions and the osmotic activity of the bile acid salts. Koloid Zeit/Zeit Polymere 244:246-252, 1971.

f Fontell, K. Micellar behavior in solutions of bile-acid salts. II. Light scattering by the aqueous solutions. Kolloid Zeit/Zeit Polymere 244:253-257, 1971.

g Fontell, K. Micellar behavior in solutions of bile-acid salts. IV. An x-ray study of the aqueous solutions. Kolloid Zeit/Zeit Polymere 246:710-718, 1971.

h Forker, E.L. Two sites of bile formation as determined by mannitol and erythritol clearance in the guinea pig. J. Clin. Invest. 46:1189-1195, 1967.

i Forker, E.L. Bile formation in guinea pigs: Analysis with inert solutes of graded molecular radius. Am. J. Physiol. 215:56-62, 1968.

j Forker, E.L. The effect of estrogen in bile formation in the rat. J. Clin. Invest. 48:654-663, 1969.

k Forker, E.L. Mechanisms of hepatic bile formation. Ann. Rev. Physiol. 39:323-347, 1977.

l Forker, E.L. and Luxon, B. Hepatic transport kinetics and plasma disappearance curves: Distributed modeling versus conventional approach. Am. J. Phys. 235:E648-E660, 1978.

m Forker, E.L. and Luxon, B.A. Albumin helps mediate removal of taurocholate by rat liver. J. Clin. Invest. 67:1517-1522, 1981.

n Forth, W., Rummel, W., and Glasner, H. Zur resorptionshemmenden Wirkung von Gallensauren. Naunyn-Schmeidebergs Arch. Parmak. 254:364-380, 1966.

o de Fossey, M. Resultats preliminaires du traitement de la lithiase biliaire par l'acide chenodesoxycholique. M.C.D. 4(Suppl 1):15-17, 1975.

p Foster, M.G., Hooper, C.W., and Whipple, G.H. Metabolism of bile acids. III. Administration by stomach of bile, bile acids, taurine, and cholic acid to show the influence upon bile acid elimination. J. Biol. Chem. 38:379-392, 1919.

a Fouin-Fortunet, H., LeQuernec, L., Erlinger, S., Lerebours, E., and Colin, R. Hepatic alterations during total parenteral nutrition in patients with inflammatory bowel disease: A possible consequence of lithocholate toxicity. Gastroenterology 82:932-937, 1982.

b Francavilla, A., Amoruso, A., Panella, C., Doronzo, F., Sansonno, D., and Frigerio, G. Effectiveness of ursodeoxycholic acid administered in a single bedtime dose to patients with radiolucent gallstones. 16th Meeting of the EASL, Lisbon, 1981, pp 173 (abstract).

c Franz, B., and Bode, J.C. Total plasma bile acid concentration in chronic hepatitis and cirrhosis: Fasting values and effect of intraduodenal bile salt administration. Klin. Wschr. 52:522-526, 1974.

d Frazer, A.C., Schulman, J.H., and Stewart, H.C. Emulsification of fat in the intestine of the rat and its relation to absorption. J. Physiol. 103:306-316, 1944.

e Frazer, A.C. and Sammons, H.G. The formation of mono- and diglycerides during the hydrolysis of triglycerides by pancreatic lipase. Biochem. J. 39:122-128, 1945.

f Frazer, A.C. The physical chemistry of intestinal adsorption of fats. J. Colloid and Interface Science 29:314, 1969.

g Freedman, B. Gas-liquid chromatography of hydroxy fatty esters: comparison of trifluoroacetyl and trimethlysilyl derivatives. J. Am. Oil Chemists' Soc. 44:113-116, 1967.

h Freeman, C.P. Properties of fatty acids in dispersions of emulsified bile salt and the significance of these properties in fat absorption in the pig and the sheep. Brit. J. Nutr. 23:249-263, 1969.

i Freeman, J.B., Meyer, P.D., and DenBesten, L. Effects of freezing and incubation on biliary lipid analysis. Proc. Soc. Exptl. Biol. Med. 147:31-34, 1974.

j Freeman, J.B., Cohen, W.N., and DenBesten, L. Cholecystokinin cholangiography and analysis of duodenal bile in the investigation of pain in the right upper quadrant of the abdomen without gallstones. Surg. Gyn. & Obst. 140:371-376, 1975.

k Freeman, J.B., Meyer, P.D., Printen, K.J., Mason, E.E., and DenBesten, L. Analysis of gallbladder bile in morbid obesity. Am. J. Surg. 129:163-166, 1975.

l Frenkel, M. Lithogenic bile. Ned. Tijdschr. Geneeskd. 118:1939-1945, 1974.

m Freston, J.W., Bouchier, I.A.D., and O'Grady, M. Studies on experimental cholelithiasis in rabbits. Gut 2:716-717, 1966.

a Freston, J.W. and Bouchier, I.A.D. The influence of total vagotomy in dihydrocholesterol-induced cholelithiasis. Gastroenterology 57:670-678, 1969.

b Fried, A.A., Petrow, V., and Lack, L. The synthesis of diazo halo and sulfoxy-bile acid derivatives: Potential affinity labels. Steroids 34:171-185, 1979.

c Friedman, G., Kannel, W., and Dawber, T. The epidemiology of gallbladder disease: Observations in the Framingham Study. J. Chron. Dis. 19:273-292, 1966.

d Frigerio, G. A series of controlled multicenter trials as a wide-phase study of ursodeoxycholic acid for radiolucent gallstone dissolution. Ital. J. Gastroenterol. 13:294, 1981.

e Frigerio, G. Ursodeoxycholic acid (UDCA) in the treatment of dyspepsia: Report of a multicenter controlled trial. Curr. Ther. Res. 26:214-224, 1979.

f Frohling, W. and Stiehl, A. Bile salt glucuronides: Identification and quantitative analysis in the urine of patients with cholestasis. Europ. J. Clin. Invest. 6:67-74, 1976.

g Fromm, H. and Hofmann, A.F. Breath test for altered bile acid metabolism. Lancet 2:621-625, 1971.

h Fromm, H., Thomas, P.J., and Hofmann, A.F. Sensitivity and specificity in tests of distal ileal functions: Prospective comparison of bile acid and vitamin B_{12} absorption in ileal resection patients. Gastroenterology 64:1077-1090, 1973.

i Fromm, H., Eschler, A., Tollner, D., Canzler, H., and Schmidt, F.W. In vivo dissolving of gallstones. The effect of chenodeoxycholic acid. Dtsch. med. Wschr. 100:1619-1624, 1975.

j Fromm, H. and Hofmann, A.F. The importance of bile acids in human disease. With 20 figures. Ergebnisse der Inn. Med. Kinderheilkunde. (Adv. Intern. Med. & Pediat.) 37:143-192, 1975.

k Fromm, H., Holz-Slomczyk, M., Zobl, H., Schmidt, E., and Schmidt, F.W. Studies of liver function and structure in patients with gallstones before and during treatment with chenodeoxycholic acid. Acta Hepato-Gastroent. 22:359-369, 1975.

l Fromm, H., Erbler, H.C., Eschler, A., and Schmidt, F.W. Alterations of bile acid metabolism during treatment with chenodeoxycholic acid. Studies of the role of the appearance of ursodeoxycholic acid in the dissolution of gallstones. Klin. Wschr. 54:1125-1131, 1976.

a Fromm, H., Amin, P., Klein, H., and Kupke, I. Use of a simple enzymatic assay for cholesterol analysis in human bile. J. Lipid Res. 21:259-261, 1980.

b Fromm, H., Farivar, S., Hofmann, A.F., Carlson, G.L. and Amin, P. Metabolism in man of 7-ketolithocholic acid: Precursor of cheno- and ursodeoxycholic acids. Am. J. Phys. 239:G161-G166, 1980.

c Frommer, D.J. Defective biliary excretion of copper in Wilson's disease. Gut 15:125-129, 1974.

d Fry, R.J.M. and Staffeldt, E. Effect of a diet containing sodium deoxycholate on the intestinal mucosa of the mouse. Nature 203:1396-1398, 1964.

e Fuchs, K., Schubert, S., Bellman, H., and Wohlgemuth, B. Gesichtpunkte zur Pathogenese der Cholelithiasis unter modernen Lebensbedingungen. Dt. Z. Verdau 39:166-172, 1979.

f Fujihira, E., Kaneta, S., and Ohshima, T. Strain difference in mouse cholelithiasis and the effect of taurine on the gallstone formation in C_{27}BL/C mice. Biochem. Med. 19:211-217, 1978.

g Fujisawa, K., Kitahara, T., Ogura, K., Kurihara, N., and Kameda, H. Studies on the metabolic fate of chenodeoxycholic acid in human. Gastroenterology 79:1105, 1980 (abstract).

h Fukuda, H. and Iritani, N. The binding of cholic acid to protein in rat serum and liver. J. Biochem. 90:1757-1762, 1981.

i Funatsu, K. and Phillips, M.J. Dissolution of human cholesterol gallstones in vitro with bile salts. a scanning and stereoscanning electron microscopic study. Lab. Invest. 40:166-171, 1979.

j Furusawa, T., Nakama, T., Itoh, H., and Hisadome, T. Reappraisal of cholesterol solubilization in bile salt-lecithin solution and the stability of bile. Gastroenterol. Jap. 12:253-262, 1977.

k Gadacz, T.R., Allan, R.N., Mack, E., and Hofmann, A.F. Impaired lithocholate sulfation in the rhesus monkey: A possible mechanism for chenodeoxycholate toxicity. Gastroenterology 70:1125-1129, 1976 (Letter to Editor).

l Gadacz, T.R. Efficacy of Capmul and the dissolution of biliary stones. J. Surg. Res. 26:378-380, 1979.

m Gadacz, T.R. The effect of monooctanoin on retained common duct stones. Surgery 89:527-531, 1981.

n Gaginella, T.S., Bass, P., Perrin, J.H., and Vallner, J.J. Effect of bile salts on partitioning behavior and GI absorption of a quaternary ammonium compound, Isopropamide Iodide. J. Pharm. Sci. 62:1121-1125, 1973.

a Gaginella, T.S., Perrin, J.H., Vallner, J.J., and Bass, P. Effect of bile salts on partitioning and oral toxicity of a bisquaternary ammonium drug, Decamethonium Bromide. J. Pharm. Sci. 63:790-792, 1974.

b Gaginella, T.S., Stewart, J.J., Gullikson, G.W., Olsen, W.A., and Bass, P. Inhibition of small intesatinal mucosal and smooth muscle cell function by ricinoleic acid and other surfactants. Life Sciences 16:1595-1606, 1975.

c Gainsborough, H. Gallstone dissolution by chenodeoxycholic acid. Lancet 1: 42, 1973 (Letter to Editor).

d Galapeaux, E.A., Templeton, R.D., and Borkon, E.L. The influence of bile on the motility of the dog's colon. Am. J. Physiol. 121:130-136, 1938.

e Galeazzi, R., Bonazzi, P., Calaresu, C., and Orlandi, F. Effect of combined administration of chenodeoxycholic acid (CDCA) and ethinyl oestradiol (EE) on biliary secretion in rat. Ital. J. Gastroenterol. 13:214, 1981 (abstract).

f Galivan, J. Stabilization of cholic acid uptake in primary cultures of hepatocytes by dexamethasone and tocopherol. Archiv. Biochem. & Biophys. 214:850-852, 1982.

g Gallagher, K., Mauskopf, J., Walker, J.T., and Lack, L. Ionic requirements of the active ileal bile salt transport system. J. Lipid Res. 17:572-577, 1976.

h Galloway, S.J., Casarella, W.J., and Seaman, W.B. The nonoperative treatment of retained stones in the common bile duct. Surg. Gyn. & Obst. 137: 55-58, 1973.

i Gans, J.H. and Cater, M.R. Effect of catecholamines on bile acid metabolism in dogs. Fed. Proc. 27:573, 1968 (abstract).

j Garbutt, J.T., Heaton, K.W., Lack, L., and Tyor, M.P. Increased ratio of glycine to taurine-conjugated bile salts in patients with ileal disorders. Gastroenterology 56:711-720, 1969.

k Garbutt, J.T., Lack, L., and Tyor, M.P. The enterohepatic circulation of bile salts in gastrointestinal disorders. Am. J. Med. 51:627-636, 1971.

l Garbutt, J.T., Lack, L., and Tyor, M.P. Physiological basis of alterations in the relative conjugation of bile acids with glycine and tuarine. Am. J. Clin. Nutr. 24:218-228, 1971.

m Garbutt, J.T. and Kenney, T.J. Effect of cholestyramine on bile acid metabolism in normal men. J. Clin. Invest. 51:2781-2789, 1972.

n Garbutt, J.T., Curry, S.B., and Stevens, R.D. Biliary lipid composition in black American males. Gastroenterology 64:857, 1973 (abstract).

o Gardner, B. Experiences with the use of intracholedochal heparinized saline for the treatment of retained common duct stones. Ann. Surg. 177:240-244, 1971.

a Gardner, B., Ostrowitz, A., and Masur, R. Reappraisal of the possible role of heparin in dissolution of gallstones: A clinical extension of laboratory studies in removal of retained common duct stones. Surgery 69:854-857, 1971.

b Gardner, B., Masur, R., Path, J., and Ostrowitz, A. Effect of taurocholic acid and BSP on conjugation patterns and suspension stability of human and rat bile. Am. J. Surg. 125:204-210, 1973.

c Gasbarrini, G., Bonvicini, F., Riario-Sforza, G., Ianiro, G., Bernardi, M., Corazza, G.R., DiCosmo, C., Cassiani, R., and Gabriele, P. Laboratory and clinical investigations after ursodeoxycholic acid treatment. Preliminary observations on uric acid excretion in bile. Ital. J. Gastroenterol. 10 (Suppl 1):70-72, 1978.

d Gatmaitan, O., Yotsuyanagi, T., and Higuchi, W.I. Mechanisms for interface-controlled transport of cholesterol in micellar sodium cholate-lecithin and micellar sodium cholate-lecithin-sodium oleate systems. J. Colloid Interface Sci. 61:499, 1977.

e Gebhardt, J., Heueck, A., Leuschner, U., and Wurbs, D. Die direkte Auflosung von Gallengangssteinen. Z. Gastroenterol. XIX (9), 1981 (abstract 12).

f Geistfeld, B., Bond, M., and St. Clair, R. Cholelithiasis in a male rhesus monkey (Macaca Mulatta) fed a cholesterol-containing diet. J. Med. Primatol. 6:237-244, 1977.

g Gelrud, L., Gregory, D., Vlahcevic, Z., Schwartz, C., and Swell, L. Effect of ethanol and ethanol-related diseases on biliary lipid metabolism. Biochem. & Pharm. Ethanol 1:445-458, 1979.

h George, P. Disorders of the extrahepatic bile ducts. Clin. Gastroenterol. 2:127-146, 1973.

i Gerok, W. Gallensaurestoffwechsel und Lyse der Gallensteine. Med. Welt 29:53-56, 1978.

j Gerok, W. and Matern, S. Pathogenetische Bedeutung der Gallensauren. Klin. Wochenschr. 59:575-589, 1981.

k Gerolami, A., Crotte, C., Mule, A., Varette, Y., and Sarles, H. Lithiase biliaire experimentals de la souris. Action comparee de l'acids cholique et de l'acide taurocholique associes ou non a du cholesterol. Biol. Gastroenterol. 1:23-32, 1971.

l Gerolami, A., Crotte, C., Mule, A., et al. Experimental gallstones in the mouse. Mechanism of action of dehydrocholic acid. Rev. Eur. Etud. Clin. Biol. 17:500-502, 1972.

m Gerolami, A., Montet, J-C., Vigne, J-L., Grangier, M., and Mule, A. Metabolism of dehydrocholic acid. Chromatographic study of its derivatives in the bile "In vitro" study of their ability to form mixed micelles. Biol. Gastronenterol. 5:265-272, 1972.

a Gerolami, A., Crotte, C., Grangier, M., and Mule, A. Bile secretion of mice treated with chenodeoxycholic acid. Biol. Gastroenterol. 6:169-170, 1973.

b Gerolami, A. and Montet, J-C. Pathogenie de la lithiase biliaire. Secretion des lipides biliaires et cholelithiase cholesterolique. Biol. Gastroenterol. 6:63-71, 1973.

c Gerolami, A. and Sarles, H. b-Sitosterol and chenodeoxycholic acid in the treatment of cholesterol gallstones. Lancet 2:721, 1975 (Letter to Editor).

d Gerolami, A., Sarles, H., Brette, R., Paraf, A., Ratureau, J., Debray, C., Bermann, C., Etienne, J.P., Chaput, J.C., and Petite, J. Test therapeutique controle avec l'acide chenodesoxycholique. Biol. Gastroenterol. 8:12-20, 1975.

e Gerolami, A., Sarles, H., Brette, R., Paraf, A., Ratureau, J., Debray, C., Bermann, C., Etienne, J.P., Chaput, J.C., and Petite, J. Controlled trial of chenodeoxycholic therapy for radiolucent gallstones. A multicenter study. Digestion 16:299-307, 1977.

f Gerolami, A., Montet, J., Marteau, C., Reynier, M., and Crotte, C. Mechanismes d'action de l'acide chenodesoxycholique et l'acide ursodesoxycholique dans le traitement de la lithiase biliaire. Gastroenterol. Clin. Biol. 4:588-599, 1980.

g Gerskowitch, V.P., Allan, J.G., and Russell, R.I. Increased faecal excretion of bile acids in post-vagotomy diarrhoea. Brit. J. Surg. 60:912, 1973 (abstract).

h Gerskowitch, V.P. and Russell, R.I. The physiology of bile acids in duodenum and jejunum. Scot. Med. J. 18:138-141, 1973.

i Gianni, L. DiPadova, F., Nicolin, A., Curti, R., Fargion, S., DiPadova, C., and Podda, M. Bile acid induced inhibition of lymphoproliferase response to mitogens. Rendiconti 9:240, 1977 (abstract).

j Gibson, G.E. and Forker, E.L. SC-2644 and taurocholate: Different effects on apparent BSP Tm in the dog. Gastroenterology 64:162, 1973 (abstract).

k Gilat, T., Raton, J., Gelman-Malachi, E., Papo, J., Tietz, A., and Peled, Y. A trial of gallstone dissolution using low doses of chenic acid. Giorn. Gastroent. End. 2:9-16, 1979.

l Giller J. and Phillips, S.F. The contribution of the colon to electrolyte and water conservation in man. J. Lab. Clin. Med. 81:733-746, 1973.

m Gilmore, I.T. and Thompson, R.P.H. Direct measurement of the first-pass extraction of bile acids by the liver in man. Gut 19:A971, 1978 (abstract).

n Gilmore, I.T. Studies on the clearance of bile acids from blood. M.D. Thesis, University of Cambridge, 1979.

a Gilmore, I.T., Stokes, K., Hofmann, A.F., Gurantz, D., and Lorenzo, D. Differing acute effects of chenodeoxycholyl conjugates and ursodeoxycholyl conjugates on biliary phospholipid and cholesterol secretion in gallstone patients. Gastroenterology 79:1020, 1980 (abstract).

b Gilmore, I.T. and Thompson, R.P.H. Plasma clearance of oral and intravenous cholic acid in subjects with and without chronic liver disease. Gut 21:123-127, 1980.

c Gilmore, I.T., Barnhart, J.L., Hofmann, A.F., and Erlinger, S. Effects of individual taurine-conjugated bile acids on biliary lipid secretion and sucrose clearance in the unanesthetized dog. Am. J. Physiol. 242:G40-G46, 1982.

d Girard, R.M. and Legros, G. Retained and recurrent bile duct stones. Surgical or nonsurgical removal? Ann. Surg. 193:150-154, 1981.

e Glasinovic, J-C., Dumont, M., Duval, M., and Erlinger, S. Hepatocellular uptake of taurocholate in the dog. J. Clin. Invest. 55:419-426, 1975.

f Glasser, J., Weiner, I.M., and Lack, L. Comparative physiology of intestinal taurocholate transport. Am. J. Physiol. 208:359-362, 1965.

g Gleich, G.J. and Hofmann, A.F. Use of cholestyramine to control diarrhea associated with acquired hypogammaglobulinemia. Am. J. Med. 51:281-286, 1971.

h Glenn, F. The baboon and experimental cholelithiasis. Arch. Surg. 100:105, 1970.

i Glenn, F. Postcholecystectomy choledocholithiasis. Surg. Gyn. & Obst. 134:249-252, 1972.

j Glueck, C., Jandacek, R.J., Subbiah, M.T.R., Gallon, L., Yunker, R., Allen, C., Hogg, E., and Laskarzewski, P.M. Effect of sucrose polyester on fecal bile acid excretion and composition in normal man. Am. J. Clin. Nutr. 33:2177-2181, 1980.

k Go, V.L.W., Hofmann, A.F., and Summerskill, W.H.J. Pancreozymin bioassay in man based on pancreatic enzyme secretion: Potency of specific amino acids and other digestive products. J. Clin. Invest. 49:1558-1564, 1970.

l Go, V.L.W., Hofmann, A.F., and Summerskill, W.H.J. Simultaneous measurements of total pancreatic, biliary, and gastric outputs in man using a perfusion technique. Gastroenterology 58:321-328, 1970.

m Go, V.L.W., Poley, J.R., Hofmann, A.F., and Summerskill, W.H.J. The disturbances in fat digestion induced by acidic jejunal pH due to gastric hypersecretion in man. Gastroenterology 58:638-646, 1970.

n Goddard, P. and Hill, M.J. Degradation of steroids by intestinal bacteria. IV. The aromatisation of ring A. Biochim. Biophys. Acta 280:336-342, 1972.

a Goebell, H. Die Epidemiologie des Gallensteinleidens. Akt. Ernahrung 3:95-102, 1977.

b Goh, E. and Heimberg, M. Stimulation of hepatic cholesterogenesis by fatty acids. Gastroenterology 65:542, 1973 (abstract).

c Goldstein, J.L. and Brown, M.S. Binding and degradation of low-density lipoproteins by cultured human fibroblasts. J. Biol. Chem. 249:5153-5162, 1974.

d Goldstein, J.L., Dana, S.E., and Brown, M.S. Esterification of low density lipoprotein cholesterol in human fibroblasts and its absence in homozygous familial hypercholesterolemia. Proc. Nat. Acad. Sci. 71:4288-4292, 1974.

e Goldstein, L.I. and Schoenfield, L.J. Pathogenesis and medical treatment of gallstones. Adv. Intern. Med. 20:131-135, 1974.

f Goldstein, L.I., Bonorris, G.G., Coyne, M.J., and Schoenfield, L.J. Persistent effects of chenodeoxycholic acid on biliary lipids in the hamster. J. Lab. Clin. Med. 85:1032-1041, 1975.

g Good, L.I., Edell, S.L., Soloway, R.D., Trotman, B.W., Mulhern, C., and Arger, P.A. Ultrasonic properties of gallstones. Effect of stone size and composition. Gastroenterology 77:258-263, 1979.

h Goodchild, M.C., Murphy, G.M., Howell, A.M., Nutter, S.A., and Anderson, C.M. Aspects of bile acid metabolism in cystic fibrosis. Arch. Dis. Childh. 50:769-778, 1975.

i Gorbach, S.L. and Tabaqchali, S. Bacteria, bile, and the small bowel. Gut 10:963-972, 1969.

j Gordon, B.A., Kuksis, A., and Beveridge, J.M.R. The effect of dietary fat on bile acid metabolism in man. Canad. J. Biochem. 42:897-905, 1964.

k Gordon, E.R., Dadoun, M., Goresky, C.A., Chan, T-H., Perlin, A.S. The isolation of an azobilirubin b-D-monoglucoside from dog gallbladder bile. Biochem. J. 143:97-105, 1974.

l Gordon, E.R., Goresky, C.A., Chan, T-H., and Perlin, A.S. The isolation and characterization of bilirubin diglucuronide, the major bilirubin conjugate in bile. Biochem. J. 155:477-486, 1976.

m Gordon, S.G. and Kern, F., Jr. The absorption of bile salt and fatty acid by hamster small intestine. Biochem. Biophys. Acta 153:372-378, 1968.

n Gordon, S.G., Miner, P., and Kern, F., Jr. Characteristics of conjugated bile salt absorption by hamster jejunum. Biochim. Biophys. Acta 248:333-342, 1971.

o Gordon, S.J., Buelow, R.G., Haeffner, L.J., Schaedler, R.W. and Kowlessar, O.D. Diarrheal states associated with low deoxycholic acid. Gastroenterology 64:736, 1973 (abstract).

a Gordon, S.J., Kinsey, M.D., Magen, J.S., Joseph, R.E., and Kowlessar, O.D. Structure of bile acids associated with secretion in the rat cecum. Gastroenterology 77:38-44, 1979.

b Goresky, C.A. Initial distribution and rate of uptake of sulfobromophthalein in the liver. Am. J. Physiol. 20:713-726, 1964.

c Goresky, C.A., Bach, G.G., and Nadeau, B.E. The uptake of materials by the intact liver: Transport and net removal of galactose. J. Clin. Invest. 52:991-1009, 1973.

d Goresky, C.A., Haddad, H.H., Kluger, S.W., and Nadeau, B.E. The enhancement and maximal bilirubin excretion with taurocholate-induced increments in bile flow. Canad. J. Physiol. Pharmacol. 52:389-403, 1974.

e Goresky, C.A. The hepatic uptake process: Its implications for bilirubin transport. In Jaundice. CA Gorsky, MM Fisher, eds. Plenum Press, New York, 1975, pp 159-174.

f Goresky, C.A. and Fisher, M.M. Jaundice. Plenum Press, New York, 1975.

g Goresky, C.A. Hepatic membrane carrier transport processes: Their involvement in bilirubin uptake. In Chemistry and Physiology of Bile Pigments. Chapter 23, Publishing House, U.S. Government, Washington, D.C., 1976, pp 240-256.

h Gorin, J.P. and Souciet, G. Les acides biliaires. Nouv. Presse Med. 1:1425-1430, 1972.

i Gosink, B.B. and Leopold, G.R. Ultrasound andt the gallblader. Semin. Roentgenol. 11:185-189, 1976.

j Goswami, S.K. and Frey, C.F. Manganous chloride spray reagent for cholesterol and bile acids on thin-layer chromatograms. J. Chromatog. 53:389-390, 1970.

k Goswami, S.K. and Frey, C.F. Spray detection of bile acids on thin-layer chromatograms. J. Chromatog. 47:126-127, 1970.

l Goswami, S.K. and Frey, C.F. A novel method for the separation and identification of bile acids and phospholipids of bile on thin-layer chromatograms. J. Chromatog. 89:87-91, 1974.

m Goto, J., Hasegawa, M., Kato, H., and Nambara, T. A new method for simultaneous determination of bile acids in human bile without hydrolysis. Clin. Chim. Acta 87:141-147, 1978.

n Goto, J., Kato, H., Saruta, Y., and Nambara, T. Studies on steroids. CLXX. Separation and determination of bile acid 3-sulfates in human bile by high-performance liquid chromatography. J. Chromatogr. 226:13-24, 1981.

a Gotz, R., Raedsch, R., Walker, S., Stiehl, A., and Kommerell, B. Conjugation of chenodeoxycholic acid and lithocholic acid with taurine and glycine by isolated hepatocytes. 16th Meeting of the EASL, Lisbon, 1981 (abstract).

b Grabowski, G., McCoy, K.E., Williams, G.C., Dempsey, M.E., and Hanson, R.F. Evidence for carrier proteins in bile acid synthesis: The effect of squalene and sterol carrier protein and albumin in the activity of 12a-hydroxylase. Biochem. Biophys. Acta 441:380-390, 1976.

c Gracey, M., Papadimitiou, J., Burke, V., Thomas, J., and Bower, G. Effects on small intestinal function and structure induced by feeding a deconjugated bile salt. Gut 14:519-528, 1973.

d Gracie, W.A. and Ransohoff, D.F. The natural history of silent gallstones: The innocent gallstone is not a myth. Gastroenterology 80:1161, 1981 (abstract).

e Graham, J., Bird, R., and Northfield, T.C. Novel mechanism of action for chenodeoxycholic acid in gallstone dissolution. Gut 22:A432, 1981 (abstract).

f Grant, N. Estrogens and gallstones. N. Engl. J. Med. 290:912, 1974 (Letter to Editor).

g Gray, R. Disappearing gallstones: Report of two cases. Brit. J. Surg. 61:101-103, 1974.

h Greco, A.V., Mingrone, G., and Passi, S. Bile acid content of gallbladder bile and stones in type IIb and IV hyperlipoproteinemia. Clin. Chim. Acta 116:81-89, 1981.

i Green, H.O., Moritz, J., and Lack, L. Binding of sodium taurocholate by bovine serum albumin. Biochim. Biophys. Acta 231:550-552, 1971.

j Greenberger, N.J. and Skillman, T.G. Medium-chain triglycerides: Physiologic considerations and clinical implications. N. Engl. J. Med. 280:1045, 1969.

k Greenwell, B.E. Prospects for chenodiol therapy. Ann. Intern. Med. 95: 659-660, 1981 (letter).

l Gregg, J.A. New solvent systems for thin-layer chromatography of bile acids. J. Lipid Res. 7:579-581, 1966.

m Gregg, J.A. and Poley, J.R. Excretion of bile acids in normal rabbits. Am. J. Physiol. 211:1147-1151, 1966.

n Gregg, J.A. Urinary excretion of bile acids in patients with hepatocellular disease and obstructive jaundice. Am. J. Clin. Path. 49:404-409, 1968.

a Gregory, D.H., Vlahcevic, Z.R., and Swell, L. Determination of the cholesterol saturation of human bile and its relevance to gallstone formation. Am. J. Dig. Dis. 19:268-270, 1974.

b Gregory, D.H., Vlahcevic, Z.R., Schatzki, P., and Swell, L. Mechanism of secretion of biliary lipids. I. Role of bile canalicular and microsomal membranes in the synthesis and transport of biliary lecithin and cholesterol. J. Clin. Invest. 55:105-114, 1975.

c Gregory, D.H., Vlahcevic, Z.R., Prugh, M.F., and Swell, L. Mechanism of secretion of biliary lipids: Role of a microtubular system in hepatocellular transport of biliary lipids in the rat. Gastroenterology 74: 93-100, 1978.

d Greim, H., Trulzsch, D., Czygan, P., Rudick, J., Hutterer, F., Schaffner, F., and Popper, H. Mechanism of cholestasis. VI. Bile acids in human livers with or without biliary obstruction. Gastroenterology 63:846-850, 1972.

e Greim, H., Trulzsch, D., Roboz, J., Czygan, P., Hutterer, F., Schaffner, F., and Popper, H. Mechanism of cholestasis. V. Bile acids in normal rat livers and in those after bile duct ligation. Gastroenterology 63:837-845, 1972.

f Greim, H., Czygan, P., Schaffner, F., and Popper, H. Determination of bile acids in needle biopsies of human liver. Biochem. Med. 8:280-286, 1973.

g Greim, H., Trulzsch, D., Czygan, P., Hutterer, F., Schaffner, F., and Popper, H. Bile acid formation by liver microsomal systems. Annals N.Y. Acad. Sci. pp 139-147, 1973.

h Greim, H. and Czygan, P. Gallensauren in der Leber und im Serum bei verschiedenen Lebererkrankungen. Verh. Dtsch. Ges. Inn. Med. 80:443-445, 1974.

i Grodins, F.S., Berman, A.L., and Ivy, A.C. Observations on the toxicities and choleretic activities of certain bile salts. J. Lab. Clin. Med. 27:181-186, 1941.

j Gronwall, R., Engelking, L.R., Anwer, M.S., Erichsen, D.F., and Klentz, R.D. Bile secretion in ponies with biliary fistulas. Am. J. Vet. Res. 36: 653-654, 1975.

k Grozinger, K.H. Cholesterol in the blood and bile. Fortschr. Med. 98: 1261-1264, 1980.

l Grundy, S.M., Ahrens, E.H., Jr., and Miettinen, T.A. Quantitative isolation and gas-liquid chromatographic analysis of total fecal bile acids. J. Lipid Res. 6:397-410, 1965.

m Grundy, S.M., Hofmann, A.F., Davignon, J., and Ahrens, E.H., Jr. Human cholesterol synthesis is regulated by bile acids. J. Clin. Invest. 45: 1018-1019, 1966 (abstract).

a Grundy, S.M. and Ahrens, E.H., Jr. Measurements of cholesterol turnover, synthesis and absorption in man, carried out by isotope kinetic and sterol balance methods. J. Lipid Res. 10:91-107, 1969.

b Grundy, S.M., Ahrens, E.H., Jr., and Davignon, J. The interaction of cholesterol absorption and cholesterol synthesis in man. J. Lipid Res. 10:304-314, 1969.

c Grundy, S.M. and Ahrens, E.H., Jr. The effects of unsaturated dietary fats on absorption, excretion, synthesis, and distribution of cholesterol in man. J. Clin. Invest. 49:1135-1152, 1970.

d Grundy, S.M., Ahrens, E.H., Jr., and Salen, G. Interruption of the enterohepatic circulation of bile acids in man: Comparative effects of cholestyramine and ileal exclusion on cholesterol metabolism. J. Lab. Clin. Med. 78:94-121, 1971.

e Grundy, S.M. Treatment of hypercholesterolemia by interference with bile acid metabolism. Arch. Intern. Med. 130:638-648, 1972.

f Grundy, S.M. Working conference on gallstones. Gastroenterology 63:201-203, 1972.

g Grundy, S.M., Ahrens, E.H., Jr., Salen, G., Schreibman, P.H., and Nestel, P.J. Mechanism of action of clofibrate on cholesterol metabolism in patients with hyperlipidemia. J. Lipid Res. 13:531-551, 1972.

h Grundy, S.M. and Metzger, A.L. A physiological method for estimation of hepatic secretion of biliary lipids in man. Gastroenterology 62:1200-1217, 1972.

i Grundy, S.M., Metzger, A.L., and Adler, R.D. Mechanisms of lithogenic bile formation in American Indian women with cholesterol gallstones. J. Clin. Invest. 51:3026-3043, 1972.

j Grundy, S.M., Duane, W.C., Adler, R.D., Aron, J.M., and Metzger, A.L. Biliary lipid output in young women with cholesterol gallstones. Metabolism 23:67-73, 1974.

k Grundy, S.M. Effects of polyunsaturated fats on lipid metabolism in patients with hypertriglyceridemia. J. Clin. Invest. 55:269-282, 1975.

l Grundy, S.M., Mok, H.Y.I., and von Bergmann, K. Regulation of biliary cholesterol secretion in man. Proc. of the Symp. on Lipoprotein Metabolism in Heidelberg. H Greten, ed., 1975, pp 112-118.

m Grundy, S.M. and Mok, H.Y.I. Determination of cholesterol absorption in man by intestinal perfusion. J. Lipid Res. 18:263-271, 1977.

n Grundy, S.M. Biliary lipids, gallstones, and treatment of hyperlipidaemia. J. Clin. Invest. 9:179-180, 1979.

o Gumucio, J. and Valdivieso, V. Studies on the mechanisms of the ethynyl estradiol impairment of bile flow and bile salt excretion in the rat. Gastroenterology 61:339-344, 1971.

a Gumucio, J.J., Accatino, L., Macho, A.M., and Contreras, A. Effect of phenobarbital on the ethynyl estradiol-induced cholestasis in the rat. Gastroenterology 65:651-657, 1973.

b Gurantz, D., Gilmore, I.T., Hofmann, A.F., and DiPietro, R.A. Acute effects of individual bile acids given enterally on biliary lipid secretion in the hamster. Gastroenterology 78:1307, 1980 (abstract).

c Gurantz, D., Gilmore, I.T., Hofmann, A.F., and Kozmary, S. Biliary lipid secretion in the hamster: greater cholesterol secretion induced by unconjugated bile acids. Hepatology 1:513, 1981 (abstract).

d Gustafsson, B.E. and Norman, A. Comparison of bile acids in intestinal contents of germfree and conventional rats. Proc. Soc. Exptl. Biol. Med. 110:387, 1962.

e Gustafsson, B.E., Midtvedt, T., and Norman, A. Isolated fecal microorganisms capable of 7a-dehydroxylating bile acids. J. Exptl. Med. 123:413-432, 1966.

f Gustafsson, B.E., Midtvedt, T., and Norman, A. Metabolism of cholic acid in germ-free animals after the establishment in the intestinal tract of deconjugating and 7a-dehydroxylating bacteria. Acta Path. Microbiol. Scand. 72:433-443, 1968.

g Gustafsson, B.E. and Norman, A. Physical state of bile acids in intestinal contents of germ-free and conventional rats. Scand. J. Gastroenterol. 3:625-631, 1968.

h Gustafsson, B.E. and Norman, A. Influence of the diet on the turnover of bile acids in germ-free and conventional rats. Brit. J. Nutr. 23:429-442, 1969.

i Gustafsson, B.E., Einarsson, K., and Gustafsson, J-A. Influence of cholesterol feeding on liver microsomal metabolism of steroids and bile acids in conventional and germ-free rats. J. Biol. Chem. 250:8496-8502, 1975.

j Gustafsson, B.E., Angelin, B.O., Bjorkhem, I., Einarsson, K., and Gustafsson, J. Effects of feeding chenodeoxycholic acid on metabolism of cholesterol and bile acids in germ-free rats. Lipids 16:228-233, 1981.

k Guzelian, P. and Boyer, J.L. Glucose reabsorption from bile--evidence for a biliohepatic circulation. J. Clin. Invest. 53:526-535, 1974.

l Hacki, W. and Paumgartner, G. Assessment of bile salt independent bile formation by injection of taurocholate. In The Liver. Quantitative Aspects of Structure and Function. G Paumgartner, R Preisig, eds. S Karger Verlag, Basel, 1973, pp 360-367.

m Haeffner, L., Gordon, S.J., Magen, J.S., and Kowlessar, O.D. Evaluation of the 3a-hydroxysteroid dehydrogenase assay for ursodeoxycholic acid, and 7 oxo- and 12 oxo-bile acids. J. Lipid Res. 21:477-480, 1980.

a Hagerman, L.M. and Schneider, D.L. In vitro binding of mixed micellar solutions of fatty acids and bile salts by cholestyramine. Proc. Soc. Exptl. Biol. Med. 143:89-92, 1973.

b Hall, R.C., Fast, D., and Tepperman, J. Rabbit gallbladder absorbs cholic faster than chenodeoxycholic acid. Deconjugation unrelated to absorption. Gastroenterology 64:858, 1973 (abstract).

c Halloran, L.G., Schwartz, C.C., Vlahcevic, Z.R., Gregory, D.H., and Swell, L. Effect of chenodeoxycholic acid administration on bile acid and cholesterol synthesis in man. Surg. Forum XXVI:439-442, 1975.

d Hammarsten, O. Ueber dehydrocholalsaure, ein neues oxydation produkt der cholalsaure. Ber. D. Dtsch. Chem. Ges. 14:71-76, 1881.

e Hamprecht, B., Nussler, C., Waltinger, G., and Lynen, F. Influence of bile acids on the activity of rat liver 3-hydroxy-3-methylglutaryl coenzyme A reductase. I. Effect of bile acids in vitro and in vivo. Europ. J. Biochem. 18:10-14, 1971.

f Hamprecht, B., Roscher, R., Waltinger, G., and Nussler, C. Influence of bile acids on the activity of rat liver 3-hydroxy-3-methylglutaryl coenzyme A reductase. II. Effect of cholic acid in lymph fistula rats. Europ. J. Biochem. 18:15-19, 1971.

g Handelsman, B., Bonorris, G.G., Marks, W., and Schoenfield, L.J. Enrichment of bile with taurine-conjugated ursodeoxycholic acid in hamsters. Hepatology 1:24A, 1981 (abstract).

h Hanson, R.F. The formation and metabolism of 3a,7a-dihydroxy-5b-cholestan-26-oic acid in man. J. Clin. Invest. 50:2051-2055, 1971.

i Hanson, R.F., Klein, P.D., and Williams, G.C. Bile acidf formation in man: Metabolism of 7a-hydroxy-4-cholesten-3-one in bile fistula patients. J. Lipid Res. 14:50-53, 1973.

j Hanson, R.F., Isenberg, J.N., Williams, G.C., Hachey, D., Szczepanik, P., Klein, P.D., and Sharp, H.L. The metabolism of 3a,7a,12a-trihydroxy-5b-cholestan-26-oic acid in two siblings with cholestasis due to intrahepatic bile duct anomalies. An apparent inborn error of cholic acid synthesis. J. Clin. Invest. 56:577-587, 1975.

k Hanson, R.F. and Duane, W.C. A possible alternative to cholecystectomy. Cholesterol gallstones - The search of a cause yields a new treatment. Nod. Med. of Austral. pp 9-13, Feb., 1976.

l Hanson, R.F., Sharp, H.L., and Williams, G.C. The metabolism of 3a,7a,12a-trihydroxy-5b-cholestan-26-oic acid (THCA) into cholic acid: An enzyme assay using homogenates of human liver. J. Lipid Res. 17:294-296, 1976.

a Hanson, R.F., Szczepanik, P.A., Klein, P.D., Johnson, E., and Williams, G.C. Formation of bile acids in man. Metabolism of 7a-hydroxy-4-cholesten-3-one in normal subjects with an intact enterohepatic circulation. Biochim. Biophys. Acta 431:335-346, 1976.

b Hanson, R.F., Williams, G.C., Hachey, D., and Sharp, H.L. Hepatic lesions and hemolysis following administration of 3a,7a,12a-trihydroxy-5b-cholestan-26-oyl taurine to rats. Gastroenterology 70:983, 1976 (abstract).

c Hansson, K. Pancreatitis and free bile acids. Acta Chir. Scand. 126:338, 1963.

d Hardison, W.G.M. and Rosenberg, I.H. Bile salt deficiency in the steatorrhea following resection of the ileum and proximal colon. N. Engl. J. Med. 277:337-343, 1967.

e Hardison, W.G.M. and Rosenberg, I.H. The effect of neomycin on bile salt metabolism and fat digestion in man. J. Lab. Clin. Med. 74:564-573, 1969.

f Hardison, W.G.M. Metabolism of sodium dehydrocholate by the rat liver: Its effect on micelle formation in bile. J. Lab. Clin. Med. 77:811-820, 1971.

g Hardison, W.G.M. and Apter, J.T. Micellar theory of biliary cholesterol excretion. Am. J. Physiol. 222:61-67, 1972.

h Harman, C.G., Englert, E., Jr., and Wales, E.E., Jr. Deconjugation of bile salts in the gallbladder during experimental cholelithiasis. Gastroenterology 58:299, 1970 (abstract).

i Harries, J.T. and Sladen, G.E. The effects of different bile salts on the absorption of fluid, electrolytes, and monosaccharides in the small intestine of the rat in vivo. Gut 13:596-603, 1972.

j Hart, J.T. and Scott, I. Bran and blood-lipids. Lancet 1:175, 1974 (Letter to Editor).

k Hartley, G.S. Aqueous solutions of paraffin-chain salts. A study in micelle formation. In Actualites Scientifiques et Industrielles. Hermann & Cie, Paris, 1936.

l Hartley, G.S. Solutions of soap-like substances. In Prog. and Chem. in Fats and Other Lipids. RT Holman, WO Lundberg, and T Malkin, ed. Pergamon, Vol 3, pp 20-55, 1955.

m Hartmann, W., Paulini, K., and Goebell, H. Light an electron microscopy of human liver before and during chenodeoxycholic acid therapy. Hepato-Gastroenterol. 27:91-98, 1980.

n Hasik, J., Hryniewiecki, L., and Grala, T. Minimalne zapotrzebowanie na bialko u chorych z kamica zolciowa leczonych kwasem chenodezoksycholowym. Polskie Archiwum Med. Wewnetrznej 65:451-458, 1981.

o Haslewood, E.S. and Haslewood, G.A.D. Preparation of the 3-monosulphates of cholic acid, chenodeoxycholic acid and deoxycholic acid. Biochem. J. 155:401-404, 1976.

a Haslewood, G.A.D. Metabolism of steroids. IV. Ketonic acids derived from cholic acid. Biochem. J. 38:108, 1944.

b Haslewood, G.A.D. and Wootton, V. Comparative studies of bile salts. I. Preliminary survey. Biochem. J. 47:584-597, 1950.

c Haslewood, G.A.D. The biological significance of chemical differences in bile salts. Biol. Rev. 39:537, 1964.

d Haslewood, G.A.D. Bile Salts. Methuen & Co., London, 1967.

e Haslewood, G.A.D. Bile salt evolution. J. Lipid Res. 8:535-550, 1967.

f Haslewood, G.A.D., Murphy, G.M., and Richardson, J.M. A direct enzymic assay for 7a-hydroxy bile acids and their conjugates. Clin. Sci. 44:95-98, 1973.

g Haslewood, G.A.D. The Biological Importance of Bile Salts. North-Holland Publishing Co., Amsterdam, 1978.

h Hatanaka, H., Kawaguchi, A., Hayakawa, S., and Katsuki, H. Structural specificity of bile acid for inhibition of sterol synthesis in cell-free extracts of yeast. Biochim. Biophys. Acta 270:397-406, 1972.

i Hattori, T. and Hayakawa, S. Isolation and characterization of a bacterium capable of 7a-dehydroxylating cholic acid from human faeces. Microbiol. 1:287-294, 1969.

j Haubrich, W.S. Getting rid of gallstones without surgery. JAMA 231:747-748, 1975.

k Hauser, E., Baumgartner, E., and Meyer, K. Zur Kenntnis der Chenodesoxy cholsaure (3a,7a-dihydroxy-5b-cholsaure). Helv. Chim. Acta 43:1595, 1960.

l Hauton, J.C., Laurent, B., Gerolami, S., Antandrea, A., Greusard, C., Fafond, H., Tessier, N., and Sarles, H. Etude preliminaire d'une fraction peptidique extraite avec les lipides neutres du plasma. Clin. Chim. Acta 17:171, 1967.

m Hayakawa, S. Microbiological transformation of bile acids. In Advances in Lipid Research. R Paoletti, D Kritchevsky, ed. Academic Press, London-New York, Vol 11, 1973, pp 143-192.

n Hayes, J.D., Strange, R.C., and Percy-Robb, I.W. Identification of two lithocholic acid-binding proteins. Separation of ligandin from glutathione S-transferase B. Biochem. J. 181:699-708, 1979.

o Hayward, A.F., Freston, J.W., and Bouchier, I.A.D. Changes in the ultrastructure of the gallbladder epithelium in rabbits with experimental gallstones. Gut 9:550-556, 1968.

p Heath, T.C., Caple, I.W., and Redding, P.M. Effect of the enterohepatic circulation of bile salts on the flow of bile and its content of bile salts and lipids in sheep. Quart. J. Exptl. Physiol. 55:93-103, 1970.

a Heaton, K.W., Austad, W.I., Lack, L., and Tyor, M.P. Enterohepatic circulation of C^{14}-labelled bile salts in disorders of the distal small bowel. Gastroenterology 55:5-16, 1968.

b Heaton, K.W. and Lack, L. Ileal bile salt transport: Mutual inhibition in an in vivo system. Am. J. Physiol. 214:585-590, 1968.

c Heaton, K.W. The importance of keeping bile salts in their place. Gut 10:857-863, 1969.

d Heaton, K.W. and Read, A.E. Gallstones in patients with disorders of the terminal ileum and disturbed bile salt metabolism. Brit. Med. J. 3:494-496, 1969.

e Heaton, K.W. Abnormal bile or faulty gall bladder? Brit. Med. J. 1:289, 1971 (Letter to Editor).

f Heaton, K.W. Bitter humour: The development of ideas about bile salts. J. Royal Coll. Phys. 6:83-97, 1971.

g Heaton, K.W., Heaton, S.T., and Barry, R.E. An in vivo comparison of two bile salt-binding agents, cholestyramine and lignin. Scand. J. Gastroenterol. 6:281-286, 1971.

h Heaton, K.W. Bile salts in health and disease. Edinburgh, Churchill Livingstone, 1972.

i Heaton, K.W. The epidemiology of gallstones and suggested aetiology. Clin. Gastroenterol. 2:67-83, 1973 (review).

j Heaton, K.W. Gallstones and dietary carbohydrate. _In_ Plant Foods for Man 1:33-44, 1973 (review).

k Heaton, K.W. Gallstone formation. _In_ Ninth Symp. on Adv. Med. JG Walker, ed. Pitman, London, 1973, pp 363-378.

l Heaton, K.W. and Pomare, E.W. Effect of bran on blood lipids and calcium. Lancet 1:49-50, 1974.

m Heaton, K.W. Bile formation. _In_ Topics in Gastroenterology 2, SC Truelove, J Trowell, eds. Blackwell, Oxford, 1975, pp 209-226.

n Heaton, K.W. Bile salts and fiber. _In_ Fiber Deficiency and Colonic Disorders. RW Reilly, JB Kirsner, ed. Plenum, New York, 1975, pp 27-37.

o Heaton, K.W. Gallstones and cholecystitis. _In_ Refined Carbohydrate Foods and Disease: Some Implications of Dietary Fibre. DP Burkitt, HC Trowell, eds. Academic Press, London, 1975, op 173-194.

p Heaton, K.W. Les effets d'un regime a base fibres cellulosiques sue le metabolisme des sels biliaires et sur la composition de la bile. M.C.D. 4(Suppl 1):27-29, 1975.

a Heaton, K.W. Bile salts and diarrhea. In Topics in Paediatric Gastroenterology. JA Dodge, ed. Pitman, London, 1976, pp 115-128.

b Heaton, K.W. Clinical aspects of bile acid metabolism. In Recent Advances in Gastroenterology 3, IAD Bouchier, ed. Churchill Livingstone, Edinburgh, 1976, pp 199-230.

c Heaton, H.W. Disturbances of bile acid metabolism in intestinal disease. Clin. Gastroenterol. 6:69-89, 1977.

d deHeer, K., Werner, B., Sauer, H.D., and Kloppel, G. Effect of cholestyramine and chenodeoxycholic acid on liver cirrhosis. An experimental study in rats. Z. Exp. Chir. 13:105-113, 1980.

e Hefti, M.L. Cholelithiasis: Therapeutic litholysis. Praxis 67:1225-1231, 1978.

f Hegardt, F.G. and Dam, H. The solubility of cholesterol in aqueous solution of bile salts and lecithin. Z. Ernahr. 10:223-233, 1971.

g Hegsted, D.M., Andrus, B., Gotsis, A., and Portman, O.W. The quantitative effects of cholesterol, cholic acid and type of fat on serum cholesterol and vascular sudanophilia in the rat. J. Nutr. 63:273-288, 1957.

h Heikura, S., Simila, S., Finni, K., Maentausta, O., and Janne, O. Cholic acid and chenodeoxycholic acid concentrations in serum during infancy and childhood. Acta Paediatr. Scand. 69:659-662, 1980.

i Heirwegh, K.P.M., van Hees, G.P., Leroy, P., Van Roy, F.P., and Jansen, F.H. Heterogeneity of bile pigment conjugates as revealed by chromatography of their ethyl anthranilate azopigments. Biochem. J. 120:877-890, 1970.

j Hellenius, A. and Simons, K. Solubilization of membranes by detergents. Biochim. Biophys. Acta 415:29-79, 1975.

k Heller, F. and Bouchier, I.A.D. Cholesterol and bile salt studies on the bile of patients with cholesterol gallstones. Gut 14:83-88, 1973.

l Heller, F. and Harvengt, C. Cholesterolic gallstones. Pathophysiology and treatment. Acta Gastroenterol. Belg. 40:392-405, 1978.

m Hellstrom, K. and Sjovall, J. Metabolism of chenodeoxycholic acid in the rabbit. Bile acids and steroids 104. Acta Chem. Scand. 14:1763-1769, 1960.

n Hellstrom, K. On the origin of lithocholic and ursodeoxycholic acids in man. Bile acids and steroids 106. Acta Physiol. Scand. 51:218, 1961.

o Hellstrom, K. and Sjovall, J. Conjugation of bile acids in patients with hypothyroidism. J. Athero. Res. 1:205, 1961.

p Hellstrom, K. and Einarsson, K. Bile acid metabolism in hyperlipoproteinaemia. Clin. Gastroenterol. 6:103-128, 1977.

a Hepner, G.W., Hofmann, A.F., and Thomas, P.J. Metabolism of steroid and amino acid moieties of conjugated bile acids in man. I. Cholyl glycine (glycocholic acid). J. Clin. Invest. 51:1889-1897, 1972.

b Hepner, G.W., Hofmann, A.F., and Thomas, P.J. Metabolism of steroid and amino acid moieties of conjugated bile acids in man. II. Glycine-conjugated dihydroxy bile acids. J. Clin. Invest. 51:1898-1905, 1972.

c Hepner, G.W. and Hofmann, A.F. Cholic acid therapy for constipation: A controlled trial. Mayo Clin. Proc. 48:356-358, 1973.

d Hepner, G.W. and Hofmann, A.F. Different effects of free and conjugated bile acids and their keto derivatives on (Na^+, K^+)-stimulated and Mg^{2+} ATPase in rat intestinal mucosa. Biochim. Biophys. Acta 291:237-245, 1973.

e Hepner, G.W., Sturman, J.A., Hofmann, A.F., and Thomas, P.J. Metabolism of steroid and amino acid moieties of conjugated bile acids in man. III. Cholyl taurine (taurocholic acid). J. Clin. Invest. 52:433-440, 1973.

f Hepner, G.W. Breath analysis: gastroenterological applications. Gastroenterology 67:1250-1256, 1974.

g Hepner, G.W., Hofmann, A.F., Malagelada, J-R., Szczepanik, P.A., and Klein, P.D. Increased bacterial degradation of bile acids in cholecystectomized patients. Gastroenterology 66:556-564, 1974.

h Hepner, G.W. Altered bile acid metabolism in vegetarians. Am. J. Dig. Dis. 20:935-940, 1975.

i Hepner, G.W. Effect of decreased gallbladder stimulation on enterohepatic cycling and kinetics of bile acids. Gastroenterology 68:1574-1581, 1975.

j Hepner, G.W. and Quarfordt, S.H. Kinetics of cholesterol and bile acids in pateints with cholesterol cholelithiasis. Gastroenterology 69:318-325, 1975.

k Hepner, G.W. and Vessell, E.S. Normal antipyrine metabolism in patients with cholesterol cholelithiasis: Evidence that the disease is not due to generalized hepatic microsomal dysfunction. Am. J. Dig. Dis. 20:9-12, 1975.

l Hepner, G.W. and Vessell, E.S. Assessment of aminopyrine metabolism in man by breath analysis after oral administration of ^{14}C-aminopyrine. N. Engl. J. Med. 291:1384-1388, 1975.

m Hepner, G.W. The effect of phenobarbital on biliary lipid metabolism and hepatic microsomal drug metabolism in patients with cholesterol cholelithiasis. Am. J. Dig. Dis. 21:370-375, 1976.

n Hepner, G.W. and Demers, L.M. The dynamics of the enterohepatic circulation of the glycine conjugates of cholic, chenodeoxycholic, deoxycholic, and sulfolithocholic acid in man. Gastroenterology 72:499-501, 1977.

o Herndon, J.H., Jr. Pathophysiology of pruritus associated with elevated bile acid levels in serum. Arch. Intern. Med. 130:632-637, 1972.

a Herzog, R.J. Gallstone migration and pancreatitis. N. Engl. J. Med. 290:1201, 1974 (Letter to Editor).

b Heubi, J.E., Balastreri, W.E., Partin, J.C., Schubert, W.K., and McGraw, C.A. Refractory infantile diarrhea due to primary bile acid malabsorption. J. Pediat. 94:546-551, 1979.

c Heuman, R., Norrby, S., Sjodahl, R., Tiselius, H., and Tagesson, C. Altered gallbladder bile composition in gallstone disease. Scand. J. Gastroenterol. 15:581-586, 1980.

d Heywood, R., Palmer, A.K., Foll, C.V., and Lee, M.R. Pathological changes in fetal Rhesus monkey induced by oral chenodeoxycholic acid. Lancet 2:1021, 1973 (Letter to Editor).

e Higashi, H., Setoguchi, T., and Katsuki, T. Interconversion between chenodeoxycholic and ursodeoxycholic in anaerobic cultures of intestinal bacteria and reduction of 7-ketolithocholic acid to both bile acids. Acta Hepatolog. 19:803, 1978.

f Higashi, S., Setoguchi, T., and Katsuki, T. Conversion of 7-ketolithocholic acid to ursodeoxycholic acid by human intestinal anaerobic microorganisms: Interchangeability of chenodeoxycholic acid and ursodeoxycholic acid. Gastroenterol. Jpn. 14:417-424, 1979.

g Higuchi, W.I., Prakongpan, S., Surpuriya, V., and Young, F. Retarding effect of lecithin on the dissolution rate of cholesterol monohydrate in bile acid media. Science 178:633-634, 1972.

h Higuchi, W.I., Prakongpan, S., and Young, F. Dissolution rates of cholesterol monohydrate crystals and human cholesterol gallstones in bile acid-lecithin solutions: Enhancing effect of added alkyl quaternary ammonium salts. J. Pharm. Sci. 62:1207-1208, 1973.

i Higuchi, W.I., Prakongpan, S., and Young, F. Mechanisms of dissolution of human cholesterol gallstones. J. Pharm. Sci. 62:945-948, 1973.

j Higuchi, W.I., Sjuib, F., Mufson, D., Simonelli, A.P., and Hofmann, A.F. Dissolution kinetics of gallstones: Physical model approach. J. Pharm. Sci. 62:942-945, 1973.

k Higuchi, W.I., Surpuriya, V., Prakongpan, S., and Young, F. Participation of micelle at crystal-solution interface in rate-determining step for cholesterol gallstone dissolution in unsaturated bile media. J. Pharm. Sci. 62:695, 1973.

l Higuchi, W.I., Su, C.C., Park, J.Y., Alkan, M.H., and Gulari, E. Mechanism of cholesterol gallstone dissolution: analysis of the kinetics of cholesterol monohydrate dissolution in taurocholate/lecithin solution by the Mazer, Benedek and Carey model. J. Phys. Chem. 85:127, 1981.

m Hikasa, Y., Nagase, M., Tanimura, H., Shioda, R., Setoyama, M., Kobayashi, N., Mukaihara, S., Kamata, T., Naruyama, K., Kato, H., Mori, K., and Soloway, R.D. Epidemiology and etiology of gallstones. Arch. Jap. Chir. 49:555-571, 1980.

a Hill, M.J. and Aries, V.C. Faecal steroid composition and its relationship to cancer of the large bowel. J. Path. 104:129-139, 1971.

b Hill, M.J., Crowther, J.S., Drasar, B.S., Hawksworth, G., Aries, V., and Williams, R.E.O. Bacteria and aetiology of cancer of large bowel. Lancet 1:95-100, 1971.

c Hill, M.J. Bacteria and the etiology of colonic cancer. Cancer 34:815-818, 1974.

d Hill, M.J. The role of colon anaerobes in the metabolism of bile acids and steroids and its relation to colon cancer. Cancer, 1975 (December).

e Hill, M.J., Drasar, B.S., Williams, R.E.O., Meade, T.W., Cox, A.G., Simpson, J.E.P., and Morson, B.C. Faecal bile acids and clostridia in patients with cancer of the large bowel. Lancet 1:535-538, 1975.

f Hill, M.J. The role of unsaturated bile acids in the etiology of large bowel cancer. In Origins of Human Cancer, Cold Spring Harbor Laboratory, London, 1977, pp 1627-1640.

g Hirameth, S.V. and Elliott, W.H. Bile acids. LXIV. Synthesis of 5a-cholestane-3a,7a,25-triol and esters of new 5a-bile acids. Steroids 38:465-475, 1981.

h Hirano, S. and Masuda, N. Epimerization of the 7-hydroxy group of bile acids with 7a- and 7b-hydroxysteroid dehydrogenase activity, respectively. J. Lipid Res. 22:1060-1068, 1981.

i Hirano, S., Masuda, N., and Oda, H. In vitro transformation of chenodeoxycholic acid and ursodeoxycholic acid by human intestinal flora, with particular reference to the mutual conversion between the two bile acids. J. Lipid Res. 22:735-743, 1981.

j Hirano, S., Masuda, N., Oda, H., and Mukai, H. Transformation of bile acids by Clostridium perfringens. Appl. Environ. Microbiol. 42:394-399, 1981.

k Hisadome, T., Nakama, T., Itoh, H., and Furusawa, T. Physical-chemical properties of chenodeoxycholic acid and ursodeoxycholic acid. Gastroenterol. Jpn. 15:257-263, 1980.

l Hisatsugu, T., Takeda, K., and Tamura, T. Disintegrating effect of hexametaphosphate on specific inorganic cholecystolith. Jap. J. Clin. Med. 29:2329-2337, 1971.

m Hislop, I.G., Hofmann, A.F., and Schoenfield, L.J. Determinants of the rate and site of bile acid absorption in man. J. Clin. Invest. 46:1070-1071, 1967 (abstract).

n Ho, K.J. Comparative studies on the effect of cholesterol feeding on biliary composition. Am. J. Clin. Nutr. 29:705-709, 1976.

a Ho, K-J. Circadian distribution of bile acids in the enterohepatic circulatory system in rats. Am. J. Physiol. 230:1331-1335, 1979.

b Ho, K-J., Ho, C., Hsu, S., and Chen, J. Bile acid pool size in relation to functional status of gallbladder and biliary lipid composition in Chinese. Am. J. Clin. Nutr. 33:1026-1032, 1980.

c Ho, K-J. and Ho, L-H. Inhibitory effect of bile acids on the activity of human b-glucuronidase at its optimal pH (41170). Proc. Soc. Exptl. Biol. Med. 167:304-309, 1981.

d Ho, N.F.H. and Higuchi, W.I. Theoretical model studies of intestinal drug absorption. IV. Bile acid transport of premicellar concentrations across diffusion layer-membrane barrier. J. Pharm. Sci. 63:686-690, 1974.

e Hoffman, N.E., Simmonds, W.J., and Morgan, R.G.H. A comparison of absorption of free fatty acid and c-glyceryl ether in the presence and absence of a micellar phase. Biochim. Biophys. Acta 231:487-495, 1971.

f Hoffman, N.E. and Hofmann, A.F. Metabolism of steroid and amino acid moieties of conjugated bile acids in man. IV. Description and validation of a multicompartmental model. Gastroenterology 67:887-897, 1974.

g Hoffman, N.E., Hofmann, A.F., and Thistle, J.L. Effect of bile acid feeding on cholesterol metabolism in gallstone patients. Mayo Clin. Proc. 49:236-239, 1974.

h Hoffman, N.E., Donald, D.E., and Hofmann, A.F. Effect of primary bile acids on bile lipid secretion from perfused dog liver. Am. J. Physiol. 229:714-720, 1975.

i Hoffman, N.E., Iser, J.H., and Smallwood, R.A. Hepatic bile acid transport: Effect of conjugation and position of hydroxyl groups. Am. J. Physiol. 229:298-302, 1975.

j Hoffman, N.E., Sewell, R.B., and Smallwood, R.A. Bile acid structure and biliary lipid secretion. II. A comparison of three-hydroxy and two-keto bile acids. Am. J. Phys. 3:E637-E640, 1978.

k Hoffman, N.E. and Hofmann, A.F. Metabolism of steroid and amino acid moieties of conjugated bile acids in man. V. Equations for the perturbed enterohepatic circulation and their application. Gastroenterology 72:141-148, 1977.

l Hofmann, A.F. Thin-layer adsorption chromatography of free and conjugated bile acids on silicic acid. J. Lipid Res. 2:127-128, 1962.

m Hofmann, A.F. and Borgstrom, B. Physico-chemical state of lipids in intestinal content during their digestion and absorption. Fed. Proc. 21:43-50, 1962.

n Hofmann, A.F. The behavior and solubility of monoglycerides in dilute, micellar bile salt solution. Biochim. Biophys. Acta 70:306-316, 1963.

a Hofmann, A.F. The function of bile salts in fat absorption: The solvent properties of dilute micellar solutions of conjugated bile salts. Biochem. J. 89:57-68, 1963.

b Hofmann, A.F. The preparation of chenodeoxycholic acid and its glycine and taurine conjugates. Acta Chem. Scand. 17:173-186, 1963.

c Hofmann, A.F. The role of bile salts in fat absorption: The solvent properties of dilute micellar solutions of conjugated bile salts. Biochem. J. 89:57-78, 1963.

d Hofmann, A.F. The function of bile salts in fat absorption. Thesis, University of Lund, 1964.

e Hofmann, A.F. Thin-layer chromatography of bile acids and their derivatives. In New Biochemical Separations. Morris, James eds. London:Van Nostrand, 1964, pp 283-294.

f Hofmann, A.F. and Borgstrom, B. The intraluminal phase of fat digestion in man: The lipid content of the micellar and oil phases of intestinal content obtained during fat digestion and absorption. J. Clin. Invest 43:247-257, 1964.

g Hofmann, A.F. and Mosbach, E.H. Identification of allodeoxycholic acid as the major component of gallstones induced in the rabbit by 5a-cholestan-3b-ol. J. Biol. Chem. 239:2813-2821, 1964.

h Hofmann, A.F. Clinical implications of physicochemical studies on bile salts. Gastroenterology 48:484-494, 1965.

i Hofmann, A.F. A physicochemical approach to the intraluminal phase of fat absorption. Gastroenterology 50:56-64, 1966.

j Hofmann, A.F. Efficient extraction of polar anionic lipids with tetraheptyl ammonium chloride, a liquid ion exchanger. J. Lipid Res. 8:55-58, 1967.

k Hofmann, A.F. The syndrome of ileal disease and the broken enterohepatic circulation: Cholerheic enteropathy. Gastroenterology 52:752-757, 1967.

l Hofmann, A.F. and Small, D.M. Detergent properties of bile salts: Correlation with physiological function. Ann. Rev. Med. 18:333-376, 1967.

m Hofmann, A.F. Functions of bile in the alimentary canal. In Handbook of Physiology. CF Code, ed. Washington, D.C.: American Physiological Society. Vol 5, Chap 117, 2507-2533, 1968.

n Hofmann, A.F., Bokkenheuser, V.D., Hirsch, R.L., and Mosbach, E.H. Experimental cholelithiasis in the rabbit induced by cholestanol feeding: Effect of neomycin treatment on bile composition and gallstone formation. J. Lipid Res. 9:244-253, 1968.

o Hofmann, A.F., Szczepanik, P.A., and Klein, P.D. Rapid preparation of tritium labeled bile acids by enolic exchange on basic alumina containing tritiated water. J. Lipid Res. 9:707-713, 1968.

a Hofmann, A.F. Relationship between the molecular structure of bile salts in their physiologic functions. In Bile Salt Metabolism. Schiff, Carey, and Dietschy, ed. Thomas, Springfield, Chap 15, 1969, 160-169.

b Hofmann, A.F., Mosbach, E.H., and Sweeley, C.C. Bile acid composition of bile from germ-free rabbits. Biochim. Biophys. Acta 176:204-207, 1969.

c Hofmann, A.F., and Poley, J.R. Cholestyramine treatment of diarrhea associated with ileal resection. N. Engl. J. Med. 281:397-402, 1969.

d Hofmann, A.F. Gallensaurenstoffwechsel. Therapiewoche 40:2388-2392, 1970.

e Hofmann, A.F., Schoenfield, L.J., Kottke, B.A., and Poley, J.R. Methods for the description of bile acid kinetics in man. In Methods in Medical Research. Olson, ed. (Chicago:Yearbook Medical Publishers) pp 149-180, 1970.

f Hofmann, A.F. Bile acid metabolism and liver disease. In Alcohol and the Liver. Int'l Symp, Freiburg, Oct., 1970, F.K. Schattauer, Stuttgart, 1971, pp 421-433.

g Hofmann, A.F. and Fromm, H. New breath test for bile acid deconjugation. N. Engl. J. Med. 285:686-687, 1971 (Editorial).

h Hofmann, A.F. and Kern, F., Jr. The significance of bile acids in gastrointestinal and hepatic disease. Disease-A-Month (Yearbook Medical Publishers) Nov., 1971, pp 1-38.

i Hofmann, A.F. Bile acid malabsorption caused by ileal resection. Arch. Intern. Med. 130:597-605, 1972.

j Hofmann, A.F. and Danzinger, R.G. The physiological and clinical significance of ileal resection. In Surgical Annual. Nyhus, Cooper, eds. Appleton-Century-Crofts, New York, 1972, pp 305-326.

k Hofmann, A.F., Danzinger, R.G., Hoffman, N.E., Klein, P.D., Berngruber, O.W. and Szczepanik, P.A. Validation and comparison of deuterium/tritium and carbon 13/14 in clinical studies of bile acid metabolism. In Proc. Seminar on the Use of Stable Isotopes in Clinical Pharmacology. PD Klein and LJ Roth, eds. Conf 711115. National Technical Information Service, Springfield, Virginia, 1972, pp 37-52.

l Hofmann, A.F. and Poley, J.R. Role of bile acid malabsorption in the pathogenesis of diarrhea and steatorrhea in patients with ileal resection. I. Response to cholestyramine or replacement of dietary long chain triglyceride by medium chain triglyceride. Gastroenterology 62:918-934, 1972.

m Hofmann, A.F., Klein, P.D., Thistle, J.L., Hachey, D.L., Hoffman, N.E., LaRusso, N.F., Thomas, P.J., and Szczepanik, P.A. Studies on the cause and treatment of gallstones using deuterium labeled bile acids. In Proc of First Internat'l Conf on Stable Isotopes in Chemistry, Biology, and Medicine. PD Klein and SV Peterson, eds. Conf 730525. National Technical Information Service, Springfield, Virginia, 1973, pp 369-379.

a Hofmann, A.F. and Mekhjian, H.S. Bile acids and the intestinal absorption of fat and electrolytes in health and disease. In Bile Acids. Nair, Kritchevsky, eds. Plenum Press, New York, Vol 2, 1973, pp 103-152.

b Hofmann, A.F., Northfield, T.C., and Thistle, J.L. Can a cholesterol-lowering diet cause gallstones? N. Engl. J. Med. 288:46-47, 1973 (Editorial).

c Hofmann, A.F. and Thomas, P.J. Bile acid breath test: Extremely simple, moderately useful. Ann. Intern. Med. 29:743-744, 1973.

d Hofmann, A.F. Gallstones: The age of dissolution draws near. Med. Times 102:113-123, 1974.

e Hofmann, A.F. Pathogenesis and treatment of cholesterol gallstones. Verh. Deutsch. Gesell. f. Inn. Med. 80:407-412, 1974.

f Hofmann, A.F. and Hoffman, N.E. Measurement of bile acid kinetics by isotope dilution in man. Gastroenterology 67:314-323, 1974.

g Hofmann, A.F., Korman, M.G., and Krugman, S. Sensitivity of serum bile acid assay for detection of liver damage in viral hepatitis type B: Prospective study in five patients. Am. J. Dig. Dis. 19:908-910, 1974.

h Hofmann, A.F. and Paumgartner, G. Chenodeoxycholic Acid Therapy of Gallstones. F.K. Schattauer Verlag, Stuttgart, New York, 1974, 60 p.

i Hofmann, A.F. and Thistle, J.L. An algorithm for monitoring and managing drug hepatotoxicity. Gastroenterology 67:309-313, 1974.

j Hofmann, A.F. and Thistle, J.L. Chenodeoxycholic acid: Cost. N. Engl. J. Med. 290:406, 1974 (Letter to Editor).

k Hofmann, A.F. and Thistle, J.L. Chenodeoxycholic acid: Possible intestinal injury. N. Engl. J. Med. 290:405-406, 1974 (Letter to Editor).

l Hofmann, A.F. and Thistle, J.L. Chenodeoxycholic acid: The Mayo Clinic experience. Hosp. Prac. 9:41-48, 1974.

m Hofmann, A.F. The enterohepatic circulation of bile acids in man. Second NATO Adv. Study Inst. on the Biliary System. August, 1975, Aalborg, Denmark, pp 92-99, (abstract).

n Hofmann, A.F. and Paumgartner, G. Chenodeoxycholic Acid Therapy of Gallstones: Update 1975. F.K. Schattauer Verlag, Stuttgart-New York, 1975.

o Hofmann, A.F. and Thistle, J.L. Treating gallstones: Does chenic acid have a place? Inn. Med. 2:19-21, 1975 (Editorial).

p Hofmann, A.F. The enterohepatic circulation of bile acids in man. In Stollerman/Advances in Internal Medicine. Yearbook Medical Publishers, New York, 21:501-534, 1976.

a Hofmann, A.F. Fat digestion: The interaction of lipid digestion products with micellar bile acid solutions. In Lipid Absorption: Biochemical and Clinical Aspects. K Rommel and H Geobell, eds. MTP Press, Lancaster, 1976, pp 3-18.

b Hofmann, A.F., LaRusso, N.F., Korman, M.G., Calcraft, B.J., Cowen, A.E., Hoffman, N.E., and Schalm, S.W. Physiological meaning and diagnostic sensitivity of serum cholate levels. In Liver. R Preisig, J Bircher, and G Paumgartner, eds. Editio Cantor, Aulendorf, 1976, pp 259-267.

c Hofmann, A.F. Bile acids, diarrhea, and antibiotics: Data, speculation, and a unifying hypothesis. J. Inf. Diseases 135:S126-S136, 1977.

d Hofmann, A.F. The enterohepatic circulation of bile acids in man. Clin. Gastroenterol. 6:3-24, 1977.

e Hofmann, A.F. Metabolisme entero-hepatique des acides biliaires. Med. Chir. Dig. 6:1-5, 1977.

f Hofmann, A.F. Neue Aspekte und klinische Bedeutung der Gallensauren. Der Internist 18:1-6, 1977.

g Hofmann, A.F. Desaturation of bile and cholesterol gallstone dissolution with chenodeoxycholic acid. Am. J. Clin. Nutr. 30:993-1000, 1977.

h Hofmann, A.F. The enterohepatic circulation of conjugated bile acids in healthy man: Quantitative description and functions. In Cholesterol Metabolism and Lipolytic Enzymes. J Polonovski, ed. Masson Publishing U.S.A., Inc., New York, 1977, pp 69-86.

i Hofmann, A.F. Fat absorption and malabsorption: Physiology, diagnosis, and treatment. Viewpoints 9(4) September, 1977.

j Hofmann, A.F. and Klein, P.D. Characterization of bile acid metabolism in man using bile acids labeled with stable isotopes. In Stable Isotopes. TA Baillie, ed. University Park Press, Baltimore, 1978, pp 189-204.

k Hofmann, A.F., Thistle, J.L., Klein, P.D., Szczepanik, P.A., and Yu, P.Y.S. Chenotherapy for gallstones. II. Induced changes in bile composition and gallstone response. JAMA 239:1145-1147, 1978.

l Hofmann, A.F. The enterohepatic circulation of bile acids, including the history of ursodeoxycholic acid. Med. Chir. Dig. 9:619, 1980.

m Hofmann, A.F. The medical treatment of cholesterol gallstones. A major advance in preventive gastroenterology. Am. J. Med. 69:4-7, 1980.

n Hofmann, A.F. Pharmacology of chenic and ursodeoxycholic acid. Ital. J. Gastroenterol. 12:344, 1980 (abstract).

o Hofmann, A.F. The uncommon pharmacology of chenodeoxycholic acid: The first regulator of biliary cholesterol levels in man. Europ. J. Clin. Invest. 10:257-258, 1980.

a Hofmann, A.F., Schmack, B., Thistle, J.L., and Babayan, V.K. Clinical experience with monooctanoin for dissolution of bile duct stones: An uncontrolled multicenter trial. Dig. Dis. Sci. 26:954-955, 1981 (letter).

b Hofmann, A.F., Grundy, S.M., Lachin, J.M., Lan, S.P., Baum, R.A., Hanson, R.F., Hersh, T., Hightower, N.C. Jr., Marks, J.W., Mekhjian, H., Schaefer, R.A., Soloway, R.D., Thistle, J.L., Thomas, F.B., Tyor, M.P., and the National Cooperative Gallstone Study Group. Pretreatment biliary lipid composition in white patients with radiolucent gallstones in the National Cooperative Gallstone Study (NCGS). Gastroenterology (in press)

c Holan, K.R., Holzbach, R.T., Hsieh, J.Y., Welch, D.K., and Turcotte, J.G. Effect of oral administration of essential phospholipid, b-glycerophosphate, and linoleic acid on biliary lipids in patients with cholelithiasis. Digestion 19:251-258, 1979.

d Holan, K.R., Holzbach, R.T., Hermann, R.E., Cooperman, A.M., and Claffey, W.J. Nucleation time: A key factor in the pathogenesis of cholesterol gallstone disease. Gastroenterology 77:611-617, 1979.

e Holasek, A. Ueber den Ursprung des Kotfettes. II. Versuche an Ratten mit Gallengangverschluss. Hoppe-Seyler's Zeit. Physiol. Chem. 298:219, 1954.

f Holland, C. and Heaton, K.W. Increasing frequency of gallbladder operations in the Bristol clinical area. Brit. Med. J. 3:672-675, 1972.

g Holland, W.W. and Whitehead, T.P. Value of new laboratory tests in diagnosis and treatment. Lancet 2:391-394, 1974.

h Holsti, P. Cirrhosis of the liver induced in rabbits by gastric instillation of 3-monohydroxycholanic acid. Nature 186:250, 1960.

i Holsti, P. Bile acids as a cause of liver injury: Cirrhogenic effect of chenodeoxycohlic acid in rabbits. Acta Path. Microbiol. Scand. 54:479, 1962.

j Holt, P.R. Intestinal absorption of bile salts in the rat. Am. J. Physiol. 207:1, 1964.

k Holt, P.R. Competitive inhibition of intestinal bile salt absorption in the rat. Am. J. Physiol. 210:635-639, 1966.

l Holt, P.R. Medium chain triglycerides: Their absorption, metabolism and clinical applications. In Progress in Gastroenterology. Greene and Stratton, 1968, pp 227.

m Holt, P.R. Studies of Medium Chain Triglycerides in Patients with Differing Mechanisms for Fat Malabsorption. 1st Edition, University of Pennsylvania Press, Philadelphia, 1968, pp 97-107.

n Holt, P.R. The roles of bile acids during the process of normal fat and cholesterol absorption. Arch. Intern. Med. 130:574-583, 1972.

o Holub, K. The problem of gallstone dissolution. Zentralbl. Chir. 102:833-838, 1977.

a Holzbach, R.T. and Marsh, M. Dietary cholelithiasis. Lancet 2:936-937, 1970.

b Holzbach, R.T. Lithogenic bile in young Indian women. N. Engl. J. Med. 284:1040-1041, 1971 (Letter to Editor).

c Holzbach, R.T., Marsh, M.E., and Hallberg, M.C. The effect of pregnancy on lipid composition of guinea pig gallbladder bile. Gastroenterology 60:288-293, 1971.

d Holzbach, R.T., Marsh, M., Olszewski, M., and Holan, K. Cholesterol solubility in bile: Evidence that supersaturated bile is frequent in healthy man. J. Clin. Invest. 52:1467-1479, 1973.

e Holzbach, R.T. The solubility and nucleation of cholesterol in bile. Gastroenterology 66:323-325, 1974 (Letter to Editor).

f Holzbach, R.T. and Marsh, M. Transient liquid crystals in human bile analogs. Mol. Cryst. and Liq. Cryst. 28:217-223, 1975.

g Holzbach, R.T., Corbusier, C., Marsh, M., and Naito, H.K. The process of cholesterol cholelithiasis induced by diet in the prairie dog: A physicochemical characterization. J. Lab. Clin. Med. 87:987-998, 1976.

h Holzbach, R.T., Oh, S.Y., McDonnell, M.E., and Jamieson, A.M. Hydrodynamic size measurements of pure bile salt and bile salt mixed-lipid micelles by quasielastic laser light scattering: Comparison with relative saturability for dissolved cholesterol. Gastroenterology 70:971, 1976 (abstract).

i Holzbach, R.T., Oh, S.Y., McDonnell, M.E., and Jamieson, A.M. Quasielastic laser spectrometry studies of pure bile salt and bile salt-mixed lipid micellar systems. Proc. Mittal Symp., Plenum Press (in press).

j Holzbach, R.T. and Corbusier, C. Liquid crystals and cholesterol nucleation during equilibration in supersaturated bile analogs. Biochim. Biophys. Acta 528:436-444, 1978.

k Holzbach, R.T., Marsh, M.E., Freedman, M.R., Fazio, V.W., Lavery, I.C., and Jagelman, D.A. Portal vein bile acids in patients with severe inflammatory bowel disease. Gut 21:428-435, 1980.

l Horak, W., Waldram, R., Davis, M., Manthorpe, D.J., and Williams, R. Effect of amylobarbitone on bile acid kinetics in man. Digestion 10:324, 1974 (abstract).

m Horak, W., Waldram, R., Murray-Lyon, I.M., Schuster, E., and Williams, R. Kinetics of ^{14}C-cholic acid in fulminant hepatic failure, a prognostic test. Gastroenterology 71:809-813, 1976.

n Horak, W., Knoflach, P., Schuster, E., Kemenesi, W., and Grabner, G. Plasma disappearance and conjugation of ^{14}C-cholic acid in patients with obstructive jaundice. In Bile Acid Metabolism in Health and Disease. G Paumgartner and A Steihl, eds., MTP Press, Lancaster, 1977, pp 247-251.

a Horak, W., Polterauer, P., Renner, F., Rauhs, R., Mulbacher, R., Funovics, J., and Weidhofer, J. Effect of chenodeoxycholic acid (CDCA), ursodeoxycholic acid (UDCA) and cholic acid (CA) on bile lipids in the baboon. Abstraktband 14:50, 1979 (abstract).

b Horak, W., Polterauer, P., Renner, F., Rauhs, R., Muhlbacher, F., Funovics, J., and Weidhofer, J. Effect of different bile acids on cholesterol and phospholipid secretion in the isolated perfused baboon liver. VI Internat'l Bile Acid Meeting, Freiburg, 1980, pp 145 (abstract).

c Hordinsky, B.Z. Terpenes in the treatment of gallstones. Min. Med. 54:649-652, 1971.

d Horlick, S.E., Lakshminarayanaiah, N., Trotman, B.W., Kahn, M.J., Wirt, G.D., Bernstein, S.E. Calcium binding properties of bile salts: A possible protective role in pigment gallstone disease. Hepatology 1:518, 1981 (abstract).

e Horsburgh, D.S., Metzger, H.N., and Tumen, H.J. Diagnostic biliary drainage. A plea for a seldom-used diagnostic procedure. Am. J. Dig. Dis. 18:966-970, 1973.

f Hoshita, N., Shefer, S., Cheng, F.W., Dayal, B., Batta, A.K., Tint, G.S., Salen, G., and Mosbach, E.H. Biosynthesis of chenodeoxycholic acid: Side chain hydroxylation of 5b-cholestane-3a,7a-diol by subcellular fractions of guinea pig liver. Lipids 13:961-965, 1978.

g Hoshita, T., Kono, M., Matsumoto, M., Uchiyama, M., and Kuramoto, T. Metabolism of bile acids. I. Absorption, distribution, excretion, and metabolism of ursodeoxycholic acid. Pharm. Soc. Japan 94:1196-1205, 1974.

h Hoshita, T., Harada, N., Morita, I., and Kihira, K. Comparative biochemical studies of bile acids and bile alcohols. XX. Intestinal absorption of bile alcohols. J. Biochem. (Tokyo) 90:1363-1369, 1981.

i Hosono, H. and Iwasaki, M. Acute toxicity and hemolysis studies of ursodeoxycholic acid in rats and mice. Kiso to Rinsho (Clinical Report) 9:3159-3166, 1975.

j Howe, E.E., Bosshardt, D.K., Gilfillan, J., Hunt, V.M., and Huff, J.W. The hypolipemic properties of 5b-cholanic acid in the mouse and rat. Arch. Biochem. Biophys. 129:264-272, 1969.

k Howell, J.I., Lucy, J.I., Pirola, R.C., and Bouchier, I.A.D. Macromolecular assemblies of lipid in bile. Biochim. Biophys. Acta 210:1-6, 1970.

l Hrabak, P. Gallensauren und Cholelithiasis. Bad Berka (DDR) Jan., 1975.

m Hrabak, P., Doskova, M., Skorepa, J., and Souckova, E. Dissolution of biliary calculi with chenodeoxycholic acid: Our first experience. Cas. Lek. Cesk. 116:1337-1342, 1977.

n Hrabak, P. Chenodeoxycholic acid in conservative treatment for cholelithiasis. Mechanism of lithogenic bile formation and therapeutical indices. Cas. Lek. Cesk. 117:1577-1582, 1978.

a Hrabak, P., Doskova, M., Souckova, E., Konecny, K., and Holaskova, M. Konzervativni lecba cholelitiazy kyselinou chenodesoxycholovou. Biotransformace kyseliny chenodesoxycholove a vyznam tvorby sulfatu kyseliny litocholove. Cas. Lek. Ces. 118:1078-1082, 1979.

b Hraback, P., Doskova, M., and Souckova, E. Cholelithiasis treated with chenodeoxycholic acid. An analysis of changes in the pattern of bile acids. Cas. Lek. Cesk. 120:817-823, 1981.

c Hsia, S.L., Matschiner, J.T., Mahowald, T.A., Elliot, W.H., Doisy, E.A., Jr., Thayer, S.A., Doisy, E.A. Bile acids. X. Characterization and partial synthesis of acid IV. J. Biol. Chem. 230:597-601, 1958.

d Hubel, K.A. Gallstone migration. Gastroenterology 67:385-386, 1974 (Editorial).

e Huijbregts, A., van Berge Henegouwen, G.P., Hectors, M.P.C., van Shaik, A., and van der Werf, S.D. Effects of a standardized wheat bran preparation on biliary lipid composition and bile acid metabolism in young healthy males. Europ. J. Clin. Invest. 10:451-458, 1980.

f Huijbregts, A.W.M., van Shaik, A., van Berge Henegouwen, G.P., and van der Werf, S.D. Serum lipids, biliary lipid composition, and bile acid metabolism in vegetarians as compared to normal controls. Europ. J. Clin. Invest. 10:443-449, 1980.

g Huijbregts, A.W.M., Cox, T.M., Hermsen, J., van Berge Henegouwen, G., van Schaik, A., and Chadwick, V. Micellar solubilization of intestinal lipids after ursodeoxycholic acid therapy in short bowel patients and healthy controls. Neth. J. Med. 24:108-113, 1981.

h Hummel, J.P. and Dreyer, W.J. Measurement of protein-binding phenomena by gel filtration. Biochim. Biophys. Acta 63:530-532, 1962.

i Hunt, G.R.A. A comparison of Triton X-100 and the bile salt taurocholate as micellar ionophores or fusogens in phospholipid vesicular membranes. A ^{1}H NMR method using the lanthanide probe ion Pr^{3+}. FEBS Lett. 119:132-136, 1980.

j Hunt, G.R.A. and Jawaharlal, K. A ^{1}H-NMR investigation of the mechanism for the ionophore activity of the bile salts in phospholipid vesicular membranes and the effect of cholesterol. Biochim. Biophys. Acta 601: 678-684, 1980.

k Hunt, R.D., Leveille, G.A., and Sauberlich, H.E. Dietary bile acids and lipid metabolism. II. The ductular cell reaction induced by lithocholic acid. Proc. Soc. Exptl. Biol. Med. 113:139-142, 1963.

l Hunt, R.D., Leveille, G.A., and Sauberlich, H.E. Dietary bile acids and lipid metabolism. III. Effects of lithocholic acid in mammalian species. Proc. Soc. Exptl. Biol. Med. 115:277-280, 1964.

a Hunt, R.D. Proliferation of bile ductules (the ductular cell reaction) induced by lithocholic acid. Fed. Proc. 24:431, 1965 (abstract).

b Hunt, T. Cholagogues and choleretics. Practitioner 206:51-55, 1971.

c Hurst, A.P. Constipation and allied intestinal disorders. 2nd Edition. Oxford University Press, London, 1919, 440 pp.

d Hutterer, F., Bacchin, P.G., Denk, H., Schenkman, J.B., Schaffner, F., and Popper, H. Mechanism of cholestasis. II. Effect of bile acids on the microsomal electron transfer system in vitro. Life Sci. 9(II):1159-1166, 1970.

e Hutterer, F., Bacchin, P.G., Raisfeld, I.H., Schenkman, J.B., Schaffner, F., and Popper, H. Alteration of microsomal biotransformation in the liver in cholestasis. Proc. Soc. Exptl. Biol. Med. 133:702-717, 1970.

f Hutterer, F., Denk, H., Bacchin, P.G., Schenkman, J.B., Schaffner, F., and Popper, H. Mechanism of cholestasis. I. Effect of bile acids on microsomal cytochrome P-450 dependent biotransformation system in vitro. Life Sci. 9:877-887, 1970.

g Hwang, K-K. and Kelsey, M.I. Evidence of epoxide hydrase activity in human intestinal microflora. Cancer Biochem. Biophys. 3:31-35, 1978.

h Hylemon, P.B. and Stellwag, E.J. Bile acid biotransformation rates of selected gram-positive and gram-negative intestinal anaerobic bacteria. Biochem. Biophys. Res. Comm. 69:1088-1094, 1976.

i Hylemon, P.B., Cacciapuoti, A.F., White, B.A., Whitehead, T.R., and Fricke, R.J. 7a-Dehydroxylation of cholic acid by cell extracts of Eubacterium species V.P.I. 12708. Am. J. Clin. Nutr. 33:2507-2510, 1980.

j Hyon, U. and Yoshida, M. Bile acid secretion following release of biliary obstruction. Gastroenterologia Japonica 14:553-564, 1979.

k Iga, T. and Klaassen, C.D. Hepatic extraction of bile acids in rats. Biochem. Pharmacol. 31:205-209, 1982.

l Igimi, H. Experimental studies on dissolution of cholesterol stones. Fukuoka Acta Med. 42:55-66, 1972.

m Igimi, H. Ursodeoxycholate - a common bile acid in gallbladder bile of Japanese subjects. Life Sciences 18:993-1000, 1976.

n Igimi, H., Hisatsugu, T., and Nishimura, M. The use of d-limonene prepara tion as a dissolving agent of gallstones. Am. J. Dig. Dis. 21:926-939, 1976.

o Igimi, H., Noriyuki, T., Yuichi, I., and Hidehiko, S. Ursodeoxycholic acid--in vitro cholesterol solubility changes of composition of human gallbladder bile after oral treatment. Life Sci. 21:1373-1380, 1977.

a Igimi, H. and Carey, M.C. Cholesterol monohydrate (ChM) gallstones dissolved faster in chenodeoxycholate (CDC)-rich bile than in ursodeoxycholate (UDC)-rich bile. Gastroenterology 78:1186, 1980 (abstract).

b Igimi, H. and Carey, M.C. pH-solubility relations of chenodeoxycholic and ursodeoxycholic acids: Physical-chemical basis for dissimilar solution and membrane phenomena. J. Lipid Res. 21:72-89, 1980.

c Igimi, H. and Carey, M. Cholesterol gallstone dissolution in bile: Dissolution kinetics of crystalline (anhydrate and monohydrate) cholesterol with chenodeoxycholate, ursodeoxycholate, and their glycine and taurine conjugates. J. Lipid Res. 22:254-270, 1981.

d Iida, T. and Chang, F.C. Potential bile acid metabolites. 3. A new route to chenodeoxycholic acid. J. Org. Chem. 13:2786-2788, 1981.

e Iida, T., Taneja, H.R., and Chang, F.C. Potential bile acid metabolites. IV. Inversion of 7a-hydroxyl; ursodeoxycholic acid. Lipids 16:863-865, 1981.

f Ikawa, S. Metabolism of 3b,7b-dihydroxy-5-cholen-(24-^{14}C)-oic acid in the rat. J. Biochem. 82:1093-1102, 1977.

g Ikeda, MN., Nanba, S., Hayakawa, S., and Ohmori, S. Colorimetric determination of glycine conjugates of bile acids. J. Clin. Chem. Clin. Biochem. 18:407-411, 1980.

h Imrie, C.W. and Whyte, A.S. Patients with gallstones. Lancet 2:1149, 1972 (Letter to Editor).

i Infante, R., Bouma, M-E., Lageron, A., and Levy, V-G. Toxicologic study of chendeoxycholic acid. Therapie 32:401-402, 1977.

j Ingelfinger, F.J. Gallstones and estrogens. N. Engl. J. Med. 290:51-52, 1974 (Editorial).

k International Symposium on Ursodeoxycholic Acid, Paris, 1980. Med. Chir. Dig. 9:619-635, 1980.

l Isaacs, P.E.T., Iser, J.H., Murphy, G.M., and Dowling, R.H. Serum bile acids (SBA's) and plasma bile acid disappearance (PBAD) as tests of liver function: A study in controls, patients with liver disease and gallstone patients before and after chenodeoxycholic acid (CDCA) treatment. Gut 17:822, 1976 (abstract).

m Isaksson, B. On the lipid constituents of normal bile. Acta Soc. med. Upsalien 56:177-195, 1951.

n Isaksson, B. A method for spectrophotometric determination of chenodeoxycholic acid in bile. Acta Chem. Scand. 6:889-897, 1954.

o Isaksson, B. On the dissolving power of lecithin and bile salts for cholesterol in human bladder bile. Acta Soc. med. Upsalien 59:296-306, 1954.

a Isaksson, B. On the lipid constituents of bile from human gallbladder containing cholesterol gallstones. A comparison with normal human bladder bile. Acta Soc. med. Upsal. 59:277, 1953-1954.

b Isaksson, B. On the lipids and bile acids in normal and pathological bladder bile: A study of the main cholesterol dissolving components of human bile. MD Dissertation, University of Gothenburg, Lund, Sweden, 1954.

c Iser, J.H., Dowling, R.H., Mok, H.Y.I., and Bell, G.D. Chenodeoxycholic acid treatment of gallstones - a follow-up report and analysis of factors influencing response to therapy. N. Engl. J. Med. 293:378-383, 1975.

d Iser, J.H., Murphy, G.M., and Dowling, R.H. Is intermittent chenodeoxycholic acid therapy feasible for dissolving gallstones? The speed of change in biliary lipids and bile acids after starting and stopping treatment. Gut 16:840, 1975 (abstract).

e Iser, J., Jones, D., Murphy, G.M., and Dowling, R.H. Congenital bile acid (BA) deficiency associated with intractable constipation in a 28-year-old woman. Gut 17:821, 1976 (abstract).

f Iser, J.H., Murphy, G.M., and Dowling, R.H. Chenodeoxycholic acid (CDCA) treatment of gallstones: A follow-up at five years. Gut 17:822, 1976 (abstract).

g Iser, J.H., Packer, J.S., Smallwood, R.A., and Hoffman, N.E. Hepatic transport of taurocholic acid in the rat: Development of a mathematical model. Clin. Exptl. Pharm. Phys. 3:29-36, 1976.

h Iser, J.H., Murphy, G.M., and Dowling, R.H. Speed of change in biliary lipids and bile acids with chenodeoxycholic acid--is intermittent therapy feasible? Gut 18:7-15, 1977.

i Iser, J.H., Maton, P.N., Murphy, G.M., and Dowling, R.H. Resistance to chenodeoxycholic acid (CDCA) treatment in obese patients with gall stones. Brit. Med. J. 1:1509-1512, 1978.

j Iser, J. and Sali, A. Chenodeoxycholic acid: A review of its pharmacological properties and therapeutic use. Drugs 21:90-119, 1981.

k Iser, J. Medical treatment of gallstones. Aust. Fam. Physician 10:492-494, 1981.

l Ishikawa, S., Iizuka, A., and Yanaura, S. Choleretic properties of chenodeoxycholic acid (CDCA) and dehydrocholic acid (DHCA) in rats. Hippon Yakurigaku Zasshi 76:25-32, 1980.

m Isselbacher, K.J. Mechanisms of absorbtion of long and medium chain triglycerides. _In_ Medium Chain Triglycerides, JR Senior, ed. Univ. Pennsylvania Press, Philadelphia, 1968, pp 21-34.

n Isselbacher, K.J. A medical treatment for gallstones? N. Engl. J. Med. 286:40-42, 1972 (Editorial).

a Isselbacher, K.J. Chenodiol for gallstones: Dissolution or disillusion? Ann. Intern. Med. 95:377-379, 1981.

b Itoh, S., Onishi, S., Isobe, K., Manabe, M., and Inukai, K. Foetomaternal relationships of serum bile acid pattern estimated by high pressure liquid chromatography. Biochem. J. 204:141-145, 1982.

c Ivey, K.J., DenBesten, L., and Bell, S. Absorption of bile salts from human gastric mucosa. J. Appl. Physiol. 29:806-808, 1970.

d Iwamura, K., Shimura, S., Koike, H., Yanagisawa, F., Mokino, K., Kimura, K., and Sadatsuki, T. Clinical and pathological findings of the liver in patients with cholelithiasis. Gastroenterol. Jpn. 7:184, 1972 (abstract).

e Iwamura, K. and Ueno, F. Clinical studies on gallstone dissolution by chenodeoxycholic acid. Tokai J. Clin. Exptl. Clin. Med. 3:97-106, 1978.

f Iwamura, K. Clinical studies on cheno- and ursodeoxycholic acid treatment for gallstone dissolution. Hepato-Gastroenterol. 27:26-34, 1980.

g Iwasaki, M. Liver diseases and endotoxin. I. Effect of bile acid on endotoxin. Jap. J. Gastroenterol. 78:1240, 1981.

h Iwasaki, T. Uber die Konstitution der Urso-desoxycholsaure. Z. Physiol. Chem. 244:181-193, 1936.

i Iwata, T. and Yamasaki, K. Enzymatic determination and thin-layer chromatography of bile acids in blood. J. Biochem. 56:424-431, 1964 (Tokyo).

j Jablonski, P. and Owen, J.A. The clinical chemistry of bromsulfophthalein and other cholephilic dyes. Adv. Clin. Chem. 12:309-385, 1969.

k Jacobsen, J.G. and Smith, L.H., Jr. Biochemistry and physiology of taurine and taurine derivatives. Physiol. Rev. 48:424-511, 1968.

l James, O.F.W., Agnew, J.E., and Bouchier, I.A.D. Assessment of the ^{14}C-glycocholic acid breath test. Brit. Med. J. 2:191-195, 1973.

m James, O.F.W., Cullen, J., and Bouchier, I.A.D. Chenodeoxycholic acid therapy for gallstones: Effectiveness, toxicity and influence on bile acid metabolism. Quart. J. Med. 44:349-367, 1975.

n Jansen, M.A., Olson, J.R., and Fujimoto, J.M. Taurolithocholate-induced increase in the intrabiliary pressure generated during retrograde intrabiliary infusion of saline in rats: Antagonism by taurocholate and glycocholate. Toxicol. Appl. Pharmacol. 54:9-19, 1980.

o Jansson, R. and Svanvik, J. Effects of intravenous secretin and cholecystokinin on gallbladder net water absorption and motility in the cat. Gastroenterology 72:639-643, 1977.

a Jansson, R., Steen, G., and Svanvik, J. Effects of intravenous vasoactive intestinal peptide (VIP) on gallbladder function in the cat. Gastroenterology 75:47-50, 1978.

b Jarrett, L.N., Balfour, T.W., Bell, G.D., Knapp, D.R., and Rose, D.H. Intraductal infusion of mono-octanoin: Experience in 24 patients with retained common duct stones. Lancet 1:68-70, 1981.

c Javitt, N.B. Clinical aspects of bile acid metabolism. Schw. med. Wschr. 98:269, 1968.

d Javitt, N.B. and Emerman, S. Effect of sodium taurolithocholate on bile flow and bile acid excretion. J. Clin. Invest. 47:1002-1014, 1968.

e Javitt, N.B. Symposium on bile salts. Foreward. Am. J. Med. 51:565-567, 1971.

f Javitt, N.B. Pathways of bile acid synthesis. In Bile Acids in Human Diseases. II. Bile Acid Meeting, Freiburg. P Back and W Gerok, eds. F.K. Schattauer Verlag, Stuttgart-New York, 1972, pp 17-21.

g Javitt, N.B. Excretion of monohydroxy bile acid ester sulfates in the rat. In The Liver: Quantitative Aspects of Structure and Function. Karger, New York, 1973, pp 355-359.

h Javitt, N.B., Morrissey, K.P., Siegel, E., Goldberg, H., Gartner, L.M., Hollander, M., and Kok, E. Cholestatic syndromes in infancy: Diagnostic value of serum bile acid pattern and cholestyramine administration. Pediat. Res. 7:119-125, 1973.

i Javitt, N.B. Bile salts and liver disease in childhood. Postgrad. Med. 50:354-361, 1974.

j Javitt, N.B. Timing of cholestyramine doses in cholestatic liver disease. N. Engl. J. Med. 290:1328-1329, 1974 (Letter to Editor).

k Javitt, N.B., Lavy, U., and Kok, E. Neonatal cholestatic jaundice: Diagnostic and therapeutic approach. VI Meeting Int'l. Assn. for Study of Liver. Acapulco, Mexico, Oct., 1974 (abstract).

l Javitt, N.B. Chenodeoxycholic acid: The next phase. Hosp. Prac. 10:11-12, 1975 (Editorial).

m Javitt, N.B. Diagnostic value of serum bile acids. Clin. Gastroenterol. 6:219-226, 1977.

n Javitt, N.B. The cheno cooperative study: Its meaning for gallstone treatment. Hosp. Prac. pp 8 & 13, January, 1982.

o Javor, T., et al. Effects of phenobarbital treatment on biliary excretion in man. Drug Met. Disp. 1:424-427, 1973.

a Jazrawi, R.P., Bridges, C., Joseph, A., and Northfield, T.C. Effect of artificial depletion of bile acid pool on hepatic and gallbladder bile in man. Gut 21:A895, 1980 (abstract).

b Jeannin, J.F., Chessebeuf, M., Martin, M.S., Lagneau, A., and Martin, F. Proliferative effect of lithocholic acid on rat liver cells in culture. Biomedicine 31:207-209, 1979.

c Johansson, G. On the metabolism of lithocholic acid in chicken and rabbit. Acta Chem. Scand. 20:240, 1966.

d Johansson, G. Effect of cholestyramine and diet on hydroxylations in the biosynthesis and metabolism of bile acids. Europ. J. Biochem. 17:292, 1970.

e Johns, W.H. and Bates, T.R. Quantification of the binding tendencies of cholestyramine. I. Effect of structure and added electrolytes on the binding of unconjugated and conjugated bile-salt anions. J. Pharm. Sci. 58:179-183, 1969.

f Johns, W.H. and Bates, T.R. Quantification on the binding tendencies of cholestyramine. II. Mechanism of interaction with bile salt and fatty acid anions. J. Pharm. Sci. 59:329-333, 1970.

g Johnson, D.B., Tyor, M.P., and Lack, L. The use of 7a-^{3}H- and 7a, 7b,-^{3}H-cholesterol in the enzymic assay of cholesterol 7a-hydroxylase. J. Lipid Res. 17:353, 1976.

h Johnson, J., Ellis, A.L., and Riegel, C. Studies of gallbladder function. XIV. Absorption of sodium tetraiodophenolphthalein from normal and damaged gallbladder. Am. J. Med. Sci. 193:483-488, 1937.

i Johnston, C.G. and Nakayama, F. Solubility of cholesterol and gallstones in metabolic material. Arch. Surg. 75:436-442, 1957.

j Johnston, J.M. The mechanism of fat absorption. In Handbook of Physiology. T.H. Wilson, ed. Williams & Wilkins, Baltimore, Vol 3, 1968, pp 1353-1375.

k Johnston, S.A. and McBain, J.W. Freezing points of solutions of typical colloidal electrolytes, soaps, sulphonates, sulphates, and bile salt. Proc. Roy. Soc. 181:119-133, 1942.

l Jones, D.C., Lofland, H.B., Clarkson, T.B., St. Clair, R.W. Plasma cholesterol concentrations in squirrel monkeys as influenced by diet and phenotype. J. Food Sci. 40:2-7, 1975.

m Jones, D.C., Melchoir, G.W., and Reeves, M.J.W. Quantitative analysis of individual bile acids by gas-liquid chromatography. An improved method. J. Lipid Res. 17:273-277, 1976.

n Jones, M.B., Weinstock, S., Koretz, R.L., Lewin, K.J., Higgins, J., and Gitnick, G.L. Clinical value of serum bile acid levels in chronic hepatitis. Dig. Dis. Sci. 26:978-983, 1981.

a Jorge, A.D. and Sanchez, D. Wirkung der Chenodesoxycholsaure auf Cholesteringallensteine. Leber Magen Darm 8:365-369, 1978.

b Jorge, A., Milutin, C., Gutierrez, L. and Burgos, M. Ultrastructure of the liver in patients with cholesterol stones receiving chenodeoxycholic acid. Leber Magen Darm 9:200-204, 1979.

c Jorge, A. and Sanchez, D. El efecto del acido quenodesoxicolico en la litiasis cholesterinica. Acta Gastroenterol. Lat. Am. 10:269-276, 1980.

d Jorge, A., Sanchez, D., and Findor, J.A. Litiasis vesicular colesterinica. In Temas de Terapeutica Clinica II. FG Lasala, CL Sagasta, and CR Gherardi, eds. Libreria Akadia, Buenos Aires, 1981, pp 320-325.

e Josephson, B. and Rydin, A. The resorption of the bile acids from the intestine. Biochem. J. 30:2224-2228, 1936.

f Josephson, B. Elimination of cholic acids. IV. In patients with liver diseases. J. Clin. Invest. 18:343-350, 1939.

g Josephson, B. The circulation of the bile acids in connection with their production, conjugation, and excretion. Physiol. Rev. 21:463-486, 1941.

h Juniper, K., Jr. and Burson, E.N., Jr. Biliary tract studies. II. The significance of biliary crystals. Gastroenterology 32:175-208, 1957.

i Juniper, K., Jr. Physicochemical characteristics of bile and their relation to gallstone formation. Am. J. Med. 39:98-107, 1965.

j Kaess, H. Auflosung von Gallensteinen. Int. Praxis 15:755-756, 1975.

k Kajiyama, G., Mizuno, T., Yamada, K., Maruhashi, A., Matsura, C., and Miyoshi, A. Effect of chenodeoxycholic acid and its conjugates on cholesterol gallstone dissolution in hamsters. Caracas, 33, Nov., 1975.

l Kajiyama, G. and Maruhashi, A. Symposium on pathophysiology of biliary tract diseases with special emphasis on gallstone disease. VI. Basic and clinical studies on bile acid preparations for the treatment of gallstones. Nippon Naika Gakkai Zasshi 66:1201-1205, 1977.

m Kajiyama, G., Maruhashi, A., Mizuno, T., Yamada, K., Kawamoto, T., Fujiyama, M., Kubota, S., Sasaki, S., Oyamada, K., Nakao, S., and Miyoshi, A. Treatment of gallstones with chenodeoxy- acid and ursodeoxycholic acid. The influence of presence or absence of hyperlipidemia on gallstone dissolution. Hiroshima J. Med. Sci. 28:67-71, 1979.

n Kajiyama, G., Kawamoto, T., Fujiyama, M., Maruhashi, A., and Miyoshi, A. Effect of the purified unsaponifiable fraction of soybean in combination with ursodeoxycholic acid on cholesterol saturation of bile and stone dissolution in gallstone patients. Hiroshima J. Med. Sci. 30:71-83, 1981.

a Kakis, G., Phillips, M.J., and Yousef, I.M. The respective roles of membrane cholesterol and of sodium potassium adenosine triphosphatase in the pathogenesis of lithocholate-induced cholestasis. Lab. Invest. 43:73-81, 1980.

b Kakis, G. and Yousef, I.M. Mechanism of cholic acid protection in lithocholate-induced intrahepatic cholestasis in rats. Gastroenterology 78:1402-1411, 1980.

c Kallberg, M. and Tobiasson, P. Determination of cholic and chenodeoxycholic acid in serum: Evaluation of two commercial radioimmunoassay methods. J. Clin. Chem. Clin. Biochem. 18:491-495, 1980.

d Kallner, A. On the biosynthesis and metabolism of allodeoxycholic acid in the rat. Acta Chem. Scand. 21:315-321, 1967.

e Kallner, A. On the reduction of 3-keto bile acids in vitro. Archiv. Kemi 26:553-565, 1967.

f Kallner, A. Bile acids in bile of cod, Gadus callarias. Hydroxylation of deoxycholic acid and chenodeoxycholic acid in homogenates of cod liver. Bile acids and steroids 200. Acta Chem. Scand. 22:2361-2370, 1968.

g Kallner, M. Bile acid kinetics in normal- and hyperlipemic man. Opuscula Medica 35(Suppl.):1-351, 1974.

h Kallner, M. The effect of chenodeoxycholic acid feeding on bile acid kinetics and fecal neutral steroid excretion in patients with hyperlipoproteinemia types II and IV. J. Lab. Clin. Med. 86:595-604, 1975.

i Kamata, T. Experimental study on hepatic HMG-CoA reductase activity in relation to the formation and dissolution of cholesterol gallstones. Nippon Geka Hokan 49:477-495, 1980.

j Kameda, H. Gallstone disease in Japan. Gastroenterology 46:109-114, 1964.

k Kameda, H. Gallstones: Composition, structural characteristics and geographic distribution. Rec. Adv. Gastroenterol. 4:117-124, 1967.

l Kameda, H. and the Tokyo Cooperative Gallstone Study Group. Efficacy and indications of ursodeoxycholic acid treatment for dissolving gallstones. Gastroenterology 78:542-548, 1980.

m Kanagalingam, K. and Strause, E. Influence of lithocholic acid on 2-aminothracene-induced alterations in DNA synthesis in rat tissues in vivo. Cancer Biochem. Biophys. 4:159-166, 1980.

n Kanazawa, T., Shimazaki, A., Sato, T., and Hoshino, T. Studies on the synthesis of ursodeoxycholic acid. Nippon Kaguku Zasshi 76:297-301, 1955.

o Kang-Jey, H. and Taylor, C.B. Control mechanisms of cholesterol biosynthesis. Arch. Path. 90:83-92, 1970.

a Kaplowitz, N. and Javitt, N.B. Quantitative analysis of unconjugated and conjugated bile acid in duodenal fluid by densitometry after paper electrophoresis. J. Lipid Res. 14:224-228, 1973.

b Kaplowitz, N., Kok, E., and Javitt, N.B. Postprandial serum bile acid for the detection of hepatobiliary disease. JAMA 225:292-293, 1973.

c Kappert, F.W. Medikament oder Operation? med. (Praxis) 8:23-25, 1981.

d Karbach, Y.I. Separation of taurochenodeoxycholic acid from goose bile and preparation of chenodeoxycholic acid. Lab. Delo. 378, 1969. C.A. 71:877-886, 1969.

e Karlaganis, G. and Paumgartner, G. Analysis of bile acids in serum and bile by capillary gas-liquid chromatography. J. Lipid Res. 19:771-774, 1978.

f Karlaganis, G. and Paumgartner, G. Determination of bile acids in serum by capillary gas-liquid chromatography. Clin. Chim. Acta 92:19-26, 1979.

g Kawai, S. Die Ueberfuhrung von Cholsaure in Anthropodesoxycholsaure. Z. Physiol. Chem. 214:71, 1933.

h Kawamoto, T., Yamada, K., Mizuno, T., Matsuura, Ch., Fujiyama, M., Kubota, S., Maruhashi, A., Kajiyama, G., and Miyoshi, A. The effect of chenodeoxycholic acid (CDC) on cholesterol gallstone in hamsters. 5th Asian-Pacific Cong. of Gastroenterol. Singapore, pp 155, May, 1976 (abstract).

i Kawasaki, H., Yamanishi, Y., Kishimoto, Y., Hirayama, C., Ikawa, S., Kuchiba, K., and Kondo, T. Abnormality of oral ursodeoxycholic acid tolerance test in the Dubin-Johnson syndrome. Clin. Chim. Acta 112:13-19, 1981.

j Kay, R.E. and Entenman, C. Stimulation of taurocholic acid synthesis and biliary excretion of lipids. Am. J. Physiol. 200:855-859, 1961.

k Kay, R.M., Cohen, Z., Siu, K.P., Petrunka, C.N., and Strasberg, S.M. Ileal excretion and bacterial modification of bile acids and cholesterol in patients with continent ileostomy. Gut 21:128-132, 1979.

l Kay, R.M. Effects of diet on the fecal excretion and bacterial modification of acidic and neutral steroids, and implications for colon carcinogenesis. Cancer Res. 41:3774-3777, 1981.

m Kaye, M.D., Struthers, J.E., Jr., Tidball, J.S., DeNiro, E., and Kern, F., Jr. Factors affecting plasma clearance of ^{14}C cholic acid in patients with cirrhosis. Clin. Sci. Molec. Med. 45:147-161, 1973.

n Keane, R.M., Gadacz, T.R., Birmingham, W., Winchurch, R.A., and Munster, A.M. Raised bile acid levels depress human lymphocyte function. Br. J. Surg. 68:809, 1981 (abstract).

o Keclick, M. Treatment of cholelithiasis with chenodeoxycholic acid. Vnitri Lek. 21:177-182, 1975 (Russ).

a Keeling, J.W., Lamabadusuriya, S.P., and Harries, J.T. The effects of pure and micellar solutions of different bile salts on mucosal morphology in rat jejunum in vivo. J. Path. 118:157-163, 1976.

b Kellogg, T.F. The biliary bile acids of the Channel catfish, Ictalurus punctatus, and the blue catfish, Ictalurus furcatus. Comp. Biochem. Physiol. 50B:109-111, 1975.

c Kelsey, M. and Sexton, S. The biosynthesis of ethyl esters of lithocholic acid and isolithocholic acid by rat intestinal microflora. J. Steroid Biochem. 7:641-647, 1976.

d Kelsey, M. and Thompson, R. The biosynthesis of ethyl lithocholate by fecal microorganisms. J. Steroid Biochem. 7:117-124, 1976.

e Kelsey, M.I. and Sexton, S.A. Isolation and purification of lithocholic acid metabolites produced by the intestinal microflora. J. Chromatog. 133:327-334, 1977.

f Kelsey, M., Muschik, G., and Sexton, S. The metabolism of lithocholic acid-3a-sulfate by human intestinal microflora. Lipids 13:152-157, 1978.

g Kelsey, M. and Pienta, R. Transformation of hamster embryo cells by cholesterol-a-epoxide and lithocholic acid. Cancer Letters 6:143-149, 1979.

h Kelsey, M.I., Molina, J.E., and Hwang, K. A comparison of lithocholic acid metabolism by intestinal microflora in subjects of high- and low-risk colon cancer populations. Frontiers Gastrointest. Res. 4:38-50, 1979.

i Kelsey, M., Molina, J., Huang, S., and Hwang, K. The identification of microbial metabolites of sulfolithocholic acid. J. Lipid Res. 21:751-759, 1980.

j Kelsey, M.I., Hwang, K.K., Huang, S.K., and Shaikh, B. Characterization of microbial metabolites of sulfolithocholic acid by high-performance liquid chromatography. J. Steroid Biochem. 14:205-211, 1981.

k Kelsey, M.I. and Pienta, R.J. Transformation of hamster embryo cells by neutral sterols and bile acids. Toxicology Lett. 9:177-182, 1981.

l Kempi, V. and van der Linden, W. Effect of cholestyramine on the synthesis-ratio of cholic- and chenodeoxycholic acid in hamsters. Int. J. Clin. Pharm. 4:424-428, 1971.

m Kempi, V. and van der Linden, W. On the bile acid composition of hamsters and mice fed an atherogenic diet. Int. J. Clin. Pharm. 4:183-186, 1971.

n Kenney, T.J. and Garbutt, J.T. Effect of cholestyramine on bile acid metabolism in normal man. Gastroenterology 58:966, 1970 (abstract).

o Kern, F., Jr. and Borgstrom, B. The effect of a conjugated bile salt on oleic acid absorption in the rat. Gastroenterology 49:623, 1965.

a Kern, F., Jr. Clinical aspects of bile acid metabolism. Rendic. Gastroenterol. 7:205-212, 1975.

b Kern, F., Jr. and Davis, R.A. The effect of ethinyl estradiol on bile acid synthesis and cholesterol excretion in the rat. In The Liver: Quantitative Aspects of Structure and Function. R Preisig, J Bircher, G Paumgartner, eds. Dr. Madaus & Co., Koln, 1975, pp 432-438.

c Kern, F., Jr., Eriksson, H., and Sjovall, J. Effect of ethinyl estradiol on bile acid metabolism by male and female rats. In Advances in Bile Acid Research. S Matern, J Hackenschmidt, P Back, and W Gerok, eds. F.K. Schattauer Verlag, Stuttgart-New York, 1975, pp 181-183.

d Kern, F., Jr., Everson, G.T., DeMark, B., McKinley, C., Showalter, R., Erfling, W., Braverman, D.Z., Szczepanik-van Leeuwen, P., and Klein, P.D. Biliary lipids, bile acids, and gallbladder function in the human female. J. Clin. Invest. 68:1229-1242, 1981.

e Key, P.H., Bonorris, G.G., Marks, J.W., and Schoenfield, L.J. Mechanism of cholesterol desaturation of bile by chenodeoxycholic acid in gallstone patients. Gastroenterology 74:1161, 1978 (abstract).

f Key, P.H., Bonorris, G.G., Marks, J.W., Chung, A., and Schoenfield, L.J. Biliary lipid synthesis and secretion in gallstone patients before and during treatment with chenodeoxycholic acid. J. Lab. Clin. Med. 95:816-826, 1980.

g Khan, A.A., Freston, J.W., Harman, C.G., and Englert, E. The influence of lecithin in solubilizing bile cholesterol in canine cholelithiasis. Gastroenterology 58:967, 1970 (abstract).

h Kibe, A., Wake, C., Kuramoto, T., and Hoshita, T. Effect of dietary taurine on bile acid metabolism in guinea pigs. Lipids 15:224-229, 1980.

i Kienzle, H.F. and Klee, W.E. Microradiography of gallstones. Z. Gastroenterol. 19:667-672, 1981.

j Kihira, K., Morioka, Y., and Hoshita, T. Synthesis of (22R and 22S)-3a,7a, 22-trihydroxy-5b-cholan-24-oic acids and structure of haemulcholic acid, a unique bile acid isolated from fish bile. J. Lipid Res. 22:1181-1187, 1981.

k Kikuchi, H. The metabolic sequence for the occurrence of an anomalous bile acid, 12-ketochenodeoxycholic acid, found in the bile of hepatobility diseased patients. J. Biochem. 72:165-172, 1972.

l Kikuchi, H., Kuramoto, T., Hoshita, T., and Yamamoto, S. Effect of vitamin K on the excretion of cholesterol and degradation products in rats. Life Sci. 13:933-943, 1973.

m Killenberg, P.G. and Gordan, G.T. Purification and characterization of bile acid-CoA: Amino acid N-acyl transferase from rat liver. J. Biol. Chem. 253:1005-1010, 1978.

a Kimura, T. Cytotoxicity of bile acids on cultured cells. Japan. J. Gastroenterol. 77:185-194, 1980.

b Kimura, T., Shimamaura, M., Yamaguchi, A., Katayama, T., Kurita, T., and Tanaka, A. Solubilization of cultured cell membrane by bile acids. Acta Hepatica Japonica 22:717, 1981 (abstract).

c King, J.E., Oshiba, S., and Schoenfield, L.J. Bile secretion in isolated hamster liver. J. Appl. Physiol. 28:495-500, 1970.

d King, J.E. and Schoenfield, L.J. Cholestasis induced by sodium taurolithocholate in isolated hamster liver. J. Clin. Invest. 50:2305-2312, 1971.

e King, J.E. and Schoenfield, L.J. Lithocholic acid, cholestasis, and liver disease. Mayo Clin. Proc. 47:725-730, 1972.

f Kinsey, M.D., Donowitz, M., Wartofsky, L., Boehm, T.M., and Collin, D.P. The correlation between pruritus and elevated serum chenodeoxycholic acid (CDC) levels in hyperthyroidism. Gastroenterology 70:902, 1976 (abstract).

g Kinugasa, T., Uchida, K., Kadowaki, M., Takasa, H., Nomura, Y., and Saito, Y. Effect of bile duct ligation on bile acid metabolism in rats. J. Lipid Res. 22:201-207, 1981.

h Kipling, J.J. Adsorption from Solutions of Non-Electrolytes. Academic Press, 1965, 328 pp.

i Kipshidze, N.N. and Lezhawa, D.Z. Diagnostic significance of determining bile acids and cholesterol in bile. Ter. Arkh. 43:61-66, 1971 (Russ).

j Kirby, J., Heaton, K.W., and Burton, J.L. Pruritic effect of bile salts. Brit. Med. J. 4:693-695, 1974.

k Kirkpatrick, R.B., Lack, L., and Killenberg, P.G. Identification of the 3-sulfate isomer as the major product of enzymatic sulfation of chenodeoxycholate conjugates. J. Biol. Chem. 255:10157-10159, 1980.

l Kirwan, W.O., Smith, A.N., McConnell, A.A., Mitchell, W.D., and Eastwood, M.A. Action of different bran preparations on colonic function. Brit. Med. J. 4:187-189, 1974.

m Kirwan, W.O., Smith, A.N., Mitchell, W.D., Falconer, J.D., and Eastwood, M.A. Bile acids and colonic motility in the rabbit and the human. Part I. The rabbit. Gut 16:894-902, 1975.

n Kitani, K. and Kanai, S. Biliary transport maximum of tauroursodeoxycholate is twice as high as that of taurocholate in the rat. Life Sciences 29: 269-275, 1981.

o Kitani, K. and Kanai, S. Tauroursodeoxycholate prevents taurocholate induced cholestasis. Hepatology 1:33b, 1981 (abstract).

a Kivilaakso, E., Fromm, D., and Silen, W. Effect of bile salts and related compounds on isolated esophageal mucosa. Surgery 87:280-285, 1980.

b Klaassen, C.D. Does bile acid secretion determine canalicular bile production in rats? Am. J. Physiol. 220:667-673, 1971.

c Klaassen, C.D. Gas-liquid chromatographic determination of bile acids in bile. Clin. Chim. Acta 35:225-229, 1971.

d Klaassen, C.D. Comparison of the choleretic properties of bile acids. Europ. J. Pharm. 23:270-275, 1973.

e Klaassen, C.D. Bile flow and composition during bile acid depletion and administration. Canad. J. Phys. & Pharmacol. 52:334-348, 1974.

f Klaassen, C.D. Biliary excretion of metals. Drug Met. Rev. 5:165-196, 1976.

g Klaassen, C.D. Independence of bile acid and Ouabain hepatic uptake: studies in the newborn rat. Proc. Soc. Exptl. Biol. Med. 157:66-69, 1978.

h Klapdor, R., Schliewe, J., and Valerius, H. Zur Physiologie der Gallenexkretion beim Zwergschwein. Res. exp. Med. 166:241-244, 1975.

i Klapdor, R. and Humke, R. About the efficiency of the duodenal drainage with the double balloon tube technique using polyethylene glycol as duodenal marker. Acta Hepato-Gastroenterol. 23:250, 1976 (abstract).

j Kleeberg, J. Dissolution of bile stones by oral preparations. Harefuah 84:99-100, 1973.

k Knodell, R.G., Cheney, H.C., and Ostrow, J.D. Effects of phototherapy on hepatic function in human alcoholic cirrhosis. Gastroenterology 70:1112-1116, 1976.

l Knodell, R.G., Kinsey, M.D., Boedeker, E.C., and Collin, D.P. Deoxycholate metabolism in alcoholic cirrhosis. Gastroenterology 71:196-201, 1976.

m Knoebel, L.K. and Ryan, J.M. Digestion and mucosal absorption of fat in normal and bile-deficient dogs. J. Phys. 204:509-514, 1963.

n Knoebel, L.K. Intestinal absorption in vivo of micellar and nonmicellar lipid. Am. J. Physiol. 223:255-261, 1972.

o Koch, H., Rosch, W., Schenk, J., and Demling, L. Endoscopic papillotomy. MMW 121:587-590, 1979.

p Koch, M.M., Jezequel, A.M., Capurso, L., Freddara, U., Lorenzini, I., and Orlandi, F. The ultrastructure of hepatocytes in cholesterol cholelithiasis patients: A quantitative study before and during chenodeoxychoic acid (CDCA) therapy. Rendic. Gastroenterol. 9:243, 1977 (abstract).

a Koch, M.M., Giampieri, M.P., Lorenzini, I., Jezequel, A.M., and Orlandi, F. Effect of chenodeoxycholic acid on liver structure and function in man: A sterological and biochemical study. Digestion 20:8-21, 1980.

b Koch, M.M., Giampieri, M.P., Lorenzini, I., Jezequel, A., and Orlandi, F. Effect of ursodeoxycholic acid on liver structure in man. Quantitative data. Gastroenterol. Clin. Biol. 4:560-568, 1980.

c Kok, E., Burstein, S., Javitt, N.B., Gut, M., and Byon, C.Y. Bile acid synthesis. Metabolism of 3b-hydroxy-5-cholenoic acid in the hamster. J. Biol. Chem. 256:6155-6159, 1981.

d Kopp, E. Verminderter Gallensaurepool bei Patienten mit Gallensteinen. Schw. med. Wschr. 101:1563, 1971 (abstract).

e Kordac, V., Marecek, Z., Chmel, J., and Jirsa, M. Initial practical experience with the treatment of bile stones with chenodeoxycholic acid. Cas. Lek. Ces. 115:403-405, 1976.

f Korman, M.G., Hofmann, A.F., and Summerskill, W.H.J. Assessment of activity in chronic active liver disease: Serum bile acids compared with conventional tests and histology. N. Engl. J. Med. 290:1399-1402, 1974.

g Korman, M.G., LaRusso, N.F., Hoffman, N.E., and Hofmann, A.F. Development of an intravenous bile acid tolerance test: Plasma disappearance of cholylglycine in health. N. Engl. J. Med. 292:1205-1209, 1975.

h Koss, F-W., Mayer, D., and Haindl, H. Gallensauren. In Methoden der enzymatischen Analyse. 3rd Edition. HU Bergmeyer, ed. Verlag Chemie, Weinheim, 1974, pp 1934-1937.

i Kottke, B.A. Differences in bile acid excretion: Primary hypercholesterolemia compared to combined hypercholesterolemia and hypertriglyceridemia. Circulation 40:13-20, 1969.

j Krag, E. and Phillips, S.F. Active and passive bile acid absorption in man. Perfusion studies of the ileum and jejunum. J. Clin. Invest. 53:1686-1694, 1974.

k Krag, E. and Phillips, S.F. Effect of free and conjugated bile acids on net water, electrolyte, and glucose movement in the perfused human ileum. J. Lab. Clin. Med. 83:947-956, 1974.

l Krag, E. and Krag, B. Bile acid absorption and water transport in the perfused ileum of patients with regional ileitis (Crohn's Disease). Scand. J. Gastroenterol. 10:31, 1975.

m Krag, E. and Krag, B. Regional ileitis (Crohn's disease). I. Kinetics of bile acid absorption in the perfused ileum. Scand. J. Gastroenterol. 11:481, 1976.

n Krafft, F. and Biglow, H. Ueber das Verhalten der Fettsauren Alkalien und der Seifen in Gegenwart von Wasser, III. Die Seifen also Krystalloide, IV. Die Seifen als Cholloide. Berichte Dtsch. Chem. Gesellsch. 28:2566-2573, 1895.

a Krasopoulos, J.C., deBari, V.A., and Needle, M.A. The adsorption of bile salts on activated carbon. Lipids 15:365-370, 1980.

b Kratohvil, J.P. and DelliColli, H.T. Micellar properties of bile salts: Sodium taurodeoxycholate and sodium glycodeoxycholate. Canad. J. Biochem. 46:945-952, 1968.

c Kratohvil, J.P. and DelliColli, H.T. Measurements of the size of micelles: The case of sodium taurodeoxycholate. Fed. Proc. 20:1335-1342, 1970.

d Krause, D. Cholezystektomie: Immer eine personliche Entscheidung. Euromed 5:314-316, 1981.

e Kravetz, R.E. Etiology of biliary tract disease in Southwestern American Indians. Analysis of 105 consecutive cholecystectomies. Gastroenterology 46:392-398, 1964.

f Kreutzberger, A., Herz, J.E., Mantecon, R.E., and Murillo, A. Antiviral drugs. XVII. Oligocyclically N-substituted lithocholic amides. Arch. Pharm. 314:41-43, 1981.

g Kritchevsky, D. and Tepper, S.A. Influence of bile acids on serum and liver. Cholesterol of eu-, hyper-, and hypothyroid rats. Med. Pharm. Exp. 14:1-11, 1966.

h Kritchevsky, D. and Story, J.A. Binding of bile salts in vitro by non-nutritive fiber. J. Nutrition 104:458-462, 1974.

i Kritchevsky, D. and Story, J.A. In vitro binding of bile acids and bile salts. Am. J. Clin. Nutr. 28:305-306, 1975.

j Kritchevsky, D. Influence of dietary fiber on bile acid metabolism. Lipids 13:982-985, 1978.

k Kritchevsky, D., Story, J.A., and Klurfield, D.M. Dissolution of gallstones in hamsters by 3-hydroxy-3-methylglutaric acid. Experientia 34:1328, 1978 (One-page article).

l Kritchevsky, D. and Klurfield, D.M. Influence of vegetable protein on gallstone formation in hamsters. Am. J. Clin. Nutr. 32:2174-2176, 1979.

m Krog, N. and Larsson, K. Phase behavior and rheological properties of aqueous systems of industrial distilled monoglycerides. Chem. Phys. Lipids 2:129-143, 1968.

n Kroker, R., Anwer, M.S., and Hegner, D. The age dependence of bile acid metabolism in rats. Akt. Gerontol. 7:539-545, 1977.

o Kroker, R., Anwer, M.S., and Hegner, D. The lack of active bile acid transport in AS-30D ascites hepatoma cells. Naunyn-Schmiedeberg's Arch. Pharmacol. 303:287-293, 1978.

p Kroker, R., Hegner, D., and Anwer, M.S. Altered hepatobiliary transport of taurocholic acid in aged rats. Mech. Age Develop. 12:367-373, 1980.

a Krone, C.L., Theodor, E., Sleisenger, M.H., and Jeffries, G.H. Studies on the pathogenesis of malabsorption: Lipid hydrolysis and micelle formation in the intestinal lumen. Medicine 47:89-106, 1968.

b Kucerova, L., Hoenig, V., Jirsa, M., and Fabian, E. Die Bindung in vitro von Bromsulphthalein, Fettsauren, Salzen der Gallensauren und von Bilirubin an Albumin. Acta Hep.-Splen. 13:282, 1966.

c Kudchodkar, B.J., Sodhi, H.S., and Horlick, L. Absorption of dietary cholesterol in man. Metabolism 23:155-163, 1973.

d Kuenzle, C.C. Bilirubin conjugates of human bile. Biochem. J. 119:411-435, 1970.

e Kulkarni, M.S., Heidepriem, P.M., and Yielding, K.L. Production by lithocholic acid of DNA strand breaks in L1210 cells. Cancer Res. 40: 2666-2669, 1980.

f Kupfer, R.M. and Northfield, T.C. Gallstone dissolution. Brit. J. Clin. Pract. 35:137-139, 1981.

g Kupfer, R.M., Gannon, M., and Northfield, T.C. Rapid small intestinal transit in gallstone patients. Gut 22:A887, 1981 (abstract).

h Kupfer, R.M., Jazwari, R.P., and Northfield, T.C. Diurnal variation in cholesterol saturation of gallbladder bile. Gut 22:A886, 1981.

i Kurata, Y. Stereo-bile acids and bile sterols. LXI. Metabolism of lithocholic acid in hog liver preparation. J. Biochem. 55:415, 1964.

j Kurata, Y. Stereo-bile acids and bile alcohols. CII. Metabolism of lithocholic acid in mouse and dog. Hiroshima J. Med. Sci. 16:281, 1967.

k Kuriyama, K., Ban, Y., Nakashima, T., and Murata, T. Simultaneous determination of biliary bile acids in rat: electron impact and ammonia chemical ionization mass spectrometric analyses of bile acids. Steroids 34:717-728, 1979.

l Kurozumi, K., Harano, T., Yamasaki, K., and Ayaki, Y. Studies on bile acids in bear bile. J. Biochem. 74:489-495, 1973.

m Kurtz, W., Swoboda, L., and Leuschner, U. Die Verteilung nicht sulfatierter Gallensauren in Leber und Serum der Ratte nach oraler Gabe von 20 und 90 mg/kg Chenodesoxycholsaure. 10th Int'l. Cong. Gastroenterol., Budapest, June, 1976 (abstract).

n Kurtz, W., Leuschner, U., and Hellstern, A. Chenodeoxycholic acid (CDCA) accentuated sex differences in liver bile acids. Gut 20:A936, 1979 (abstract).

o Kurtz, W., Leuschner, U., and Hellstern, A. Der Einfluss der Chenodesoxycholsaure (CDC) auf den Geschlechtsdimorphismus der Lebergallensauren der Ratte. Zeit. Gastroenterol. 17:648, 1979 (abstract).

a Kurtz, W., Leuschner, U., Scholz, G., Michel, J., and Strohm, W. Differences in chenodeoxycholic acid and ursodeoxycholic acid influence on rat small intestinal wall bile acids. Ital. J. Gastroenterol. 12:331-334, 1980.

b Kurtz, W., Leuschner, U., Althoff, P., Frerichs, K., Maurer, T., and Rietbrock, N. Der Einfluss oraler Cholelitholytika auf die Resorption von Digitoxin. Z. Gastroenterol. XIX (9), 1981 (abstract).

c Kurtz, W., Leuschner, U., and Strohm, W.D. Bile acids in colorectal carcinoma patients. Gastroenterol. Japon. 16:397-398, 1981.

d Kurtz, W., Leuschner, U., Strohm, W.D., Banzer, W., and Franz, J. Unterschiedlicher Einfluss von Chenodeoxycholsaure (CDC) und Ursodeoxycholsaure (UDC) auf die Gallensauren in Kolonwand und Koloninhalt der Ratte. Z. Gastroenterol. XIX (9), 1981 (abstract 10).

e Kurtz, W., Leuschner, U., Strohm, W.D., and Kon, H. Die Gallensauren der Ileum- und Kolonmukosa bei M. Crohn und Kolonkarzinom. Z. Gastroenterol. XIX (9), 1981 (abstract 88).

f Kurtz, W., Leuschner, U., Strohm, W.D., and Kon, H. Ileal and colonic mucosal bile acids in Crohn's disease and colonic carcinoma. Internat'l Symposium on IBD, Jerusalem, 1981 (abstract).

g Kutz, K. and Schulte, A. Effectiveness of ursodeoxycholic acid in gallstone therapy. Gastroenterology 73:632-633, 1977.

h Kutz, K., Miederer, S.E., and Paumgartner, G. Case report: Chenodeoxycholic acid therapy of intrahepatic radiolucent gallstones in a patient with Caroli's syndrome. Acta Hepato-Gastroenterol. Stuttgart 25:398-401, 1978.

i Kutz, K., Both, R., Leiss, O., and von Bergmann, K. Increased risk of cholesterol gallstone formation during therapy with bezafibrate (B)? 16th Meeting of the EASL, Lisbon, 1981 (abstract).

j Kutz, K. and Schulte, A. Effect of ursodeoxycholic acid on bile supersaturated with cholesterol in patients pretreated with clofibrate. Z. Gastroenterol. 19:231-236, 1981.

k Kvietys, P.R., McLendon, J.M., and Granger, D.N. Postprandial intestinal hyperemia: Role of bile salts in the ileum. Am. J. Physiol. 241:G469-G477, 1981.

l Kwan, K.H., Higuchi, W.I., Molokhia, A.M., and Hofmann, A.F. Cholesterol gallstone dissolution rate accelerators. I. Exploratory investigations. J. Pharm. Sci. 66:1105-1108, 1977.

m Kwan, K.H., Higuchi, W.I., Molokhia, A.M., and Hofmann, A.F. Dissolution kinetics of cholesterol in simulated bile. I. Influence of bile acid type and concentration, bile acid/lecithin ratio, and added electrolyte. J. Pharm. Sci. 66:1094-1101, 1977.

a Kyd, P.A. and Bouchier, I.A.D. Absorption of water, unconjugated bilirubin, and sodium glycodeoxycholate by the rabbit gallbladder with dietary-induced gallstones. Gastroenterology 61:723-732, 1971.

b Kyd, P.A. and Bouchier, I.A.D. Cholesterol metabolism in rabbits with oleic acid-induced cholelithiasis. Proc. Soc. Exptl. Biol. Med. 141:846-849, 1972.

c Kyd, P.A. and Bouchier, I.A.D. Experimental oleic acid-induced cholelithiasis in the rabbit associated with increased biliary 5 -deoxycholic acid. Biochem. J. 128:169-172, 1972.

d Kyuichiro, O. and Taro, K. Stero-bile acid and bile sterols. XXXIX. Metabolism of lithocholic acid. J. Biochem. 50:20-23, 1961.

e Laatikainen, T.J. Fetal bile acid levels in pregnancies complicated by maternal intrahepatic cholestasis. Am. J. Obst. Gyn. 122:852-856, 1975.

f Laatikainen, T.J., Lehtonen, P.J., and Hesso, A.E. Fetal sulfated and non-sulfated bile acids in intrahepatic cholestasis of pregnancy. J. Lab. Clin. Med. 92:185-193, 1978.

g Labadie, P. Les sels biliaires. Rev. Practicine 22:3451, 1972.

h Lacassagne, A., Bun-Hoi, N., and Zajdela, F. Carcinogenic activity of apocholic acid. Nature 180:1007-1008, 1961.

i Lacassagne, A., Bun-Hoi, N., and Zajdela, F. Carcinogenic activity in situ of further steroid compounds. Nature 209:1026-1027, 1966.

j Lachin, J.M., Marks, J.W., Schoenfield, L.J., the NCGS Protocol Committee, and the National Cooperative Gallstone Study Group. Design and methodological considerations in the National Cooperative Gallstone Study: A multi-center clinical trial. Controlled Clinical Trials 2:177-229, 1981.

k Lack, L. and Weiner, I.M. In vitro absorption of bile salts by small intestine of rats and guinea pigs. Am. J. Physiol. 200:313-317, 1961.

l Lack, L. and Weiner, I.M. Intestinal absorption of bile salts and some biological implications. Gastroenterology 22:1334-1338, 1963.

m Lack, L. and Weiner, I.M. Intestinal bile salt transport: Structure-activity relationships and other properties. Am. J. Phys. 210:1142-1152, 1966.

n Lafont, H., Nalbone, G., Lairon, D., Dagorn, J-C, Domingo, N., Amic, J., and Hauton, J.C. Zone electrophoresis study of the bile lipoprotein complex. Biochimie 59:445-452, 1977.

o Lagarriga, J. and Bouchier, I.A.D. The effect of phenobarbital on cholesterol gallstones in hamsters. Gut 14:956-961, 1973.

p Lageron, A., Levy, G., Saffroy, M., and Verthier, N. Histological and histoenzymological study of the liver. I. In gallstone without treatment. Acta Histochem. 65:1-7, 1979.

a Lageron, A., Levy, V.G., Saffroy, M., and Verthier, N. Histological and histoenzymological study of the liver. II. In gallstone treated with chenodeoxycholic acid. Acta Histochem. 65:8-14, 1979.

b Lahana, D.A. and Schoenfield, L.J. Progress in medical therapy of gallstones. Surg. Clin. N. Am. 53:1053-1062, 1973.

c Lahana, D.A., Bonorris, G.G., and Schoenfield, L.J. Gallstone dissolution in vitro by bile acids, heparin, and quaternary amines. Surg. Gyn. Obst. 138:683-685, 1974.

d Laing, R., Moeller, D., and James, D. Duodenal drainage and bile sediment analysis for detection of gall bladder disease. Gastroenterology 64:841, 1973 (abstract).

e Lamabadusuriya, S.P., Guiraldes, E., and Harries, J.T. Influence of mixtures of taurocholate, fatty acids and monoolein on the toxic effects of deoxycholate in rat jejunum in vivo. Gastroenterology 69:463-469, 1975.

f Lansford, C., Mehta, S., and Kern, F., Jr. The treatment of retained stones in the common bile duct with sodium cholate infusion. Gut 15:48-51, 1974.

g LaRusso, N.F., Korman, M.G., Hoffman, N.E., and Hofmann, A.F. Dynamics of the enterohepatic circulation of bile acids. Postprandial serum concentrations of conjugates of cholic acid in health, cholecystectomized patients, and patients with bile acid malabsorption. N. Engl. J. Med. 291:689-692, 1974.

h LaRusso, N.F., Hoffman, N.E., Hofmann, A.F., and Korman, M.G. Validity and sensitivity of an intravenous bile acid tolerance test in patients with liver disease. N. Engl. J. Med. 292:1209-1214, 1975.

i LaRusso, N.F., Hoffman, N.E., Hofmann, A.F., Northfield, T.C., and Thistle, J.L. Effect of primary bile acid ingestion on bile acid metabolism and biliary lipid secretion in gallstone patients. Gastroenterology 69:1301-1314, 1975.

j LaRusso, N.F., Thistle, J.L., Hofmann, A.F., and Fulton, R.E. Treatment of retained common bile duct stones by intraductal infusion of a cholate solution: A controlled trial. Gastroenterology 68:932, 1975 (abstract).

k LaRusso, N.F., Szczepanik, P.A., Hofmann, A.F., and Coffin, S.B. The effect of deoxycholic acid ingestion on bile acid metabolism and biliary lipid secretion in normal subjects. Gastroenterology 72:132-140, 1977.

l LaRusso, N.F., Hoffman, N.E., Korman, M.G., Hofmann, A.F., and Cowen, A.E. Determinants of fasting and postprandial serum bile acid levels in healthy man. Am. J. Dig. Dis. 23:385-391, 1978.

m LaRusso, N.F. and Fowler, S. Coordinate secretion of acid hydrolases in rat bile. J. Clin. Invest. 64:948-954, 1979.

a LaRusso, N.F. and Thistle, J.L. Ursodeoxycholic acid ingestion after ileal resection. Effect of biliary bile acid and lipid composition. Dig. Dis. & Sci. 26:705-709, 1981.

b LaRusso, N.F., Kost, L.J., Carter, J.A., and Barham, S.S. Triton WR-1339, a lysosomotropic compound, is excreted into bile and alters the biliary excretion of lysosomal enzymes and lipids. Hepatology 2:209-215, 1982.

c Lasser, E.C., Amberg, J.R., Baily, N.A., Varady, P., Lachin, J., Okun, R., and Schoenfield, L.J. Validation of a computer-assisted method for estimating the number and volume of gallstones visualized by cholecystography. Invest. Radiol. 16:342-347, 1981.

d Laurent, T.C. and Persson, H. A study of micelles of sodium taurodeoxycholate in the ultracentrifuge. Biochim. Biophys. Acta 106:616-624, 1965.

e Lauterburg, B.H. and Bircher, J. Expiratory measurement of maximal aminopyrine demethylation in vivo: Effect of phenobarbital, partial hepatectomy, portacaval shunt and bile duct ligation in the rat. J. Pharm. Expt. Ther. 196:501-509, 1976.

f Lauterburg, B.H., Newcomer, A.D., and Hofmann, A.F. Clinical value of the bile acid breath test: Evaluation of the Mayo Clinic experience. Mayo Clin. Proc. 53:227-233, 1978.

g Lavy, U., Burstein, S., and Javitt, N. Fetal bile acid metabolism: Quantitation of 26-hydroxycholesterol and 7a-hydroxycholesterol in human meconium. Gastroenterology 65:556, 1973 (abstract).

h Lawrence, A.S.C. The mechanism of detergence. Nature 103:1491-1494, 1959.

i Lawrence, A.S.C. and Pearson, J.T. Electrical properties of soap + water + amphiphile systems. Trans. Faraday Soc. 63:495, 1967.

j Layden, T.J., Schwarz, J., and Boyer, J.L. Scanning electron microscopy of the rat liver. Studies of the effect of taurolithocholate and other models of cholestasis. Gastroenterology 69:724-738, 1975.

k Layden, T.J. and Boyer, J.L. The effect of thyroid hormone on bile salt independent bile flow and Na+, K+-ATPase activity in liver plasma membrane enriched in bile canaliculi. J. Clin. Invest. 57:1009-1018, 1976.

l Lee, D., Bonorris, G., Cohen, H., Gilmore, C., Marks, J., and Schoenfield, L.J. Effect of ursodeoxycholic acid on bile acid kinetics and hepatic lipid secretion. Hepatology 1:36A, 1981 (abstract).

m Lee, S.P., LaMont, J.T., and Carey, M.C. Role of gallbladder mucus hypersecretion in the evolution of cholesterol gallstones. J. Clin. Invest. 67:1712-1723, 1981.

n Lee, S.P., Lim, T.H., and Scott, A.J. Carbohydrate moieties of glycoproteins in human hepatic and gall-bladder bile, gall-bladder mucosa and gallstones. Clin. Sci. 56:533-538, 1979.

a Lee, S.P., LaMont, J.T., and Carey, M.C. Organ culture of the prairie dog gallbladder: Increased mucus synthesis and secretion is induced by lithogenic bile. Gastroenterology 76:1183, 1979 (abstract).

b Lees, A.M., Mok, H.Y.I., Lees, R.S., McCluskey, M.A., and Grundy, S.M. Plant sterols as cholesterol-lowering agents: Clinical trials in patients with hypercholesterolemia and studies of sterol balance. Atherosclerosis 28:325-338, 1977.

c Lefevre, A.F., DeCarli, L.M., and Lieber, C.S. Effect of ethanol on cholesterol and bile acid metabolism. J. Lipid Res. 13:48-55, 1972.

d Leijd, B. Cholesterol and bile acid metabolism in obesity. Clin. Sci. 59:203-206, 1980.

e Leiss, O. and von Bergmann, K. Einfluss von Cheno- und Ursodeoxycholsaure auf biliare Lipidsekretion und Serumlipoproteinkonzentration. Dtsch. Ges. f. Inn. Med. Vol. 292, 1981 (abstract).

f Leiss, O. and von Bergmann, K. Medikamentose Auflosung von Cholesteringallensteinen. Der Informierte Arzt 19:44-47, 1981.

g Leiss, O., Bosch, T., and von Bergmann, K. Effects of bile acid feeding on lipoprotein concentration, change in cholesterol synthesis and biliary lipid secretion in patients with radiolucent gallstones. In Bile Acids and Lipids. G Paumgartner, A Stiehl, and W Gerok, eds. MTP Press, Lancaster, 1981, pp 247-253.

h Leissner, K-H., Wedel, H., and Schersten, T. Comparison between the use of oral contraceptives and the incidence of surgically confirmed gallstone disease. Scand. J. Gastroenterol. 12:893-896, 1977.

i Lenz, K. An evaluation of the "breath test" in Crohn's disease. Scand. J. Gastroenterol. 10:665-671, 1975.

j Lettre, H. Zur Stereochemie der Sterine und Gallensauren. Ber. 68:766, 1935.

k Leuschner, U. and Neuenfeldt, H.U. Elektronenmikroskopische Untersuchungen an der Rattenleber nach oraler Applikation von Chenodesoxycholsaure. Z. Gastroenterol. 1:27-34, 1975.

l Leuschner, U. Morphologische Aspekte zur Behandlung von Gallensteintragern mit Chenodesoxycholsaure. Z. Gastroenterol. 13:309-313, 1975.

m Leuschner, U., Czygan, P., and Stiehl, A. Licht- und elektronenmikroskopische Untersuchungen zur Toxizitat von sulfatierter und nicht-sulfatierter Lithocholsaure. Verh. Dtsch. Ges. Inn. Med. 81:1311-1313, 1975.

n Leuschner, U. and Neuenfeldt, H.U. Licht- und elektronenmikro-skopische Untersuchungen am Magen-Darm-Trakt der Ratte nach oraler Gabe von Chenodesoxycholsaure. Z. Gastroenterol. 13:648-653, 1975.

a Leuschner, U. Die Auflosung von Gallensteinen. Therapiewoche 26:650-654, 1976.

b Leuschner, U. Fundamentals and results of the dissolution of gallstones by chenodeoxycholic acid. The 5th Asian-Pacific Congress of Gastroenterology, Singapore, 1976, pp 156.

c Leuschner, U. Hinweise fur die Auflosung von Cholesteringallensteinen mit Chenodesoxycholsaure. DMW 101:1132-1133, 1976.

d Leuschner, U. Medikamentose Gallensteinauflosung (Zusammenfassung). Z. Gastroenterol. 14:212-220, 1976.

e Leuschner, U., Jock, C., and Kurtz, W. Morphologische Untersuchungen zur Toxizitat und therapeutischen Breite von Chenodesoxycholsaure. 82. Tagung der Dtsch. Ges. Inn. Med. Wiesbaden, April, 1976.

f Leuschner, U., Schneider, M., Loos, R., and Kurtz, W. Morphologische-tierexperimentelle Untersuchungen zur therapeutischen Breite von Chenodesoxycholsaure als Cholelitholytikum. 10th Int'l. Cong. Gastroenterol. Budapest, June, 1976 (abstract).

g Leuschner, U. Dissolution of biliary cholesterol calculi using chenodeoxycholic acid. Internist 18:114-115, 1977.

h Leuschner, U., Czygan, P., Liersch, M., Frohling, W., and Stiehl, A. Morphologische untersuchungen zur toxizitat sulfatierter und nicht-sulfateirter lithocholsaure an der perfundierten rattenleber. Z. Gastroenterol. 15:246-253, 1977.

i Leuschner, U., Reber, E., and Erb, W. Erfahrungen bei der Behandlung von Gallensteinpatienten mit Chenodesoxycholsaure. Dtsch. med. Wschr. 102:156-160, 1977.

j Leuschner, U., Schneider, M., Loos, R., and Kurtz, W. Morphologische untersuchungen zur Toxizitat oral verabreichter Chenodesoxycholsaure an Leber, Magen-Darmtrakt, niere und nebenniere der Ratte. Res. Exp. Med. 171:41-55, 1977.

k Leuschner, U. and Leuschner, M. Cholelitholyse oder Cholezystektomie? Dtsch. Med. Wschr. 104:629-634, 1979.

l Leuschner, U., Schneider, M., and Korte, L. The influence of chenodeoxycholic acid and ursodeoxycholic acid on the hepatic structure of the rat. Z. Gastroenterol. 17:244-255, 1979.

m Leuschner, U., Wurbs, D., and Landgraf, H. Dissolution of biliary duct stones with mono-octanoin. Lancet 2:103-104, 1979 (Letter to Editor).

n Leuschner, U. Gallensteinauflosung. Internist 21:607-616, 1980.

o Leuschner, U., Baumgartel, H., and Wurbs, D. Auflosung von Cholesterin-Gallengansteinen mit einer modifizierten Capmul 8210-Emulsion und EDTA-Gallensalzlosung. Leber Magen Darm 10:284-287, 1980.

a Leuschner, U. Bilanz der medikamentosen Gallenstein-Auflosung. Med. Klin. 76:232-234, 1981.

b Leuschner, U. Derzeitiger Stand der chemischen Auflosung von Gallenblasen und Gallengangssteinen. Inn. Med. 4:176-177, 1981.

c Leuschner, U. Gallengangssteine: auflosen, extrahieren oder operieren? Tips f. d. Gastroent. Praxis 8:17-18, 1981.

d Leuschner, U. and Baumgartel, H. Dissolution of bile duct stones. Lancet 1:336, 1981.

e Leuschner, U. and Baumgartel, H. Mono-octanoat: Gallensteine intraduktal gelost. Selecta 48:3484-3485, 1981.

f Leuschner, U., Baumgartel, H., and Jessen, K. Auflosung von Pigmentsteinen in der Gallenwegen. Z. Gastroenterol. XIX (9), 1981 (abstract).

g Leuschner, U., Baumgartel, H., Phillip, J., and Hagenmuller, F. Dissolution of cholesterol and pigment matrix stones in the common bile duct. Gastroenterology 80:1208, 1981 (abstract).

h Leuschner, U., Leuschner, M., and Hubner, K. Gallstone dissolution in patients with chronic active hepatitis. Gastroenterology 80:1208, 1981 (abstract).

i Leuschner, U., Leuschner, M., Strohm, W.D., and Kurtz, W. Untersuchungen zur Wirksamkeit von Ursodeoxycholsaure und Chenodeoxycholsaure bei vergleichbaren Kollectiven von Gallensteinpatienten. Z. Gastroenterol. 19:168, 1981 (abstract).

j Leuschner, U., Wurbs, D., Baumgartel, H., Helm, E.B., and Classen, M. Alternating treatment of common bile duct stones with a modified glyceryl-1-monooctanoate preparation and a bile acid-EDTA solution by nasobiliary tube. Scand. J. Gastroenterol. 16:497-503, 1981.

k Leuschner, U., Baumgartel, H., Phillip, J., Jessen, K., Hagenmuller, F., Truber, E., and Classen, M. Spulbehandlung und Endoskopie im kombinierten Einsatz bei der Therapie von Gallengangssteinen. DMW 107:285-290, 1982.

l Leveille, G.A., Sauberlich, H.E., and Hunt, R.D. Effect of dietary lithocholic acid on liver size of the chick. Poul. Sci. 41:1991-1992, 1962.

m Leveille, G.A., Sauberlich, H.E., and Hunt, R.D. Dietary bile acids and lipid metabolism. I. Influence on lipids and liver size of chicks. Proc. Soc. Exptl. Biol. Med. 114:334-337, 1963.

n Leveille, G.A., Hunt, R.D., and Sauberlich, H.E. Dietary bile acids and lipid metabolism. IV. Dietary level of lithocholic acid for chicks. Proc. Soc. Exptl. Biol. Med. 115:569-572, 1964.

o Leveille, G.A., Hunt, R.D., and Sauberlich, H.E. Dietary bile acids and lipid metabolism. V. Reversibility of the effects of lithocholic acid in chicks. Proc. Soc. Exptl. Biol. Med. 115:573-574, 1964.

a Leveille, G.A., King, N.W., Sauberlich, H.E., et al. Induction and regression of biochemical and morphologic changes induced by lithocholic acid in chickens. Am. J. Vet. Res. 119:1045-1052, 1966.

b Levy, N. New views on the lithogenesis of cholesterol gallstones. Harefuah 80:451-452, 1971.

c Levy, N., Peled, Y., Gelman-Malachi, E., and Gilat, T. Cholesterol content of gallstones in Israel. Israel J. Med. Sci. 12:1331-1332, 1976.

d Levy, V., Nusinovici, V., Rosner, D., and Darnis, F. Chenodeoxycholic acid in the prevention of migraine. N. Engl. J. Med. 299:630, 1978 (Letter to Editor).

e Levy, V.G. What can one expect for chenic acid excluding lithiasis? Med. Chir. Dig. 8:245-248, 1979.

f Lewis, K.O. Biliary lipids and incidence of gallstone disease. Lancet 2:156, 1973 (Letter to Editor).

g Lewis, K.O. The nature of the copper complexes in bile and their relationship to the absorption and excretion of copper in normal subjects and in Wilson's disease. Gut 14:221-232, 1973.

h Lewis, R. and Gorbach, S. Modification of bile acids by intestinal bacteria. Arch. Intern. Med. 130:545-549, 1972.

i Li, J.R., Dinh, D.M., and Kottke, B.A. Alteration of biliary ursodeoxycholic acid in guinea pig during early stages of cholestyramine feeding. Steroids 34:705-715, 1979.

j Lieber, M.M. The incidence of gallstones and their correlation with other diseases. Ann. Surg. 135:394-405, 1952.

k Liersch, M.E.A., Barth, C.A., Hackenschmidt, H.J., Ullmann, H.L., and Decker, K.F.A. Influence of bile salts on cholesterol synthesis in the isolated perfused rat liver. Europ. J. Biochem. 32:365-371, 1973.

l Liersch, M. and Stiehl, A. Bildung von Gallensaure-Sulfatestern in perfundierten Rattenlebern nach Gallengangsverschluss. Z. Gastroenterol. 12:131-134, 1974.

m Liersch, M., Czygan, P., and Stiehl, A. Studies on hepatic uptake and secretion of bile salt sulfates by the isolated perfused rat liver. Digestion 12:326-327, 1975.

n Liersch, M.A. and Hesse, W. Synthetic capacity and cell metabolites of bile duct obstructed rat livers. Effect of free and conjugated dihydroxy bile acids. Acta Hepato-Gastroenterol. 22:281-289, 1975.

o Lillimoe, K.D., Harmon, J.W., Gadacz, T.R., Hofmann, A.F, and Weichbrod, R. Effects of taurochenodeoxycholic and tauroursodeoxycholic acids on gastric mucosa. Gastroenterology 80:1214, 1981 (abstract).

a Lindblad, L., Lundholm, K., and Schersten, T. Mannitol clearance and biliary lipid secretion. Influence of cholic and chenic acid. Digestion 12:258, 1975.

b Lindblad, L. and Schersten, T. Incorporation rate in vitro of choline and methylmethionine into human hepatic lecithins. Scand. J. Gastroenterol. 11:587-591, 1976.

c Lindblad, L. and Schersten, T. Influence of cholic and chenodeoxycholic acid on canalicular bile flow in man. Gastroenterology 70:1121-1124, 1976.

d Lindblad, L., Lundholm, K., and Schersten, T. Bile acid concentrations in systemic and portal serum in presumably normal man and in cholestatic and cirrhotic conditions. Scand. J. Gastroenterol. 12:395-400, 1977.

e Lindblad, L., Lundholm, K., and Schersten, T. Influence of cholic and chenodeoxycholic acid on biliary cholesterol secretion in man. Europ. J. Clin. Invest. 7:383-388, 1977.

f van der Linden, W. and Norman, A. Composition of human hepatic bile. Acta Chir. Scand. 133:307, 1967.

g van der Linden, W., Bergman, F., and Nakayama, F. Effect of cholestyramine on bile composition and gallstones in hamsters and in man. Tijdschr. Gastroenterol. 12:337-347, 1969.

h van der Linden, W. and Nakayama, F. Change in bile composition in man after administration of cholestyramine (a gallstone dissolving agent in hamsters). Acta Chir. Scand. 135:433-438, 1969.

i van der Linden, W. and Sunzel, H. Early versus delayed operation for acute cholecystitis. Am. J. Surg. 120:7-13, 1970.

j van der Linden, W. Bile acid pattern of patients with and without gallstones. Gastroenterology 60:1144-1145, 1971 (Editorial).

k van der Linden, W., Nakayama, F., and Bergman, F. Effect of cholesterol biosynthesis inhibitor AY-9944 on gallstone formation in hamsters. Acta Chir. Scand. 137:355-360, 1971.

l van der Linden, W. Genetic factors in gallstone disease. Clin. Gastroenterol. 2:603-614, 1973.

m van der Linden, W. and Nakayama, F. Gallstone disease in Sweden versus Japan. Am. J. Surg. 125:267-272, 1973.

n van der Linden, W. and Nakayama, F. Occurrence of cholesterol crystals in human bile. Gut 15:630-635, 1974.

o van der Linden, W. and Nakayama, F. Effect of intravenous fat emulsion on hepatic bile. Acta Chir. Scand. 142:401-406, 1976.

a van der Linden, W. and Bergman, F. An analysis of data on human hepatic bile. Relationship between main bile components, serum cholesterol and serum triglycerides. Scand. J. Clin. Lab. Invest. 37:741-747, 1977.

b van der Linden, W. and Bergman, F. Formation and dissolution of gallstones in experimental animals. Intl. Rev. Exptl. Path. 17:173-233, 1977.

c van der Linden, J. Jr., Schwaier, A., and Weis, H.J. Tupaias (tree shrews)--a new animal model for gallstone research. III. Cholesterol metabolism under different diets and CDCA. Res. Exp. Med. 178:21-28, 1980.

d Lindstedt, S. and Norman, A. On the excretion of bile acid derivatives in feces of rats fed cholic acid-24-^{14}C and chenodeoxycholic acid-24-^{14}C. Acta Physiol. Scand. 34:1, 1955.

e Lindstedt, S. and Norman, A. The turnover of bile acids in the rat: Bile acids and steroids 39. Acta Physiol. Scand. 38:120-128, 1956.

f Lindstedt, S. The turnover of cholic acid in man. Acta Physiol. Scand. 40:1-9, 1957.

g Lindstedt, S. Bile acid and steroids. LII. Formation of deoxycholic acid from cholic acid in man. Arkiv. Kemi 11:145, 1957.

h Lindstedt, S. and Norman, A. On the metabolism of taurine conjugated 3a,7a, 12a-trihydroxy coprostanic acid in the rat. Acta Chem. Scand. 11:414, 1957.

i Lindstedt, S. and Tryding, N. On the metabolism of bishomocholic, homocholic and norcholic acid in the rat. Arkiv. Kemi 11:137, 1957.

j Lindstedt, S. and Samuelsson, B. On the interconversion of cholic and deoxycholic acid in the rat. J. Biol. Chem. 234:2026, 1959.

k Lindstedt, S. and Ahrens, E.H., Jr. Conversion of cholesterol to bile acids in man. Proc. Soc. Exptl. Biol. Med. 108:286, 1961.

l Lindstedt, S. Equilibration of dietary cholesterol and bile acids in man. Clin. Chim. Acta 7:1, 1962.

m Lindstedt, S., Avigan, J., Goodman, D.S., Sjovall, J. and Steinberg, D. The effect of dietary fat on the turnover of cholic acid and on the composition of the biliary bile acids in man. J. Clin. Invest. 44:1754-1765, 1965.

n Linos, D.A., Beard, C.M., O'Fallon, W.M., Dockerty, M.B., Beart, R.W., Jr., and Kurland, L.T. Cholecystectomy and carcinoma of the colon. Lancet 2: 379-381, 1981.

o Linscheer, W.G. Optimal micellar solubilization of oleic acid, an undesirable condition for maximal absorption. Gastroenterology 62:777, 1972 (abstract).

p Linscheer, W.G. and Raheja, K.L. Effect of glycerophosphate on lithogenic bile: A new approach to treatment of cholelithiasis. Lancet 2:551-553, 1974.

a Lippel, K. and Olson, J.A. The activity of non-lipolytic digestive enzymes of the pancreas in the presence of conjugated bile salts. Biochim. Biophys. Acta 127:243, 1966.

b Locke, S.E. Medical therapy of gallstones: Ethical aspects. N. Engl. J. Med. 289:1371-1372, 1973 (Letter to Editor).

c Loeb, P.M., Berk, R.N., Feld, G.K., and Wheeler, H.O. The biliary excretion of iodipamide. Gastroenterology 68:554-562, 1975.

d Lofland, H.B. Animal model: Cholelithiasis in Brazilian squirrel monkeys (Saimiri sciureus). Am. J. Path. 79:619-622, 1975.

e Loisy, C. Chenodeoxycholic acid and Vichy's thermal cure. Med. Chir. Dig. 7:360, 1978 (Editorial).

f Long, J.H. and Gebhart, F. On the behavior of lecithin with bile salts, and the occurrence of lecithin in bile. J. Am. Chem. Soc. 30:1312-1319, 1908.

g Loof, L. and Hjerten, S. Partial purification of a human liver sulphotransferase active towards bile salts. Biochim. Biophys. Acta 617:192-204, 1980.

h Loof, L. Enzymatic sulphation of bile salts in man. Digestion 21:297-303, 1981.

i Loomis, C., Shipley, G., and Small, D. The phase behavior of hydrated cholesterol. J. Lipid Res. 20:525-535, 1979.

j Lopez del Pino, V. and LaRusso, N.F. Dissociation of bile flow and biliary lipid secretion from biliary lysosomal enzyme output in experimental cholestasis. J. Lipid Res. 22:229-235, 1981.

k Loria, P., Bertolotti, M., Ponz de Leon, M., Iori, R., and Carulli, N. Chenodeoxycholic acid metabolism in patients with thyroid dysfunction. Il fegato 27:201-203, 1981.

l Loria, P., Iori, R., Ponz de Leon, M., Zironi, F., Pignatti, F., and Carulli, N. Effect of thyroid function on the hepatic metabolism of cholesterol and bile acids. 16th Meeting of the EASL, Lisbon, 1981 (abstract).

m Lough, A.K. and Smith, A. Influence of the products of phospholipolysis of phosphatidylcholine on micellar solubilization of fatty acids in the presence of bile salts. Br. J. Nutr. 35:89-96, 1976.

n Low-Beer, T.S., Tyor, M.P., and Lack, L. Effects of sulfation of taurolithocholic and glycolithocholic acids on their intestinal transport. Gastroenterology 56:721-726, 1969.

o Low-Beer, T.S., Schneider, R.E., and Dobbins, W.O. Morphological changes of the small intestinal mucosa of guinea pig and hamster following in vitro incubation and in vivo perfusion with unconjugated bile salts. Gut 11:486-492, 1970.

a Low-Beer, T.S., Heaton, K.W., Heaton, S.T., and Read, A.E. Gallbladder inertia and sluggish enterohepatic circulation of bile salts in adult coeliac disease. Lancet 1:991-994, 1971.

b Low-Beer, T.S., Pomare, E.W., and Morris, J.S. Control of bile salt synthesis. Nature New Biol. 238:215-216, 1972.

c Low-Beer, T.S., Pomare, E.W., and Morris, D. Selective feed-back mechanism of deoxycholic acid on synthesis of chenodeoxycholic acid in man. In Bile Acids in Human Disease. P Back and W Gerok, eds. FK Schattauer Verlag, Stuttgart, 1972, pp 125-130.

d Low-Beer, T.S., Heaton, K.W., Pomare, E.W., and Read, A.E. The effect of coeliac disease upon bile salts. Gut 14:204-208, 1973.

e Low-Beer, T.S. and Pomare, E.W. Regulation of bile salt pool size in man. Brit. Med. J. 2:338-340, 1973.

f Low-Beer, T.S., Wilkins, R.M., Lack, L., and Tyor, M.P. Effect of one meal on enterohepatic circulation of bile salts. Gastroenterology 67:490-497, 1974.

g Low-Beer, T.S., Harvey, R.F., Davies, E.R., and Read, A.E. Abnormalities of serum cholecystokinin and gallbladder emptying in coeliac disease. N. Engl. J. Med. 292:961-963, 1975.

h Low-Beer, T.S. and Pomare, E.W. Can colonic bacterial metabolites predispose to cholesterol gall stone? Brit. Med. J. 1:438-440, 1975.

i Low-Beer, T.S. Diet and bile acid metabolism. Clin. Gastroenterol. 6:165-178, 1977.

j Low-Beer, T.S. and Nutter, S. Colonic bacterial activity, biliary cholesterol saturation, and pathogenesis of gallstones. Lancet 2:1063-1065, 1978.

k Lucassen, J. Hydrolysis and precipitates in carboxylate soap solutions. J. Phys. Chem. 70:1824-1830, 1966.

l Lucke, H., Stange, G., Kinne, R., and Murer, H. Taurocholate--sodium co-transport by brush-border membrane vesicles isolated from rat ileum. Biochem. J. 174:951-958, 1978.

m Luft, H.S., Bunker, J.P., and Enthoven, A.C. Should operations be regionalized? N. Engl. J. Med. 301:1364-1369, 1979.

n Lund, J. Surgical indications in cholelithiasis: Prophylactic cholecystectomy elucidated on the basis of long-term follow-up on 526 nonoperated cases. Ann. Surg. 151:153-162, 1960.

o Lundh, G. Intestinal digestion and absorption after gastrectomy. Acta Chir. Scand. 231(Suppl.):83, 1958.

a Lutton, R.G. and Large, A.M. Gallstones: Solubility studies. Surgery 42:488, 1957.

b Lutton, C. The role of the digestive tract in cholesterol metabolism. Digestion 14:342-356, 1976.

c Lutz, F.U. Hepatotoxische Veranderungen beim Hund nach Chenodesoxycholsaure - Applikation in hohen Dosen. Ultrastrukturell-stereologische Analyse. Inauguraldissertation.

d Lynn, J., O'Brien, J., and Williams, L.F., Jr. Estriol induced changes in hepatic bile lithogenic index and flow in Rhesus monkeys. Gastroenterology 64:765, 1973 (abstract).

e Mabee, T.M., Meyer, P., DenBesten, L., and Mason, E.E. The mechanism of increased gallstone formation in obese human subjects. Surgery 79:460-468, 1976.

f Macarol, V., Morris, T.Q., Baker, K.J., and Bradley, S.E. Hydrocortisone choleresis in the dog. J. Clin. Invest. 49:1714-1723, 1970.

g Macdonald, I.A., Williams, C.N., Mahony, D.E., and Christie, W.H.M. NAD- and NADP-dependent 7a-hydroxysteroid dehydrogenases from Bacteriodes fragilis. Biochim. Biophys. Acta 384:12-24, 1975.

h Macdonald, I.A., Meier, E.C., Mahony, D.E., and Costain, G.A. 3a-, 7a- and 12a-hydroxysteroid dehydrogenase activities from Clostridium Perfringens. Biochim. Biophys. Acta 450:142-153, 1976.

i Macdonald, I.A., Williams, C.N., and Mahony, D.E. Behavior of 3a- and 7a-hydroxysteroid dehydrogenases on chenodeoxycholate substituted sepharose. Steroids 28:25-30, 1976.

j Macdonald, I. Detection of bile salts with Komarowsky's reagent and group specific dehydrogenases. J. Chromatogr. 136:348-352, 1977.

k Macdonald, I.A., Singh, G., Mahoney, D.E., and Meier, C.E. Effect of pH on bile salt degradation by mixed fecal cultures. Steroids 32:245-255, 1978.

l Macdonald, I.A., Jellett, J.F., and Mahony, D.E. 12a-Hydroxysteroid dehydrogenase from Clostridium group P strain C48-50 ATCC #29733: partial purification and characterization. J. Lipid Res. 20:234-239, 1979.

m Macdonald, I., Williams, N., and Musial, B. 3a,7a, and 12aOH group specific enzymic analysis of biliary bile acids: comparison with gas-liquid chromatography. J. Lipid Res. 21:381-385, 1980.

n Macdonald, I.A., Hutchinson, D.M., and Forrest, T.P. Formation of urso- and deoxycholic acids from primary bile acids by Clostridium Absonum. J. Lipid Res. 22:458-466, 1981.

a Macdonald, I.A. and Roach, P.D. Bile salt induction of 7a- and 7b-hydroxysteroid dehydrogenases in Clostridium Absonum. Biochim. Biophys. Acta 665:262-269, 1981.

b MacGregor, I.L., Wiley, Z.D., and Sleisenger, M.H. The role of bile acids in determining ileal flow rates in normal subjects and following ileostomy. Digestion 18:192-200, 1978.

c Machleder, H.I. Changes in bile composition after truncal vagotomy. Surg. Forum 22:376-378, 1971.

d Mack, E., Saito, C., Goldfarb, S., et al. Local toxicity of T-tube infused cholate in the rhesus monkey. Surg. Forum 28:408-409, 1977.

e Mack, E.A., Saito, C., Goldfarb, S., Crummy, A.B., Thistle, J.L., Carlson, G.L., Babayan, V.K., and Hofmann, A.F. A new agent for gallstone dissolution: Experimental and clinical evaluation. Surg. Forum 29:438-439, 1978.

f Mack, E., Crummy, A.B., and Babayan, V.K. Percutaneous transhepatic dissolution of common bile duct stones. Surgery 90:584-587, 1981.

g Mack, E., Patzer, E.M., Crummy, A.B., Hofmann, A.F., and Babayan, V.K. Retained biliary tract stones. Nonsurgical treatment with Capmul 8210, a new cholesterol gallstone dissolution agent. Arch. Surg. 116:341-344, 1981.

h Mackay, C., Crook, J.N., Smith, D.C., and McAllister, R.A. The composition of hepatic and gallbladder bile in patients with gallstones. Gut 13:759-762, 1972.

i Mackinnon, M. and Hall, P. Plasma clearance of intravenous chenodeoxycholic acid in rabbits with varying severity of hepatocellular necrosis. Hepatology 1:325-328, 1981.

j Madden, J.L. Common duct stones: Their origin and surgical management. Surg. Clin. N. Am. 53:1095-1113, 1973.

k Maddrey, W. and Boyer, J.L. The acute and chronic effects of ethanol administration on bile secretion in the rat. J. Lab. Clin. Med. 82:215-225, 1973.

l Maeda, Y., Setoguchi, T., Katsuki, T., and Ishikawa, E. Development of a solid-phase enzyme immunoassay for ursodeoxycholic acid: application to plasma disappearance of injected ursodeoxycholic acid in the rabbit. J. Lipid Res. 20:960-965, 1979.

m Maentausta, O. and Janne, O. Radioimmunoassay of conjugated cholic acid, chenodeoxycholic acid, and deoxycholic acid from human serum, with use of ^{125}I-labeled ligands. Clin. Chem. 25:264-268, 1979.

n Magne, F., Saric, J., and Balabaud, C. Metabolisme des sels biliaires, 1. La Nouvelle Presse Medicale 9:2581-2584, 1980.

a Magne, F., Saric, J., and Balabaud, C. Metabolisme des sels biliaires, 2. La Nouvelle Presse Medicale 9:2645-2649, 1980.

b Magyar, I., Loi, H.G., and Feher, T. Plasma bile acid levels and liver disease. Acta Med. Acad. Scient. Hung. 38:109-115, 1981.

c Mahowald, T.A., Matschiner, J.T., Hsia, S.L., Richter, R., and Doisy, E.A. Bile acids. II. Metabolism of deoxycholic acid-24-^{14}C and chenodeoxycholic acid-24-^{14}C in the rat. J. Biol. Chem. 225:781-793, 1957.

d Mahowald, T.A., Yin, M.W., Matschiner, J.T., Hsia, S.L., Doisy, E.A., Jr., Elliott, W.H., and Doisy, E.A. Bile acids. VIII. Metabolism of 7-ketolithocholic acid-24-C^{14} in the rat. J. Biol. Chem. 230:550-558, 1958.

e Maki, T., Saitoh, T., Yamaguchi, I., et al. Autopsy incidence of gallstones in Japan. Tohoku J. Exptl. Med. 84:37-45, 1964.

f Makino, I., Nakagawa, S., and Mashimo, K. Conjugated and unconjugated serum bile acid levels in patients with hepatobiliary diseases. Gastroenterology 56:1033-1039, 1969.

g Makino, I., Sjovall, J., Norman, A., and Strandvik, B. Excretion of 3a-hydroxy-5-cholenoic acid 3a-hydroxy-5a-cholanoic acids in urine of infants with biliary atresia. FEBS Letters 15:161-164, 1971.

h Makino, I., Nakagawa, S., Shinozaki, K., and Mashimo, K. Sulfated and non-sulfated bile acids in human serum. Lipids 7:750-752, 1972.

i Makino, I. Sulfated bile acid in urine of patients with hepatobiliary diseases. Lipids 8:47-49, 1973.

j Makino, I., Hashimoto, H., Shinozaki, K., Yoshino, K., and Nakagawa, S. Excretion of 3b-hydroxy-5-cholenoic acid in urine of patients with hepatobiliary diseases. Acta Hepat. Japonica 16:657-663, 1975.

k Makino, I., Hashimoto, H., Shinozaki, K., Yoshino, K., and Nakagawa, S. Sulfated and nonsulfated bile acids in urine, serum and bile of patients with hepatobiliary diseases. Gastroenterology 68:545-553, 1975.

l Makino, I., Shinozaki, K., Yoshino, K., and Nakagawa, S. Dissolution of cholesterol gallstones by ursodeoxycholic acid. Jap. J. Gastroenterol. 72:690-702, 1975.

m Makino, I. and Nakagawa, S. Changes in biliary lipid and biliary bile acid composition in patients after administration of ursodeoxycholic acid. J. Lipid Res. 19:723-728, 1978.

n Makino, I., Tashiro, A., Hashimoto, H., Nakagawa, S., and Yoshizawa, I. Radioimmunoassay of ursodeoxycholic acid in serum. J. Lipid Res. 19:443-447, 1978.

a Makino, S., Reynolds, J.A., and Tanford, C. The binding of deoxycholate and triton X-100 to proteins. J. Biol. Chem. 248:4926-4932, 1973.

b Malagelada, J-R., Go, V.L.W., DiMagno, E.P., and Summerskill, W.H.J. Interactions between intraluminal bile acids and digestion products on pancreatic and gallbladder function. J. Clin. Invest. 52:2160-2165, 1973.

c Malagelada, J-R., Go, V.L.W., and Summerskill, W.H.J. Differing sensitivities of gallbladder and pancreas to cholecystokinin-pancreozymin (CCK-PZ) in man. Gastroenterology 64:950-954, 1973.

d Malagelada, J-R., Go, V.L.W., Summerskill, W.H.J., and Gamble, W.S. Bile acid secretion and biliary bile acid composition altered by cholecystectomy. Am. J. Dig. Dis. 18:455-459, 1973.

e Malchior, G.W., Clarkson, T.B., Bullock, B.C., and Lofland, H.B. Cholelithiasis in non human primates - Effects of species and type of dietary fat. Circulation 45(Suppl.):19, 1972 (abstract).

f Malchow, H. Konservative Therapie der extra- und intrahepatischen Cholestase und ihrer Folgezustande. Krankenhausarzt 49:25-34, 1976.

g Malchow-Moller, A., Arffmann, S., LaRusso, N.F., and Krag, E. Enzymatic determination of total 3a-hydroxy bile acids in faeces. Validation in healthy subjects of a rapid method suitable for clinical routine purpose. Scand. J. Gastroenterol. (in press)

h Mallory, A., Kern, F., Jr., Smith, J., and Savage, D. Patterns of bile acids in microflora in the human small intestine. I. Bile acids. Gastroenterology 64:26-33, 1973.

i Mallory, A., Savage, D., Kern, F., Jr., and Smith, J.G. Patterns of bile acids in microflora in the human small intestine. II. Microflora. Gastroenterology 64:34-42, 1973.

j Mamianetti, A., Laguens, R.P., Labonia, N.A., Lopez Giavanelli, J.J., Lentino, D., and Fiordalisi, H.H. Hepatotoxicity of the ursodeoxycholic acid in hamsters. Evaluation by electronic microscopy. Acta Gastroenterol. Latin Am. 11:195-201, 1981.

k Mansbach, C.M., Garbutt, J.T., and Tyor, M.P. Bile salt and lipid metabolism in patients with ileal disease with and without steatorrhea. Am. J. Dig. Dis. 12:1089-1100, 1972.

l Mansbach, C.M., Cohen, R.S., and Leff, P.B. Isolation and properties of the mixed lipid micelles present in intestinal content during fat digestion in man. J. Clin. Invest. 56:781-791, 1975.

m Marecek, Z., Korda, C.V., Jirsa, M., and Chmel, J. Treatment of cholelithiasis using chenodeoxycholic acid. Cesk. Gastroenterol. VYZ 32:530-531, 1978.

n Marecek, Z., Jirsa, M., and Kordac, V. Zlucove kyseliny v diagnostice a leceni onemocneni jater a zlucovych cest. Cas. Lek. Ces. 120:1243-1246, 1981.

a Marigold, J.H., Coltart, D.J., and Thompson, R.P.H. Direct measurement of hepatic extraction of chenodeoxycholic and ursodeoxycholic acids in man. Clin. Sci. 61:38, 1981 (abstract).

b Marigold, J.H., Gilmore, I.T., and Thompson, R.P.H. Effects of a meal on plasma clearance of [^{14}C] glycocholic acid and indocyanine green in man. Clin. Sci. 61:325-330, 1981.

c Marigold, J.H., Bull, H.J., Gilmore, I.T., Coltart, D.J., and Thompson, R.P.H. Direct measurement of hepatic extraction of chenodeoxycholic acid and ursodeoxycholic acid in man. Clin. Sci. 63:197-203, 1982.

d Marin, G.A., Ward, N.L., Karjoo, M., and Rosato, E. Bile flow and biliary lipid changes induced by ethanol in the chronic fistula dog. Gastroenterology 65:559, 1973 (abstract).

e Marks, J.W., Conley, D.R., Capretta, T.L., Bonorris, G.G., Chung, A., Coyne, M.J., and Schoenfield, L.J. Biliary cholesterol saturation in regional enteritis. Gastroenterology 70:916, 1976 (abstract).

f Marks, J.W., Bonorris, G.G., and Schoenfield, L.J. Pathophysiology and dissolution of cholesterol gallstones. In The Bile Acids, Volume 3. PP Nair and D Kritchevsky, eds. Plenum Press, New York, 1976, pp 81-113.

g Marks, J.W., Bonorris, G., Chung, A., Coyne, M., Okun, R., Lachin, J., and Schoenfield, L. Feasibility of low-dose and intermittent chenodeoxycholic acid therapy of gallstones. Am. J. Dig. Dis. 22:856-860, 1977.

h Marks, J.W., Conley, D., Capretta, T., Bonorris, G., Chung, A., Coyne, M., and Schoenfield, L.J. Gallstone prevalence and biliary lipid composition in inflammatory bowel disease. Am. J. Dig. Dis. 22:1097-1100, 1977.

i Marks, J.W., Sherman, J.H., Bonorris, G.G., Chung, A., Coyne, M.J., and Schoenfield, L.J. Gallstone dissolution by chendeoxycholic acid and phenobarbital. Am. J. Gastroenterol. 69:160-165, 1978.

j Marks, J.W., Sue, S.O., Pearlman, B.J., Bonorris, G.G., Varady, P., Lachin, J.M., and Schoenfield, L.J. Sulfation of lithocholate as a possible modifier of chenodeoxycholic acid-induced elevations of serum transaminase in patients with gallstones. J. Clin. Invest. 68:1190-1196, 1981.

k Marteau, C., Reynier, M.O., Mule, A., Crotte, C., and Gerolami, A. Action of cholic and chendeoxycholic acid on the composition of bile in mouse. Digestion 15:227-248, 1977.

l Marteau, C., Reynier, M.O., Crotte, C., Mule, A., Mathieu, S., Gerolami, A., and Gerolami, A. Action de l'acide cholique et de l'acide chenodesoxycholique sur la secretion biliaire de la souris. Effet de l'addition du b-sitosterol. Canad. J. Physiol. Pharmacol. 58:1058-1062, 1980.

m Martensson, K.M. The incidence of gallstones in Sweden. Arch. Surg. 34:650-669, 1937.

n Martin, D.E., Wolf, R.C., and Meyer, R.K. The effect of pregnancy on biliary lipids in Rhesus monkeys. Proc. Soc. Exptl. Biol. Med. 139:115-117, 1972.

a Martin, D.E., Wolf, R.C., and Houser, W.D. Naturally occurring cholelithiasis in a Rhesus monkey and its effects on plasma biliary lipid concentrations. Am. J. Vet. Res. 34:971-974, 1973.

b Martin, M.S., Justrabo, E., Jeannin, J.F., Leclerc, A., and Martin, F. Effect of dietary chenodeoxycholic acid on intestinal carcinogenesis induced by 1,2 dimethylhydrazine in mice and hamsters. Br. J. Cancer 43:884-886, 1981.

c Martini, G.A. Was ist zur Zeit gesichert in der Cholesterin-Gallensteinauflosung? Internist 22:767-768, 1981.

d Mashige, F., Imai, K., and Osuga, T. A simple and sensitive assay of total serum bile acids. Clin. Chim. Acta 70:79-86, 1976.

e Massarrat, S. and Kumpel, W. Daily fluctuation of lithogenicity in bile in the postoperative period in cholecystectomized patients. Res. exp. Med. 166:221-227, 1975.

f Masuda, H. and Nakayama, F. Composition of bile pigment in gallstones and bile and their etiological significance. J. Lab. Clin. Med. 93:353-360, 1979.

g Mateer, J.G., Baltz, J.I., Marion, D.F., and MacMillian, J.M. Liver function tests. JAMA 121:723-728, 1943.

h Matern, S., Hackenschmidt, J., Back, P., and Gerok, W. Advances in Bile Acid Research. III. Bile Acid Meeting, Freiburg, 1974. F.K. Schattauer Verlag, Stuttgart-New York, 1975, 448 pp.

i Matern, S., Sjovall, J., Pomare, E.W., Heaton, K.W., and Low-Beer, T.S. Metabolism of deoxycholic acid in man. Med. Biol. 53:107-113, 1975.

j Matern, S. and Gerok, W. Diagnostic value of serum bile acids. Acta Hepato-Gastroenterol. 26:185-189, 1979.

k Matern, S. and Gerok, W. Pathophysiology of the enterohepatic circulation of bile acids. Rev. Physiol. Biochem. Pharmacol. 85:126-159, 1979.

l Matern, S., Tietjen, K.G., Fackler, O., Hinger, K., Herz, R., and Gerok, W. Bioavailability of ursodeoxycholic acid in man: Studies with a radioimmunoassay for ursodeoxycholic acid. In Biological Effects of Bile Acids. G Paumgartner, A Stiehl, W Gerok, eds. MTP Press, Lancaster, 1979, pp 99-102.

m Matern, S., Matern, H., and Gerok, W. Characterization of UDP-glucuronosyltransferase activity towards bile acids in liver, intestine and kidney of man. IV Internat'l Gstaad Symposium, 1981 (abstract).

n Matern, S., Schill, A., Schubert, P., Lehnert, W., Tietjen, K., Schulte-Kellinghaus, M., Liomin, E., Matern, H., and Gerok, W. Bioverfugbarkeit von Ursodesoxycholsaure bie der Gallensteinauflosung des Menschen: Massenspektrometrische Studien mit ^{13}C-markierter Ursodesoxycholsaure. Z. Gastroenterol. XIX (9), 1981 (abstract).

a Mathe, D. and Chevallier, F. Effects of single ingestion of several bile acids or cholestyramine on $^{14}CO_2$ output in [26 ^{14}C] cholesterol-fed rats. Biochimie 58:1293-1295, 1976.

b Matkovics, B. and Samuelsson, B. Formation of lithocholic acid from ursodeoxycholic acid in the rat. Acta Chem. Scand. 16:673, 1962.

c Matkovics, B. and Samuelsson, B. Synthesis and metabolism of 3a,12a-dihydroxy-d^6-cholenic acid-24-^{14}C. Acta Chem. Scand. 16:683, 1962.

d Maton, P.N., Murphy, G.M., and Dowling, R.H. Ursodeoxycholic acid treatment of gallstones. Dose-response study and possible mechanism of action. Lancet 2:1297-1301, 1977.

e Maton, P.N. and Dowling, R.H. Hepatic cholesterol synthesis in cholelithiasis: Role of HMG-CoA reductase in response to and resistance to medical therapy. In Biological Effects of Bile Acids. G Paumgartner, A Stiehl, W Gerok, eds. MTP Press, Lancaster, 1979, pp 91-98.

f Maton, P., Ellis, J.H., Higgens, M.J., and Dowling, R.H. Hepatic HMG-CoA reductase in human cholelithiasis: Effects of chenodeoxycholic and ursodeoxycholic acids. Europ. J. Clin. Invest. 10:325-332, 1980.

g Maton, P., Murphy, G., and Dowling, R. Lack of response to chenodeoxycholic acid in obese and non-obese patients. Gut 21:1082-1086, 1980.

h Matschiner, J.T., Mahowald, T.A., Eliott, W.H., Doisy, E.A., Jr., Hsia, S.L., and Doisy, E.A. Bile acids. I. Two new acids from rat bile. J. Biol. Chem. 225:771-779, 1957.

i Matschiner, J.T., Mahowald, T.A., Hsia, S.L., Doisy, E.A., Jr., Eliott, W.H., and Doise, E.A. Bile acids. IV. The metabolism of hyodeoxycholic acid-24-^{14}C. J. Biol. Chem. 225:803-810, 1957.

j Matsumoto, K. and Kameda, H. Effect of bile acids on experimental gallstones in hamsters. Saishi Igaku 30:1033-1041, 1975.

k Matsumoto, H., Masamune, O., Nunode, Y., and Ohshiba, S. Diagnostic value of oral bile acid tolerance test. Jap. J. Gastroenterol. 78:1380-1387, 1981.

l Matsushiro, T., Kobayashi, N., Suzuki, N., Yamauchi, H., and Sato, T. The effect of oral chenodeoxycholic acid on cholesterol solubility in hepatic bile. Tohoku J. Exp. Med. 124:187-196, 1978.

m Matsushiro, T., Cho, H., Nagashima, H., Omokawa, S., Yamamoto, K., Hariu, T., and Tateyama, T. Factors affecting the cholesterol dissolution ability of human bile. Tokoho J. Exp. Med. 135:51-61, 1981.

n Matzkies, F. Fortschriftliche Gastroenterologie. Sonographische Diagnostik setzt sich durch. Arztliche Praxis No. 21, p 949, 1975.

a Maudgal, D.P., Bird, R., Enyobi, V.O., Blackwood, W.S., and Northfield, T.C. Chenic acid in gallstone patients--effect of low cholesterol and of high plant sterol diets. Gut 18:419, 1977 (abstract).

b Maudgal, D.P., Bird, R., Blackwood, W., and Northfield, T.C. Low-cholesterol diet: Enhancement of effect of CDCA in patients with gall stones. Brit. Med. J. 2:851-853, 1978.

c Maudgal, D.P., Bird, R., and Northfield, T.C. Optimal timing of doses of chenic acid in patients with gall stones. Brit. Med. J. 1:922-923, 1979.

d Maudgal, D.P., Kupfer, R., Bird, R., and Northfield, T.C. Best buy bile acid treatment for gallstones. Gut 21:A897, 1980 (abstract).

e Maudgal, D.P., Kupfer, R., Zentler Munro, P., and Northfield, T. Postprandial gall-bladder emptying in patients with gallstones. Brit. Med. J. 1:141-146, 1980.

f Maudgal, D.P., Kupfer, R.M., and Northfield, T.C. Minimum effective dose of chenic acid for gallstone patients: Reduction with bedtime administration and a low cholesterol diet. Gut 23:280-284, 1982.

g Mayer, D., Haindl, H., Koss, F.W., and Lamprecht, W. Enzymatische Bestimmung von Gallensauren in Korperflossigkeiten und Geweben. Z. Anal. Chem. 243:242-248, 1968.

h Mazer, N.A., Carey, M.C., Kwasnick, R.F., and Benedek, G. Quasielastic light scattering studies of aqueous biliary lipid systems. Size, shape and thermodynamics of bile salt micelles. Biochemistry 18:3064-3075, 1979.

i Mazer, N.A., Benedek, G.B., and Carey, M.C. Quasielastic light-scattering studies of aqueous biliary lipid systems. Mixed micelle formation in bile salt-lecithin solutions. Biochemistry 19:601-615, 1980.

j Mazzariello, R. Review of 220 cases of residual biliary tract calculi treated without reoperation: An eight-year study. Surgery 73:299-306, 1973.

k Mazzella, G., Roda, A., Sama, C., Aldini, R., Roda, E., and Barbara, L. Lithocholic acid metabolism before and after CDCA therapy. Rendic. Gastroenterol. 9:234-235, 1977.

l Mazzella, G., Messale, E., Morselli, A.M., Rossi, M.R., Roda, E., Roda, A., and Barbara, L. Effect of chenodeoxycholic acid (CDCA) and ursodeoxycholic acid (UDCA) administration on bile lipid secretion in normal weight and obese gallstone patients. Ital. J. Gastroenterol. 13:281-282, 1981 (abstract).

m McBain, E.L. and Hutchinson, E. Solubilization and Related Phenomena: Physical Chemistry. Academic Press, New York, 1955, pp 84-109.

n McBain, J.W., Merrill, R.C., Jr., Vinograd, J.R. The solubilization of water-insoluble dye in dilute solutions of aqueous detergents. J. Am. Chem. Soc. 63:670-676, 1941.

a McClelland, M.J., Smallwood, R.A., and Hoffman, N.E. Binding of cholic acid to soluble proteins from rat liver. FEBS Letters 82:255-258, 1977.

b McCormick, W.C., III., Bell, C.C., Jr., Swell, L., and Vlahcevic, Z.R. Cholic acid synthesis as an index of the severity of liver disease in man. Gut 14:895-902, 1973.

c McDougall, R.M., Yakymyshyn, L., Walker, K., and Thurston, O.G. Effect of wheat bran on serum lipoproteins and biliary lipids. Canad. J. Surg. 21:433-435, 1978.

d McGovern, R.F. and Quackenbusch, F.W. Turnover of bile acids in the hypercholesterolemic rat as influenced by saturation of dietary fat. Lipids 8:466-469, 1973.

e McJunkin, B., Fromm, H., Sarva, R.P., and Amin, P. Factors in the mechanism of diarrhea in bile acid malabsorption: Fecal pH--a key determinant. Gastroenterology 80:1454-1464, 1981.

f McLean Baird, I., Walters, R.L., Davies, P.S., Hill, M.J., Drasar, B.S., and Southgate, D.A.T. The effects of two fiber supplements on gastrointestinal transit, stool weight and frequency, bacterial flora, and fecal acids in normal subjects. Metabolism 26:117-128, 1977.

g McLeod, G.M. and Wiggins, H.S. Bile salts in small intestinal contents after ileal resection and in other malabsorption syndromes. Lancet 1:873-876, 1968.

h McSherry, C.K. and Glenn, F. Surgical aspects of biliary tract disease. Am. J. Med. 51:651-658, 1971.

i McSherry, C.K., Glenn, F., and Javitt, N.B. Composition of basal and stimulated hepatic bile in baboons, and the formation of cholesterol gallstones. Proc. Nat. Acad. Sci. 68:1564-1568, 1971.

j McSherry, C.K., Javitt, N.B., DeCarvalho, J.M., and Glenn, F. Cholesterol gallstones and the chemical composition of bile in baboons. Ann. Surg. 173:569-577, 1971.

k McSherry, C.K., Morrissey, K.P., Schwarm, R.L., and Glenn, F. Hepatic function and morphology in the baboon fed chenodeoxycholic acid for one year. Gastroenterology 67:815, 1974 (abstract).

l McSherry, C.K., Morrissey, K.P., Swarm, R.L., May, P.S., Niemann, W.H., and Glenn, F. Chenodeoxycholic acid induced liver injury in pregnant and neonatal baboons. Ann. Surg. 184:490-499, 1976.

m McSherry, C.K., Deitrich, J., May, P., Niemann, W., Morrissey, K., Palmer, R., and Glenn, F. Biliary lipid metabolism in the pregnant baboon. Surg. Gyn. & Obst. 144:727-733, 1977.

n McSherry, C.K. and Glenn, F. The incidence and causes of death following surgery for nonmalignant biliary tract disease. Ann. Surg. 191:271-275, 1980.

a McSherry, C.K. The National Cooperative Gallstone Study report: A surgeon's perspective. Ann. Intern. Med. 95:379-380, 1981.

b Meihoff, W.E., and Kern, F., Jr. Bile salt malabsorption in regional ileitis, ileal resection and mannitol-induced diarrhea. J. Clin. Invest. 47:261-267, 1968.

c Meinders, A., van Berge Henegouwen, G., Willekens, F., Ruben, A., and Schwerzel, A. Biliary bile acids and lipid composition in Diabetes Mellitus. Diabetologia 19, 1980 (abstract).

d Mekhjian, H.S. and Phillips, S.F. Perfusion of the canine colon with unconjugated bile acids. Effect on water and electrolyte transport, morphology and bile acid absorption. Gastroenterology 59:120-129, 1970.

e Mekhjian, H.S., Phillips, S.F., and Hofmann, A.F. Colonic secretion of water and electrolytes induced by bile acids: Perfusion studies in man. J. Clin. Invest. 50:1569-1577, 1971.

f Melchoir, G., Lofland, H., and St. Clair, R. The effect of polyunsaturated fats on bile acid metabolism and cholelithiasis in Squirrel monkeys. Metabolism 27:1471-1484, 1978.

g Mellander, O. and Stenhagen, E. The state of bile salt solutions: I. Introduction. II. Conductivity measurements on dilute solutions of sodium taurocholate at 25°C. Acta Physiol. Scand. 4:349-361, 1942.

h Mendelsohn, D. and Mendelsohn, L. The in vitro catabolism of cholesterol: A comparison of the formation of cholest-5-en-3b-26-diol and chenodeoxycholic acid from cholesterol in rat liver. S. African J. Med. Sci. 31:121-122, 1966.

i Mendelsohn, D. and Mendelsohn, L. The in vitro catabolism of cholesterol: A comparison of the formation of 26-hydroxycholesterol and chenodeoxycholic acid from cholesterol in rat liver. Biochem. J. 7:4167-4172, 1968.

j Menger, F. and McCreery, M. Kinetic characterization of bile salt micelles. J. Am. Chem. Soc. 96:121-126, 1974.

k Menghini, G. and Pallotta, B. Marked increase in serum levels of liver enzymes in patients receiving chenic acid and phenobarbital for gallstone dissolution. Digestion 14:163-169, 1976.

l Meredith, I.J., Hilson, A., Murphy, G.M., and Dowling, R.H. An explanation for bile-acid mediated gastritis and the relief of dyspepsia with chenodeoxycholic (CDCA) and ursodeoxycholic (UDCA) acid therapy. Clin. Sci. Volume 60, 1981.

m Merrick, M.V., Eastwood, M.A., Anderson, J.R., and Ross, H.McL. Enterohepatic circulation in man of a gamma-emitting bile-acid conjugate, 23-selena-25-homotaurocholic acid (SeHCAT). J Nucl. Med. 23:126-130, 1982.

n Metreau, J-M., St. Marc Girardin, M-F., Dhumeaux, D., and Berthelot, P. Traitement de la lithiase vesiculaire par l'acide chenodesoxycholique. 25 Malades. Masson Paris 7:3437-3440, 1978.

a Metzger, A.L., Heymsfield, S., and Grundy, S.M. The lithogenic index - A numerical expression for the relative lithogenicity of bile. Gastroenterology 62:499-501, 1972 (Letter to Editor).

b Metzger, A.L., Adler, R., Heymsfield, S., and Grundy, S.M. Diurnal variation in biliary lipid composition. Possible role in cholesterol gallstone formation. N. Engl. J. Med. 288:333-336, 1973.

c Meyer, A.E. and McEwen, J.P. Bile acids and their choline salts applied to the inner surface of the isolated colon and ileum of the guinea pig. Am. J. Physiol. 153:386-392, 1948.

d Meyer, P.D., DenBesten, L., and Gurll, N.J. Effects of cholesterol gallstone induction on gallbladder function and bile salt pool size in the prairie dog model. Surgery 83:599-604, 1978.

e Midtvedt, T. and Norman, A. Bile acid transformations by microbial strains belonging to genera found in intestinal contents. Acta Path. Microbiol. Scand. 71:41-44, 1964.

f Midtvedt, T. and Norman, A. Bile acid transformations by microbial strains belonging to genera found in intestinal contents. Acta Path. Microbiol. Scand. 71:629-638, 1967.

g Midtvedt, T. and Norman, A. Anaerobic, bile acid transforming microorganisms in rat intestinal content. Acta Path. Microbiol. Scand. 72:337, 1968.

h Midtvedt, T. Microbial bile acid transformation. Am. J. Clin. Nutr. 27:1341-1347, 1974.

i Miettinen, T.A., Pelkonen, R., Nikkila, E.A., and Heinonen, O. Low excretion of fecal bile acids in a family with hypercholesterolemia. Acta Med. Scand. 182:645-650, 1967.

j Miettinen, T.A. Detection of changes in human cholesterol metabolism. Ann. Clin. Res. 2:300-320, 1970.

k Miettinen, T.A. Cholesterol production in obesity. Circulation 44:842, 1971.

l Miettinen, T.A. Relationship between faecal bile acids, absorption of fat and vitamin B_{12} and serum lipids in patients with ileal resections. Europ. J. Clin. Invest. 1:452-460, 1971.

m Miettinen, T.A. The role of bile salts in diarrhoea of patients with ulcerative colitis. Gut 12:632-635, 1971.

n Miettinen, T.A. and Peltokallio, P. Bile salt, fat, water and vitamin B_{12} excretion after ileostomy. Scand. J. Gastroenterol. 6:543-552, 1971.

o Miettinen, T.A. Biliary and faecal bile acids in patients with interrupted enterohepatic circulation. Scand. J. Gastroenterol. 9:24, 1974 (abstract).

p Miettinen, T.A. Bile acid metabolism. Handbuch exptl. Pharmakologie 41: 109-150, 1975.

a Miettinen, M., Turpeinen, O., Karvonen, M.J., Paavilainen, E., and Elosuo, R. Prevalence of cholelithiasis in men and women ingesting a serum cholesterol-lowering diet. Annals Clin. Res. 8:111-116, 1976.

b Miettinen, T.A. and Tarpila, S. Effect of pectin on serum cholesterol, fecal bile acids, and biliary lipids in normolipidemic and hyperlipidemic individuals. Clin. Chim. Acta 79:471-477, 1977.

c Miettinen, T.A. Hyperlipidemia, bile acid metabolism and gallstones. Ital. J. Gastroenterol. 10:53-55, 1978.

d Miki, M., Ueno, T., Ohto, M., and Ohno, T. Cross sectional structure, chemical composition and cholangiographic features of stones of the gallbladder. Nippon Shokakibyo Gakkai Zasshi 75:1233-1247, 1978.

e Miller, G. La therapeutique medicamenteuse des calculs biliaires. Medicine et Hygiene, Geneve, 1975.

f Miller, L.J., Gordon, S.F., Haeffner, L.J., Saukkonen, J.J., Kinsey, M.D., and Kowlessar, O.D. Bile acid abnormalities in uremic man. Gastroenterology 66:746, 1974 (abstract).

g Miller, N.E. and Nestel, P.J. Altered bile acid metabolism during treatment with phenobarbitone. Clin. Sci. Mol. Med. 45:257-262, 1973.

h Miller, N.E. and Nestel, P.J. Triglyceride-lowering effect of chenodeoxycholic acid in patients with endogenous hypertriglyceridaemia. Lancet 2:929-931, 1974.

i Miller, P., Weiss, S., Cornell, M., and Dockery, J. Specific ^{125}I-radioimmunoassay for cholylglycine, a bile acid, in serum. Clin. Chem. 27:1698-1703, 1981.

j Milstein, H.J., Bloomer, J.R., and Klatskin, G. Serum bile acids in alcoholic liver disease. Comparison with histological features of the disease. Am. J. Dig. Dis. 21:281-285, 1976.

k Minder, E. and Paumgartner, G. Disparate Na^+ requirement of taurocholate and indocyanine green uptake by isolated hepatocytes. Experientia 35: 888-890, 1979.

l Mingrone, G., Altomonte, L., Ghirlanda, G., and Greco, A.V. Comparative effects of chenodeoxycholic acid and ursodeoxycholic acid on lipid synthesis in rat liver. Exp. Path. 20:193-196, 1981.

m Miskovitz, P.F. Gallstones: A non-surgical approach. J. Prac. Nurs. 30:25-39, 1980.

n Missale, G., Camarri, E., Fici, F., Agosti, A., and Mordini, M. Preliminary results on the action of dihydroxydibutylether on the lithogenic index of patients with calculosis of the gall-bladder. Intl. J. Clin. Pharm. Ther. Toxicol. 18:42-43, 1980.

a Mitchell, W.D. and Eastwood, M.A. Faecal bile acids and neutral steroids in patients with ileal dysfunction. Scand. J. Gastroenterol. 7:29-32, 1972.

b Mitchell, W.D., Findlay, J.M., Prescott, R.J., Eastwood, M.A., and Horn, D.B. Bile acids in the diarrhoea of ileal resection. Gut 14:348-353, 1973.

c Mitchell, W.D., Findlay, J.M., Macrae, R., Eastwood, M.A., and Anderson, R. Factors affecting bile acid metabolism in cholerrheic enteropathy. Digestion 11:135-146, 1974.

d Mitropoulos, K.A. and Myant, N.B. The formation of lithocholic acid, chenodeoxycholic and a- and b-muricholic acids from cholesterol incubated with rat-liver mitochondria. Biochem. J. 103:472-479, 1967.

e Mitropoulos, K.A. and Myant, N.B. The formation of lithocholic acid, chenodeoxycholic acid, and other bile acids from 3b-hydroxychol-5-enoic acid in vitro and in vivo. Biochim. Biophys. Acta 144:430-439, 1967.

f Mitropoulos, K.A., Suzuki, M., Myant, N.B., and Danielsson, H. Effects of thyroidectomy and thyroxine treatment on the activity of 12a-hydroxylase and of some components of microsomal electron transfer chains in rat liver. FEBS Letters 1:13-15, 1968.

g Mitropoulos, K.A. and Myant, N.B. Conversion of cholesterol into naturally occurring bile acids in vitro. In Bile Salt Metabolism. L Schiff, JB Carey, Jr., J Dietschy, eds. Charles C. Thomas, Springfield, 1969, pp 115-126.

h Mitropoulos, K.A., Avery, M.D., Myant, N.B., and Gibbons, G.F. The formation of cholest-5-ene-3b,26-diol as an intermediate in the conversion of cholesterol into bile acids by liver mitochondria. Biochem. J. 130:363-371, 1972.

i Mitropoulos, K.A. and Balasubramaniam, S. Cholesterol 7a-hydroxylase in rat liver microsomal preparations. Biochem. J. 128:1-9, 1972.

j Mitropoulos, K.A., Balasubramaniam, S., Gibbons, G.F., and Reeves, B.E.A. Diurnal variation in the activity of cholesterol 7a-hydroxylase in the livers of fed and fasted rats. FEBS Letters 27:203-206, 1972.

k Mitropoulos, K.A., Balasubramaniam, S., and Myant, N.B. The effect of interruption of the enterohepatic circulation of bile acids and of cholesterol feeding on cholesterol 7a-hydroxylase in relation to the diurnal rhythm in its activity. Biochim. Biophys. Acta 326:428-438, 1973.

l Mitropoulos, K.A., Myant, N.B., Gibbons, G.F., Balasubramaniam, S., and Reeves, B.E.A. Cholesterol precursor pools for the synthesis of cholic and chenodeoxycholic acids in rats. J. Biol. Chem. 249:6052-6056, 1974.

m Mitropoulos, K.A. The biosynthesis of bile acids and its control. In Advances in Bile Acid Research. S Matern, J Hackenschmidt, P Back, and W Gerok, ed. F.K. Schattauer Verlag, Stuttgart-New York, 1975, pp 13-24.

a Mitropoulos, K.A. Diurnal variation in bile acid biosynthesis. Second NATO Advanced Study Institute on the Biliary System. Aalborg, Denmark, August, 1975, pp 81-82 (abstract).

b Mitropoulos, K.A. and Balasubramaniam, S. The role of glucocorticoids in the regulation of the diurnal rhythm of hepatic b-hydroxy-b-methylglutaryl coenzyme-A reductase and cholesterol 7a-hydroxylase. Biochem. J. 160:49-55, 1976.

c Mitropoulos, K. and Venkatesan, S. The influence of cholesterol on the acitivity, on the isothermic kinetics and on the temperature-induced kinetics of 3-hydroxy-3-methylglutartyl coenzyme A reductase. Biochim. Biophys. Acta 489:126-142, 1977.

d Mitropoulos, K., Knight, B., and Reeves, B. 3-Hydroxy-3-methylglutaryl coenzyme a reductase. Biochem. J. 185:435-441, 1980.

e Miyai, K., Price, V.M., and Fisher, M.M. Bile acid metabolism in mammals. Ultrastructural studies on the intrahepatic cholestasis induced by lithocholic and chenodeoxycholic acids in the rat. Lab. Invest. 24:292-302, 1971.

f Miyai, K. and Richardson, A.L. Scanning electron microscopic study of hepatic ultrastructure in cholestasis and choleresis. Gastroenterology 69:848, 1975 (abstract).

g Miyake, H., Murakoshi, T., and Hisasugu, T. Studies of taurine conjugated bile acids. Fukuoka Acta Med. 53:695-702, 1962.

h Miyake, H., Yamamota, H., and Aono, K. Comparative studies on the chemical composition of gallstones in Japan, China and the United States. Fukuoka Acta Med. 54:781-826, 1963.

i Miyake, H. and Johnston, C.G. Gallstones: Ethnological studies. Digestion 1:219-228, 1968.

j Mockel, G. and Hess, W. Cholelitholyse durch Therapie mit Chenodesoxycholsaure und Beta-Sitsterin. 10. Int'l. Cong. of Gastroenterol., June, 1976, Budapest (abstract).

k Mockel, G. Erfahrungen mit der Medikamentosen Gallensteinauflosung. Hamburger Arzteblatt 35:76-79, 1981.

l Mockel, G. and Hess, W. Medikamentose Cholelitholyse, epikritscher Uberblick im Sinne des "Nil nocere". Z. Gastroenterol. XIX (9), 1981 (abstract).

m Modai, M. and Theodor, E. Intestinal contents in patients with viral hepatitis after a lipid meal. Gastroenterology 58:379-387, 1970.

n Mohr, P. and Amman, R. Problematik der medikamentosen Gallensteinauflosung. Schw. med. Wschr. 106:873-875, 1976.

o Mohr, P. Chenodeoxycholsaure und Ursodeoxycholsaure. Pharma-kritik 3:41-44, 1981.

a Mok, H.Y.I., Perry, P.M., and Dowling, R.H. Experimental expansion of the bile acid pool. Clin. Sci. 44:19P-20P, 1973.

b Mok, H.Y.I., Perry, P.M., and Dowling, R.H. The control of bile acid pool size: Effect of jejunal resection and phenobarbitone on bile acid metabolism in the rat. Gut 15:247-253, 1974.

c Mok, H.Y.I., Bell, G.D., and Dowling, R.H. Effect of different doses of chenodeoxycholic acid on bile-lipid composition and on frequency of side-effects in patients with gallstones. Lancet 2:253-257, 1974.

d Mok, H.Y.I., Bell, G.D., Whitney, B., and Dowling, R.H. Stones in the common bile duct: Non-operative management. Proc. Roy. Soc. Med. 67:658-660, 1974.

e Mok, H.Y.I., von Bergmann, K., Crouse, J.R., and Grundy, S.M. Biliary lipid metabolism in obesity. Effects of bile acid feeding before and during weight reduction. Gastroenterology 76:556-567, 1979.

f Mok, H.Y.I. and Grundy, S.M. Cholesterol and bile acid absorption during bile acid therapy in obese subjects undergoing weight reduction. Gastroenterology 78:62-67, 1980.

g Mole, B. New medical treatment of biliary calculi: Chenodeoxycholic acid. Infirm Fr. 188:5-6, 1977.

h Molino, G. and Milanese, M. Structural analysis of compartmental models for the hepatic kinetics of drugs. J. Lab. Clin. Med. 85:865-878, 1975.

i Moller, C. and Santavirta, S. Residual common duct stones. Acta Chir. Scand. 138:183-185, 1972.

j Molokhia, A.M., Higuchi, W.I., and Hofmann, A.F. Dissolution of model gallstones in vitro: Implications of T-tube infusion treatment of retained common duct stones. J. Pharm. Sci. 64:2029-2030, 1975.

k Molokhia, A.M., Hofmann, A.F., Higuchi, W.I., Tuchinda, M., Feld, K., Prakongpan, S., and Danzinger, R.G. Dissolution rates of model gallstones in human and animal biles and the importance of interfacial resistances. J. Pharm. Sci. 66:1101-1105, 1977.

l Montet, J.C., Reynier, M.O., Montet, A.M., and Gerolami, A. Distinct effects of three bile salts on cholesterol solubilization by oleate-monoolein-bile salt micelles. Biochim. Biophys. Acta 575:289-294, 1979.

m Montet, J. and Carey, M.C. Comparaison des proprietes micellaires et tensioactives des acides chenodesoxycholique (CDC) et ursodesoxycholique (UDC) et de leurs tauro (T-) et glyco (G-) conjugues en solution diluee. Gastroenterol. Clin. Biol. 4:92, 1980 (abstract).

n Moore, B. and Rockwood, D.P. On the mode of absorption of fats. J. Physiol. 21:58-84, 1897.

a Moore, B. and Parker, W.H. On the functions of the bile as a solvent. Proc. Roy. Soc. London 68:64-76, 1901.

b Moore, E.W. and Dietschy, J.M. Na and K activity coefficients in bile salts determined by glass electrodes. Am. J. Physiol. 206:1111-1117, 1964.

c Moore, R.B., Frantz, I.D. and Buchwald, H. Changes in cholesterol pool size, turnover rate, and fecal bile acid and sterol excretion after partial ileal bypass in hypercholesteremic patients. Surgery 65:98-108, 1969.

d Mordel, A.M. Results of medical treatment of biliary calculi with chenodeoxycholic acid. Med. Chir. Dig. 7:321-324, 1978.

e Morgan, R.G.H. The effect of bile salts on the lymphatic absorption by the unanaesthetized rat of intraduodenally infused lipids. Quart. J. Exp. Physiol. 49:457-465, 1964.

f Morgan, R.G.H. and Hofmann, A.F. Synthesis and metabolism of glyceryl-^{3}H-triether, a nonabsorbable oil phase marker for lipid absorption studies. J. Lipid Res. 11:223-230, 1970.

g Morgan, R.G.H. and Hofmann, A.F. Validity of ^{3}H-labeled triether, a nonabsorbable oil phase marker in the estimation of fat absorption. J. Lipid Res. 11:231-236, 1970.

h Morita, M., Ono, T., Ohto, M., Kimura, K., and Okuda, K. Bile composition and serum bile acids in patients with liver cirrhosis. Jap. J. Gastroent. 78:1953-1961, 1981.

i Morris, J.S., Low-Beer, T.S., and Heaton, K.W. Bile salt metabolism and the colon. Scand. J. Gastroenterol. 8:425-431, 1973.

j Morris, J.S. and Heaton, K.W. The fate of labelled bile salts introduced into the colon. Scand. J. Gastroenterol. 9:33-39, 1974.

k Morrissey, K.P., McSherry, Ch.K., Swarm, R.L., Nieman, W.H., and Deitrick, J.E. Toxicity of chenodeoxycholic acid in the nonhuman primate. Surgery 77:851-860, 1975.

l Morrissey, K.P. Gallstone formation and dissolution. Major Probl. Clin. Surg. 16:61-100, 1982.

m Mortola, G., Anfossi, A., Parodi, E., Cafiero, F., Pezzoli, F., and Berti Riboli, E. Terapia--Ruolo e limiti della terapia litolitica della colecistolitiasi colesterinica. Min. Med. 71:2283-2291, 1980.

n Morton, I.K.M., Saverymuttu, S.M., and Wood, J.R. Inhibition by prostaglandins of fluid transport in the isolated gallbladder of the guinea pig. Brit. J. Pharmacol. 50:460p, 1974.

o Mosbach, E.H., and Bevans, M. Biological studies of dihydrocholesterol. II. Effect of dehydrocholic acid on dihydrocholesterol-induced cholelithiasis in the rabbit. Am. Med. Assn. Arch. Path. 64:162-166, 1957.

a Mosbach, E.H., Bevans, M., Kaplan, R., and Halpern, E. Biological studies of dihydrocholesterol. III. Regression of dihydrocholesterol-induced cholecystitis and cholelithiasis in the rabbit. Am. Med. Assn. Arch. Path. 66:72-78, 1958.

b Mosbach, E.H., Bevans, M., Kaplan, R., Halpern, E., and Harris, D. Biological studies of dihydrocholesterol. IV. Effect of bile acids and other choleretic agents of dihydrocholesterol-induced cholelithiasis in the rabbit. Am. Med. Assn. Arch. Path. 67:197-203, 1959.

c Mosbach, E.H. and Bevans, M. Early pathologic and biochemical changes in rabbits fed dihydrocholesterol. Am. J. Path. 37:631-639, 1960.

d Mosbach, E.H. and Bevans, M. Biological studies of dihydrocholesterol. V. Effect of androgens upon the biologic disposition of dihydrocholesterol in the rabbit. Am. Med. Assn. Arch. Path. 75:558-563, 1963.

e Mosbach, E.H., Bokkenheuser, V., Chattopadyay, D.P., Schmidt, M., Hirsch, R.L., and Hofmann, A.F. Prevention of cholestanol-induced cholelithiasis by neomycin. Nature 208:1226-1227, 1965.

f Mosbach, E.H., Rothschild, M.A., Bekersky, I., Oratz, M., and Mongelli, J. Bile acid synthesis in the isolated, perfused rabbit liver. J. Clin. Invest. 50:1720-1730, 1971.

g Mosbach, E.H. Hepatic synthesis of bile acids. Biochemical steps and mechanism of rate control. Arch. Intern. Med. 130:478-487, 1972.

h Mosbach, E.H., Nicolau, G., and Nichols, R.W. Nature of crystalline chenodeoxycholic acid. Lancet 2:111, 1974 (Letter to Editor).

i Mosbach, E.H. and Salen, G. Bile acid biosynthesis. Pathways and regulation. Am. J. Dig. Dis. 19:920-929, 1974.

j Mosbach, E.H. Gallstones. Dissolving them with bile acids. Nurs. Care 10:24-25, 1977.

k Moskovitz, M., White, C., Barnett, R., Stevens, S., Russell, E., Vargo, D., and Floch, M.H. Diet, fecal bile acids, and neutral sterols in carcinoma of the colon. Dig. Dis. Sci. 23:746-751, 1979.

l Motson, R.W. Dissolution of common bile duct stones. Brit. J. Surg. 68:203-208, 1981.

m Mott, G.E., Pitot, H.C., and Goldfarb, S. Evidence for bile acid synthesis by transplantable hepatomas. Cancer Res. 34:1688-1693, 1974.

n Moutafis, C.D., Myant, N.B., and Tabaqchali, S. The metabolism of cholesterol after resection or by-pass of the lower small intestine. Clin. Sci. 35:537-545, 1968.

o Moutafis, C.D. and Myant, N.B. The metabolism of cholesterol in two hypercholesterolaemic patients treated with cholestyramine. Clin. Sci. 37:443-454, 1969.

a Mower, H.F., Ray, R.M., Stemmerman, G.N., Nomura, A., and Glober, G.A. Analysis of fecal bile acids and diet among the Japanese in Hawaii. J. Nutr. 108:1289-1296, 1978.

b Mufson, D., Triyanond, K., Ravin, L.J. Cholelithiasis chenotherapy: An in vitro approach. J. Pharm. Sci. 64:362-364, 1975.

c Mukerjee, P. Analysis of distribution model for micellar solubilization using thermodynamics of small systems: Nonideality of solubilization of Benzoic acid derivatives in nonionic surfactants. J. Pharm. Sci. 60:1531-1534, 1971.

d Mukerjee, P. and Cardinal, J.R. Solubilization as a method for studying self-association: Solubility of naphthalene in the bile salt sodium cholate and the complex pattern of its aggregation. J. Pharm. Sci. 65:882, 1976.

e Muller, G.E., Bockhorn, H., Fleischmann, R., and Muller, G.H. New therapeutic approach to overcome biliary sludge after liver transplantation. Transplant Proc. 13:845-847, 1981.

f Mulley, B.A. Solubility in systems containing surface active agents. Adv. Pharm. Sci. 1:86-94, 1964.

g Munk, V.I. and Rosenstein, A. Zur Lehre von der Resorption im Darm, nach Untersuchungen an einer Lymph(chylus-)fistel beim Menschen. Virchow Archiv. 123:230-279, 1891.

h Murata, T. Simultaneous determination of biliary bile acids in rat: electron impact and ammonia chemical ionization mass spectrometric analyses of bile acids. Steroids 34:717-728, 1979.

i Murphy, G.M., Jansen, F.H., and Billing, B.H. Unsaturated monohydroxy bile acids in cholestatic liver disease. Biochem. J. 129:491-494, 1972.

j Murphy, G.M. and Signer, E. Bile acid metabolism in infants and children. Gut 15:151-163, 1974.

k Murphy, G.M. Bile and bacteria. I. Bile acid metabolism. In Paediatric Gastroenterology. CM Anderson, V Burke, eds. Blackwell Scientific Publications, Oxford, 1975, pp 387-396.

l Murray, W.R., Agnew, M., and Mackay, C. Diet and bile composition in gallstone patients. Brit. J. Surg. 61:917, 1974 (abstract).

m Myant, N.B. and Eder, H.A. The effect of biliary drainage upon the synthesis of cholesterol in the liver. J. Lipid Res. 2:363-368, 1961.

n Myant, N.B. and Lewis, B. Estimation of the rate of breakdown of cholesterol in man by measurement of $^{14}CO_2$ excretion after intravenous 26-^{14}C cholesterol. Clin. Sci. 30:117-127, 1966.

o Myant, N.B. Hormonal control of cholesterol metabolism. In The Biological Basis of Medicine. Academic Press, London, 1968, pp 193-220.

a Myant, N.B. The regulation of cholesterol metabolism as related to familial hypercholesterolaemia. Sci. Basis Med. 1970, pp 230-259.

b Myant, N.B. The influence of some dietary factors on cholesterol metabolism. Proc. Nutr. Soc. 34:271-278, 1975.

c Myant, N.B. and Mitropoulos, K.A. Cholesterol 7a-hydroxylase. J. Lipid Res. 18:135-153, 1977.

d Myher, J.J., Marai, L., Kuksis, A., Yousef, I.M., and Fisher, M.M. Identification of ornithine and arginine conjugates of cholic acid by mass spectrometry. Canad. J. Biochem. 53:583-590, 1975.

e Nagase, M., Tanimura, H., Setoyama, M, and Hikasa, Y. Present features of gallstones in Japan. Am. J. Surg. 135:788-790, 1978.

f Nagase, M., Hikasa, Y., Tanimura, H., Setoyama, M., Kamata, T., Mukaihara, S., and Maruyama, K. Etiology of cholesterol gallstones. Gastroenterol. Jpn. 14:40-47, 1979.

g Nair, P.P., Gordon, M., and Reback, J. The enzymatic cleavage of the carbon-nitrogen bond in 3a,7a,12a-trihydroxy-5b-cholan-24-oylglycine. J. Biol. Chem. 242:7-11, 1967.

h Nair, P.P., Garcia-Lilis, C., and Mendeloff, A.I. Effect of lithocholic acid and antibiotics on tissue bile acids in the rat. J. Nutr. 100:698-704, 1970.

i Nair, P.P. and Kritchevsky, D. The Bile Acids, Chemistry, Physiology and Metabolism. (three volumes). PP Nair, D Kritchevsky, eds. Plenum Press, New York. Vol I: Chemistry, 1971; Vol II Physiology and Metabolism, 1973; Vol III Pathophysiology, 1976.

j Nair, P., Mendeloff, A., Vocci, M., Bankoski, J., Gorelik, M., Herman, G., and Plapinger, R. Lithocholic acid in human liver: Identification of e-lithocholyl lysine in tissue protein. Lipids 12:922-929, 1977.

k Nair, P., Solomon, R., Bankoski, J., and Plapinger, R. Bile acids in tissues: Binding of lithocholic acid to protein. Lipids 13:966-970, 1978.

l Naito, H.K., Holzbach, R.T., and Corbusier, C. Characterization of serum lipids and lipoproteins of prairie dogs fed a chow diet or cholesterol-supplemented diet. Exptl. Mol. Path. 27:81-92, 1977.

m Naitove, A. When cholecystectomy? Hosp. Pract. 121-128, June, 1978.

n Nakagaki, M. and Nakayama, F. Class separation of bile lipids by thin-layer chromatography. J. Chromatogr. 177:343-348, 1979.

o Nakagawa, S., Makino, I., Ishazaki, T., and Dohi, I. Dissolution of cholesterol gallstones by ursodeoxycholic acid. Lancet 2:367-369, 1977.

a Nakama, T., Furusawa, T., Itoh, H., and Hisadome, T. Correlation of cholesterol and bilirubin solubilization in bile salt solution. Gastroenterol. Jpn. 14:565-572, 1980.

b Nakamura, H. Studies on the mechanism of the serum cholesterol lowering effect of ursodeoxycholic acid: Hepatic cholesterol biosynthesis and fecal excretion of end products of cholesterol metabolism. Nippon Shokakibyo Gakkai Zasshi 62:55-64, 1965.

c Nakamura, T., Ohkuni, A., and Yamanaka, M. Effect of chenodeoxycholic acid (CDCA) and ursodeoxycholic acid (UDCA) to glucose transport in hamster small intestine, in vitro. Jpn. J. Gastroenterol. 77:1355-1361, 1980.

d Nakano, Y. and Nakano, K. Some cases of gallstones dissolved by bile acid preparations. J. National Council Communal. Hospitals 70:25-32, 1973.

e Nakao, K., Ohhara, H., Taki, T., Wakabayashi, T., and Ohgoh, T. Hepatotoxic effects of lithocholic acid and sulfolithocholic acid in rabbits. Yakugaku Zasshi 100:792-798, 1980.

f Nakayama, F. and Johnston, C.G. Bile constituents of the opossum, Didelphys marusialis virginiana. Proc. Soc. Exptl. Biol. Med. 95:690, 1957.

g Nakayama, F. and Blomstrand, R. Occurrence of cephalin, sphingomyelin and lysolecithin in bile. Acta Chem. Scand. 14:1211-1212, 1960.

h Nakayama, F. and Johnston, C.G. Solubility of human gallstones in primate gallbladder. Proc. Soc. Exptl. Biol. Med. 104:73-75, 1960.

i Nakayama, F. and Miyake, H. Cholesterol complexing by macromolecular fractions in human gall bladder bile. J. Lab. Clin. Med. 65:638-648, 1965.

j Nakayama, F. Cholesterol-holding capacity of bile in relation to gallstone formation. Clin. Chim. Acta 14:171-176, 1966.

k Nakayama, F. and Miyake, H. Species differences in cholesterol-complexing macromolecular fractions in bile in relation to gallstone formation. J. Lab. Clin. Med. 67:78-86, 1966.

l Nakayama, F. and Kawamura, S. Composition of biliary lecithins. Clin. Chim. Acta 55:53-58, 1967.

m Nakayama, F. Composition of gallstones and bile: Species difference. J. Lab. Clin. Med. 73:623-630, 1969.

n Nakayama, F. and Miyake, H. Changing state of gallstone disease in Japan: Composition of the stones and treatment of the condition. Am. J. Surg. 120:794-799, 1970.

o Nakayama, F. and van der Linden, W. Bile from gallbladder harbouring gallstone: Can it indicate stone formation? Acta Chir. Scand. 136:605-610, 1970.

a Nakayama, F. Studies on calculus versus milieu: Gallstone and bile. J. Lab. Clin. Med 77:366-377, 1971.

b Nakayama, F. and van der Linden, W. Bile composition: Sweden versus Japan. Its possible significance in the difference in gallstone incidence. Am. J. Surg. 122:8-12, 1971.

c Nakayama, F. and van der Linden, W. Role of gallbladder in gallstone formation. Acta Chir. Scand. 140:45-49, 1974.

d Nakayama, F. and van der Linden, W. Stratification of bile in gallbladder and gallstone formation. Surg. Gyn. Obst. 141:587-590, 1975.

e Nakayama, F., Miyazaki, K., and Koga, A. Effect of chenodeoxycholic and ursodeoxycholic acids on isolated human hepatocytes. Gastroenterology 78: 1228, 1980 (abstract).

f Nambu, M., Namihisa, T., Yamashiro, Y., Ohama, H., Maeda, M., and Ueda, H. Plasma disappearance of serum bile acids in patients with constitutional hyperbilirubinemias and constitutional ICG excretory defect. Nippon Shokakibyo Gakkai Zasshi 77:1369-1377, 1980.

g Narayan, R., Paul, R., and Balaram, P. Fluorescent probe studies of mixed micelles of phospholipids and bile salts. Biochim. Biophys. Acta 597: 70-82, 1980.

h Narisawa, T., Reddy, B.S., and Weisburger, J.H. Effect of bile acids and dietary fat on large bowel carcinogenesis in animal models. Gastroenterol. Japon. 13:206-212, 1978.

i Nassuato, G., Vassanelli, P., Lirussi, F., Giacon, L., Orlando, R., Venuti, M., and Okolicsanyi, L. Biliary excretion of simultaneously administered bilirubin and chenodeoxycholic acid in rats. Boll. Soc. Ital. Biol. Sper. 57:891-895, 1981.

j Nassuato, G., Vassanelli, P., Lirussi, F., Giacon, L., Orlando, R., Venuti, M., and Okolicsanyi, L. Biliary excretion of simultaneously administered bilirubin and chenodeoxycholic acid in rats with porta-caval shunt. Boll. Soc. Ital. Biol. Sper. 57:896-899, 1981.

k Naunyn, B. A treatise of cholelithiasis. New Sydenham Soc. Ed., London, pp 22, 1896.

l Neale, G., Lewis, B., Weaver, K., and Panveliwalla, D. Serum bile acids in liver disease. Gut 12:145-152, 1971.

m Neelon, V.J. and Lack, L. The effect of bile salts on the formation and hydrolysis of cholesterol esters by rat liver enzymes. Biochim. Biophys. Acta 487:137-144, 1977.

n Neiderhiser, D.H., Roth, H.P., Webster, L.T., Jr. Studies on the importance of lecithin for cholesterol solubilization in bile. J. Lab. Clin. Med. 68:90, 1966.

a Neiderhiser, D.H. and Roth, H.P. Cholesterol solubilization by solutions of bile salts and bile salts plus lecithin. Proc. Soc. Exptl. Biol. Med. 128: 221-225, 1968.

b Neiderhiser, D.H. and Roth, H.P. Effect of phospholipase A on cholesterol solubilization by lecithin in a bile salt solution. Gastroenterology 58: 26-31, 1970.

c Neiderhiser, D.H., Pineda, F.M., Hejduk, L.J., and Roth, H.P. Absorption of oleic acid by the guinea pig gallbladder. J. Lab. Clin. Med. 77:985-992, 1971.

d Neiderhiser, D.H., Plantner, J.J., and Carlson, D.M. The purification and properties of the glycoproteins of pig gallbladder bile. Arch. Biochem. Biophys. 145:155, 1971.

e Neiderhiser, D.H. and Roth, H.P. The effect of modifications of lecithin and cholesterol on the micellar solubilization of cholesterol. Biochim. Biophys. Acta 270:407-413, 1972.

f Neiderhiser, D.H., Morningstar, W.A., and Roth, H.P. Absorption of lecithin and lysolecithin by the gallbladder. J. Lab. Clin. Med. 82:891-897, 1973.

g Neiderhiser, D.H., Harmon, C.K., and Roth, H.P. Absorption of cholesterol by the gallbladder. J. Lipid Res. 17:117-124, 1976.

h Neiderhiser, D.H. Enzymic formation of cholesteryl ester from cholesterol by gallbladder mucosa. Lipids 16:930-933, 1981.

i Nell, G., Goerg, K.J., and Rummel, W. Effect of bile acids on the permeability of the colon. Diarrhea Disord. Intest. Transp. pp 98-104, 1981.

j Nemchausky, B.A., Layden, T.J., and Boyer, J.L. Effects of bile acids on the lipid composition and 3-dimensional structure of the bile canaliculus. _In_ The Liver. Quantitative Aspects of Structure and Function. R Preisig, J Bircher, and G Paumgartner, eds. Editio Cantor, Aulendorf, 1976, pp 386-392.

k Nervi, F., Gonzalez, A., and Valdivieso, V. Studies on cholesterol metabolism in the diabetic rat. Metabolism Clin. & Exp. 23:495-503, 1974.

l Nervi, F. and Dietschy, J. The ability of six different lipoprotein fractions to regulate the rate of hepatic cholesterogenesis in vivo. J. Biol. Chem. 250:8704, 1975.

m Nervi, F.O., Weis, H.J., and Dietschy, J.M. The kinetic characteristics of inhibition of hepatic cholesterogenesis by lipoproteins of intestinal origin. J. Biol. Chem. 250:4145, 1975.

a Nervi, F. and Dietschy, J.M. The mechanisms of and the interrelationship between bile acid and chylomicron-mediated regulation of hepatic cholesterol synthesis in the liver of the rat. J. Clin. Invest. 61:895-909, 1978.

b Nervi, F., Covarrubias, C., Valdivieso, V., Ronco, B., Solari, A., and Torccornal, J. Hepatic cholesterogenesis in Chileans with cholesterol gallstone disease. Gastroenterology 80:539-545, 1981.

c Nestel, P.J., Whyte, H.M., and Goodman, D.S. Distribution and turnover of cholesterol in humans. J. Clin. Invest. 48:982-991, 1969.

d Nestel, P.J. and Grundy, S.M. Changes in plasma triglyceride metabolism during withdrawal of bile. Metabolism 25:1259-1268, 1976.

e Newman, H.F. and Northrup, J.D. The autopsy incidence of gallstones. Int. Abst. Surg. 109:1-13, 1959.

f Newman, M. Traitement de dissolution des calculs biliaires. Hopital Information Therapeutique 2:25, 1971.

g Ng, P.Y. and Hofmann, A.F. Tissue distribution of cholylglycine-1-^{14}C in rats and hamsters with a bile fistula or bile duct ligation. Proc. Soc. Exptl. Biol. Med. 154:134-137, 1977.

h Ng, P.Y., Allan, R.N., and Hofmann A.F. Suitability of 11,12-^{3}H-chenodeoxycholic acid and 11,12-^{3}H-lithocholic acid for isotope dilution studies of bile acid metabolism in man. J. Lipid Res. 18:753-758, 1977.

i Nicolau, G., Shefer, S., Salen, G., and Mosbach, E.H. Determination of hepatic cholesterol 7_a_-hydroxylase activity in man. J. Lipid Res. 15: 146-151, 1974.

j Nicolau, G., Shefer, S., Salen, G., and Mosbach, E.H. Determination of hepatic hydroxy-3-methylglutaryl CoA reductase in man. J. Lipid Res. 15: 94-98, 1974.

k Niessen, K.H. Gallensauren im Darmsekret von Sauglingen und Kindern. Normalwerte, Lognormalverteilung und Altersabhangigkeit der Gallensaurengesamtmenge sowie des Gallensauremusters. Monatschr. Kinderheilkd. 127: 29-36, 1979.

l Nigro, N.D. and Campbell, R.L. Bile acids and intestinal cancer. _In_ The Bile Acids. Chemistry, Physiology and Metabolism. Volume 3:Pathophysiology. PP Nair, D Kritchevsky, eds. Plenum Press, New York, 1976, pp 155-168.

m Nilsson, A. and Borgstrom, B. Absorption and metabolism of lecithin and lysolecithin by intestinal slices. Biochim. Biophys. Acta 137:240-254, 1967.

n Nilsson, S. and Schersten, T. Importance of bile acids for phospholipid secretion into human hepatic bile. Gastroenterology 57:525-532, 1969.

a Nilsson, S. Synthesis and secretion of biliary phospholipids in man. An experimental study with special reference to the relevance for gallstone formation. Acta Chir. Scand. 405:1-38, 1970.

b Nilsson, S. and Schersten, T. Influence of bile acids on the synthesis of biliary phospholipids in man. Europ. J. Clin. Invest. 1:109-111, 1970.

c Nimmo, I.A., Clapp, J.B., and Strange, R.C. Lithocholic acid binding by cytosol from trout liver. Biochem. Soc. Trans. 8:371-372, 1980.

d Nittono, H. Bile acid metabolism in infants and children and its implication for hepatobiliary diseases. Indian J. Pediat. 47:549-554, 1980.

e Nogaller, A.M. and Bykov, V.B. Sovremennye predstavleniia o mekhanizme obrazoviniia zhelchnykh kamnei. Klin. Med. 49:10-14, 1971 (Russ).

f Noll, B.W., Walsh, L.B., Doisy, E.A., and Elliott, W.H. Bile acids. XXXV. Metabolism of 5a-cholestan-3b-ol in the Mongolian gerbil. J. Lipid Res. 13:71-77, 1972.

g Noll, B.W., Ziller, S.A., Doisy, E.A., and Elliott, W.H. Bile acids. XXXVII. Identification of the 3b-isomers of allocholic and allochenodeoxycholic acids as metabolites of 5a-cholestanol in the rat. J. Lipid Res. 14:229-234, 1973.

h Norcia, L.N. Absorption and biliary secretion of intrapeitoneally injected 3-methyloxycholest-5-ene-^{14}C in the rat. Lipids 8:315-320, 1973.

i Norri, T., Yamaga, N., and Yamasaki, K. Metabolism of 7b-hydroxycholesterol-4-^{14}C in rat. Steroids 15:303-326, 1970.

j Norman, A. Separation of conjugated bile acids by partition chromatography. Acta Chem. Scand. 7:1413, 1953.

k Norman, A. Influence of chemotherapeutics on the metabolism of bile acids in the intestine of rats. Acta Physiol. Scand. 33:99, 1955.

l Norman, A. Metabolism of glycine conjugated bile acids in the rat. Kungl. Fysiograf. Sallsk. Lund Forhandl. 25, Nr. 2, 1955.

m Norman, A. Preparation of conjugated bile acids using mixed carboxylic acid anhydrides. Arkiv. Kemi 8:331-342, 1955.

n Norman, A. and Grubb, R. Hydrolysis of conjugated bile acids by clostridia and enterococci: Bile acids and steroids 25. Acta Path. Microbiol. Scand. 36:537-547, 1955.

o Norman, A. and Sjovall, J. On the transformation and enterohepatic circulation of cholic acid in the rat. J. Biol. Chem 233:872, 1958.

p Norman, A. The beginning solubilization of 20-methylcholanthrene in aqueous solutions of conjugated and unconjugated bile acid salts. Acta Chem. Scand. 14:1295-1299, 1960.

a Norman, A. The conductance of conjugated and unconjugated bile acid salts in aqueous solutions. Acta Chem. Scand. 14:1300-1309, 1960.

b Norman, A. and Bergman, S. The action of intestinal microorganisms on bile acids. Bile acids and steroids 101. Acta Chem. Scand. 14:1781-1789, 1960.

c Norman, A. and Sjovall, J. Formation of lithocholic acid from chenodeoxycholic acid in the rat. Acta Chem. Scand. 14:1815-1818, 1960.

d Norman, A. and Shorb, M. In vitro formation of deoxycholic and lithocholic acid by human intestinal microorganisms. Proc. Soc. Exptl. Biol. Med. 110:552-555, 1962.

e Norman, A. Application of gel filtration of bile acids to studies of lipid-complexes in bile. Proc. Soc. Exptl. Biol. Med. 115:902, 1964.

f Norman, A. Electrophoretic behavior of bile acids and cholesterol in gallbladder and hepatic bile. Proc. Soc. Exptl. Biol. Med. 115:936, 1964.

g Norman, A. Faecal excretion products of cholic acid in man. Br. J. Nutr. 18:173-186, 1964.

h Norman, A. and Palmer, R.H. Metabolites of lithocholic acid-24-^{14}C in human bile and feces. J. Lab. Clin. Med. 63:986-1011, 1964.

i Norman, A. and Widstrom, O. Hydrolysis of conjugated bile acids by extra-cellular enzymes present in rat intestinal contents. Proc. Soc. Exptl. Biol. Med. 117:442, 1964.

j Norman, A. Metabolism of glycocholic acid in man. Scand. J. Gastroenterol. 5:231-236, 1970.

k Norman, A. and Strandvik, B. Excretion of bile acids in erythroblastosis foetalis. Acta Paediatr. Scand. 62:161-166, 1973.

l Norman, A. and Strandvik, B. Excretion of bile acids in extrahepatic biliary atresia and intrahepatic cholestasis of infancy. Acta Paediatr. Scand. 62:253-263, 1973.

m Norman, A. and Strandvik, B. Bile acid excretion after disappearance of jaundice in intrahepatic cholestasis of infancy. Acta Paediatr. Scand. 62:264-268, 1973.

n Norman, A. and Strandvik, B. Metabolism of lithocholic acid-24-^{14}C in extrahepatic biliary atresia. Acta Paediatr. Scand. 63:92-96, 1974.

o Norman, P.T. and Norum, K.R. Newly synthesized hepatic cholesterol as precursor for cholesterol and bile acids in rat bile. Scand. J. Gastroent. 11:427-432, 1976.

p Norrby, S. and Schonebeck, J. Long term results with cholecystolithotomy. Acta Chir. Scand. 136:711-713, 1970.

a Northfield, T.C. Intraluminal precipitation of bile acids in the stagnant loop syndrome. Brit. Med. J. 2:743-745, 1973.

b Northfield, T.C., Drasar, B.S., and Wright, J.T. Value of small intestinal bile acid analysis in the diagnosis of the stagnant loop syndrome. Gut 14:341-347, 1973.

c Northfield, T.C. and Hofmann, A.F. Biliary lipid secretion in gallstone patients. Lancet 1:747-748, 1973.

d Northfield, T.C. and McColl, I. Postprandial concentrations of free and conjugated bile acids down the length of the normal human small intestine. Gut 14:513-518, 1973.

e Northfield, T.C. and Hofmann, A.F. Biliary lipid output during three meals and an overnight fast. I. Relationship to bile acid pool size and cholesterol saturation of bile in gallstone and control subjects. Gut 16:1-11, 1975.

f Northfield, T.C., LaRusso, N.F., Hofmann, A.F., and Thistle, J.L. Biliary lipid output during three meals and an overnight fast. II. Effect of chenodeoxycholic acid treatment in gallstone subjects. Gut 16:12-17, 1975.

g Northfield, T.C., Kupfer, R., Maudgal, D., Zentler-Munro, P., Meller, S., Garvie, N., and McCready, R. Gall-bladder sensitivity to cholecystokinin in patients with gallstones. Brit. Med. J. 1:143-149, 1980.

h Noshi, H., Tsujii, T., Fukui, H., Matsui, T., Nishimura, Y., and Tamura, M. Influence of chenodeoxycholic acid on the metabolism of cholesterol and bile acids in the course of cholesterol gallstone formation in Squirrel monkeys. Nippon Shokakibyo Gakkai Zasshi 75:350-358, 1978.

i Nottle, P.D. and Hughes, E. Gallstones: Operate, dissolve, or leave alone? Drugs 21:302-308, 1981.

j Nystrom, E. and Sjovall, J. Separation of lipids on methylated Sephadex. Anal. Biochem. 12:235, 1965.

k Nystrom, E. and Sjovall, J. Thin-layer chromatography of bile acids on lipophilic Sephadex. Acta Chem. Scand. 21:1974, 1967.

l Nystrom, E., Haahti, E., and Sjovall, J. Liquid chromatography on lipophilic Sephadex: Column and detection techniques. In Advances in Chromatography. JC Giddings and RA Keller, eds. Marcell Dekker Inc., New York, Vol 6, 1968, pp 119.

m Nystrom, E. and Sjovall, J. Chromatography on lipophilic Sephadex. In Methods in Enzymology, Vol. 35. JM Lowenstein, ed. Academic Press, New York, 1975, pp 378.

n O'Brien, J.J., Shaffer, E.A., Williams, L.F., Small, D.M., Lynn, J., and Wittenberg, J. A physiological model to study gallbladdder function in primates. Gastroenterology 67:119-125, 1974.

a Oda, M., Price, V.M., Fisher, M.M., and Phillips, M.J. Ultrastructure of bile canaliculi, with special reference to the surface coat and the pericanalicular web. Lab. Invest. 31:314-323, 1974.

b Oda, M., Yousef, I.M., and Phillips, M.J. Isolation of bile ducts from rat liver: Technique and preliminary ultrastructural characterization. Exptl. Mol. Path. 23:214-219, 1975.

c Oddsson, E., Rask-Madsen, J., and Krag, E. Influence of bile acids on transepithelial ionic transport and electrical polarization in the human jejunum and ileum. Scand. J. Gastroenterol. 10:32-33, 1975.

d Oddsson, E., Rask-Madsen, J., and Krag, E. Effect of glycochenodeoxycholic acid on unidirectional transepithelial fluxes of electrolytes in the perfused human ileum. Scand. J. Gastroenterol. 12:199-204, 1977.

e Oddsson, E., Rask-Madsen, J., and Krag, E. Transmural ionic fluxes and electrical potential difference in the human jejunum during perfusion with a dihydroxy bile acid. Scand. J. Gastroenterol. 12:453-456, 1977.

f Oddsson, E., Rask-Madsen, J., and Krag, E. A secretory epithelium of the small intestine with increased sensitivity to bile acids in irritable bowel syndrome associated with diarrhoea. Scand. J. Gastroenterol. 13:409-416, 1978.

g O'Donnell, M.D., McGeeney, K.F., and Fitzgerald, O. Effect of free and conjugated bile salts on a-amylase activity. Enzyme 19:129-139, 1975.

h Oftebro, H., Bjorkhem, I., Stormer, F.C., and Pedersen, J.I. Cerebrotendinous xanthomatosis: Defective liver mitochondrial hydroxylation of chenodeoxycholic acid precursors. J. Lipid Res. 22:632-640, 1981.

i Ogawa, S. Biliary amylase excretion in rats, especially in relation with plasma level of the enzyme. Jap. J. Gastroenterol. 71:316-327, 1974.

j Ogura, M. and Yamasaki, K. Non-stereospecific reduction of 3-oxochol-4-enoic (24-^{14}C) acid in the rat. Steroids 9:607-622, 1967.

k Oh, S.Y. and Holzbach, R.T. Transmission electron microscopy of biliary-mixed lipid micelles. Biochim. Biophys. Acta 441:498-505, 1976.

l Oh, S.Y., McDonnell, M., Holzbach, R., and Jamieson, A. Diffusion coefficients of single bile salt and bile salt-mixed lipid micelles in aqueous solution measured by quasielastic laser light scattering. Biochim. Biophys. Acta 488:25-35, 1977.

m Ohkubo, H., Okuda, K., Iida, S., and Makino, I. Ursodeoxycholic acid oral tolerance test in patients with constitutional hyperbilirubinemias and effect of phenobarbital. Gastroenterology 81:126-135, 1981.

a Okhuysen-Young, C. and Kellogg, T.F. The effect of cecectomy on fecal bile acid and neutral steroid excretion of the rat. Comp. Biochem. Physiol. B 70B:345-347, 1981.

b Okishio, T. and Nair, P.P. Studies on bile acids. Some observations on the intracellular localization of major bile acids in rat liver. Biochemistry 5:3662, 1966.

c Okumura, M., Tanikawa, K., Chuman, Y., Koji, T., Nakagawa, S., Nakamura, Y., Iino, H., Yamasaki, S., and Hisatsugu, T. Clinical studies on dissolution of gallstones using ursodeoxycholic acid. Gastroenterol. Jpn. 12:469-475, 1977.

d Okumura, M., Hoshino, H., and Kumai, C. Chenodeoxycholic acid level in serum from patients with PCB poisoning. Fukuoka Igaku Zasshi 72:205-209, 1981.

e Okun, R., Goldenthal, E.I., Goldstein, L.I., Wazeter, F.X., Van Gelder, G.A., and Giel, R.G. Non-primate toxicology of chenodeoxycholic acid. J. Toxicol. & Environ. Health (in press).

f Olszewski, M.F., Holzbach, R.T., Saupe, A., and Brown, G.H. Liquid crystals in human bile. Nature 242:336-337, 1973.

g O'Maille, E.R.L., Richards, T.G., and Short, A.H. Acute taurine depletion and maximal rates of hepatic conjugation and secretion of cholic acid in the dog. J. Physiol. 180:67-79, 1965.

h O'Maille, E.R.L., Richards, T.G., and Short, A.H. Factors determining the maximal rate of organic anion secretion by the liver and further evidence on the hepatic site of action of the hormone secretin. J. Physiol. 186:424-438, 1966.

i O'Maille, E.R.L. The influence of conjugation of cholic acid on its uptake and secretion: Hepatic extraction of taurocholate and cholate in the dog. J. Physiol. 189:337-350, 1967.

j O'Maille, E.R.L., Richards, T.G., and Short, A.H. Observations on the elimination rates of single injections of taurocholate and cholate in the dog. Quar. J. Exp. Physiol. 54:296-310, 1969.

k O'Maille, E.R.L. and Richards, T.G. The secretory characteristics of dehydrocholate in the dog: Comparison with the natural bile salts. J. Physiol. 261:337-357, 1976.

l O'Maille, E.R.L. Bile salt secretion. Irish J. Med. Sci. 146:190-198, 1977.

m O'Maille, E.R.L. and Richards, T.G. Possible explanations for the differences in secretory characteristics between conjugated and free bile acids. J. Physiol. 265:855-866, 1979.

a O'Maille, E.R.L. The influence of micelle formation on bile salt secretion. J. Physiol. 302:107-120, 1980.

b Onishi, S., Itoh, S., and Ishida, Y. Assay of free and glycine- and taurine-conjugated bile acids in serum by high-pressure liquid chromatography by using post-column reaction after group separation. Biochem. J. 204:135-139, 1982.

c Ono, T., Ohto, M., Kawamura, K., Saisho, H., Tsuchiya, Y., Kimura, K., Yogi, Y., Karasawa, E., Itoh, F., Suzuki, Y., Morita, M., et al. Chenodeoxycholic acid therapy for the dissolution of gallstones, its efficacy and safety. Jpn. J. Gastroetnerol. 73:1232-1246, 1976.

d Ono, T., Oto, M., Kawamura, K., and Morita, M. Bile composition in patients with cholesterol gallstones and its alteration by chenodeoxycholic acid therapy. Jpn. J. Gastroenterol. 74:619-633, 1977.

e Ono, T. and Ohto, M. Dissolution of gallstones as a therapeutic measure. Nippon Rinsho (suppl.):2188-2189, 1978.

f Onstad, G.R., Schoenfield, L.J., and Higgins, J.A. Fluid transfer in the everted human gallbladder. J. Clin. Invest. 46:606-614, 1967.

g Onuki, M., Saito, H., and Hatta, Y. The kinetics of bile acids in patients with cholesterol gallstones. Japanese J. Gastroenterol. 79:956-963, 1982.

h van den Oord, A., Danielsson, H., and Ryhage, R. On the structure of the emulsifiers in gastric juice from the crab, Cancer pagurus L. J. Biol. Chem. 240:2242-2247, 1965.

i Oshiba, S. and Schoenfield, L.J. Plasminogen activator in bile stimulated by sodium taurocholate in isolated hamster livers. Proc. Soc. Exptl. Biol. Med. 133:89-92, 1970.

j Oshio, C., Miyairi, M., and Phillips, M.J. Influence of sodium taurocholate on bile canalicular contractions. Hepatology 1:535, 1981 (abstract).

k Ostrow, J.D. Absorption of bile pigments by the gallbladder. J. Clin. Invest. 46:2035-2052, 1967.

l Ostrow, J.D. Absorption by the gallbladder of bile salts, sulfobromophthalein, and iodipamide. J. Lab. Clin. Med. 74:482-494, 1969.

m Ostrow, J.D. and Murphy, N.H. Isolation and properties of conjugated bilirubin from bile. Biochem. J. 120:311-329, 1970.

n Ostrow, J.D. Absorption of organic compounds by injured gallbladder. J. Lab. Clin. Med. 78:255-264, 1971.

a Ostrow, J.D., Devers, T.J., and Gallo, D. Determinants of the solubility of unconjugated bilirubin in bile. Relationship to pigment gallstones. In International Symposium on Chemistry and Physiology of Bile Pigments. PD Berk, N Berlin, eds. Dept. of HEW, Superintendent of Documents. Government Printing Office, Bethesda, 1977, pp 404-409.

b Ostrow, J.D., Devers, T.J., and Gallo, D. Solubilization of unconjugated bilirubin by taurocholate. In The Liver: Quantitative Aspects of Structure and Function. R Preisig, J Bircher, G Paumgartner, eds. Editio Cantor, Aulendorf, 1976, pp 429-431.

c Ostrow, J., Devers, T., and Gallo, D. Determinants of the solubility of unconjugated bilirubin in bile: Relationship to pigment gallstones. Gastroenterology 79:1102, 1980 (abstract).

d Ostrower, V.S., Coan, P., Kern, F., Jr. Effect of phenobarbital on intestinal cholic acid absorption in the rat. Gastroenterology 67:1162-1168, 1974.

e Ostrower, V.S. and Kern, F., Jr. Effect of dietary fiber on bile salt absorption in patients with ileal resection. Clin. Res. 23:17a, 1975 (abstract).

f Ostrowitz, A. and Gardner, B. Studies of bile as a suspending medium and its relationship to gallstone formation. Surgery 68:329-333, 1970.

g Ostrowitz, A., Gordon, M., Patti, J., Popowitz, L., Hedayati, H., and Gardner, B. Studies of gallstone formation in the rabbit. Surg. Forum 21:393-395, 1970.

h Osuga, T. and Portman, O.W. Experimental formation of gallstones in the Squirrel monkey. Proc. Soc. Exptl. Biol. Med. 136:722-726, 1971.

i Osuga, T. and Portman, O.W. Relationship between bile composition and gallstone formation in Squirrel monkeys. Gastroenterology 63:122-133, 1972.

j Osuga, T., Portman, O.W., Mitamura, K., and Alexander, M. A morphologic study of gallstone development in the Squirrel monkey. Lab. Invest. 30:486-493, 1974.

k Osuga, T., Portman, O.W., Tanaka, N., Alexander, M., and Ochsner, A.J., III. The effect of diet on hepatic bile formation and bile acid metabolism in Squirrel monkeys with and without cholesterol gallstones. J. Lab. Clin. Med. 88:649-661, 1976.

l Osuga, T., Mitamura, K., Mashige, F., and Imai, K. Evaluation of fluorimetrically estimated serum bile acid in liver disease. Clin. Chim. Acta 75:81-91, 1977.

m Osuga, T. Ursodeoxycholic acid: Study on the dissolution of gallstones with ursodeoxycholic acid--a double blind trial. Adv. Med. (Japan) 101:922-936, 1977.

a Ota, M., Isobe, J., Tsuji, Y., Kuramoto, T., and Hoshita, T. Metabolism of bile acids. IV. Absorption, distribution, excretion and metabolism of orally administered ursodeoxycholic acid in rats. Hiroshima J. Med. Sci. 26:233-251, 1977.

b Ota, M., Matsumoto, N., Kuramoto, T., and Hoshita, T. Metabolism of bile acids. V. Metabolism of ursodeoxycholic acid in Rhesus monkey. Hiroshima J. Med. Sci. 26:253-262, 1977.

c Ota, M., Tsunoda, H., and Hoshita, T. Metabolism of bile acids. III. Metabolism of chenodeoxycholic acid. Yakugaku 98:108-118, 1978.

d Ota, M., Tsuji, Y., and Hoshita, T. Metabolism of bile acids. VI. Metabolism of chenodeoxycholic acid in female rats. Hiroshima J. Med. Sci. 27:131-138, 1978.

e Ota, M., Tsuji, Y., and Hoshita, T. Metabolism of bile acids. VII. Metabolism of ursodeoxycholic acid in female rats. Hiroshima J. Med. Sci. 27:139-145, 1978.

f Owen, R.W., Thompson, M.H., and Hill, M.J. The identification of bacterial metabolites of chenodeoxycholic acid by GC-mass spectrometry. Biochem. Soc. Trans. 9:34A, 1981 (abstract).

g Owor, R. Gallstones in the autopsy population of Mulago Hospital, Kampala. E. Afr. Med. J. 41:251-253, 1964.

h Ozaki, S., Tashiro, A., Makino, I., Nakagawa, S., and Yoshizawa, I. Enzyme-linked immunoassay of ursodeoxycholic acid in serum. J. Lipid Res. 20:240-245, 1979.

i Pacini, N., Ferrari, A., and Canzi, E. 7a-Dehydroxylation of bile acids by O_2-intolerant anaerobic intestinal microorganisms. Ann. Ist. Super Sanita 15:167-172, 1979.

j Pacini, N., Ferrari, A., Canzi, E., Albini, E., and Marca, G. Effects of administration of chenodeoxycholic acid in the rabbit. Boll. Chim. Farm. 119:113-126, 1980.

k Pageaux, J.F., Duperray, B., Anker, D., and Dubois, M. Bile acid sulfates in serum bile acid determinations. Steroids 34:73-87, 1979.

l Pageaux, J.F., Duperray, B., Dubois, M., and Pacheco, H. Isotope derivative assay of human serum bile acids. J. Lipid Res. 22:725-729, 1981.

m de Palma, R.G., Hubay, C.A., and Insull, W. The effect of T-tube drainage of cholesterol and bile acid metabolism in man. Surg. Gyn. & Obst. 123:269-273, 1966.

n Palmer, A.K. and Heywood, R. Pathological changes in the Rhesus fetus associated with the oral administration of chenodeoxycholic acid. Toxicology 2:239-246, 1974.

a Palmer, R.H., Glickman, P.B., and Kappas, A. Pyrogenic and inflammatory properties of certain bile acids in man. J. Clin. Invest. 41:1573-1577, 1962.

b Palmer, R.H. Gallstones produced experimentally by lithocholic acid in rats. Science 148:1339-1340, 1965.

c Palmer, R.H. and Hruban, Z. Production of bile duct hyperplasia and gallstones by lithocholic acid. J. Clin. Invest. 45:1255-1267, 1966.

d Palmer, R.H. The formation of bile acid sulfates: A new pathway of bile acid metabolism in humans. Proc. Nat. Acad. Sci. 58:1047-1050, 1967.

e Palmer, R.H. Toxic effects of lithocholic acid and related 5 -H steroids. _In_ Bile Salt Metabolism. Schiff, Carey, and Dietschy, eds. Thomas, Springfield, 1969, pp 184-204.

f Palmer, R.H. Bile acid sulfates. II. Formation, metabolism, and excretion of lithocholic acid sulfates in the rat. J. Lipid Res. 12:680-687, 1971.

g Palmer, R.H. and Bolt, M.G. Bile acid sulfates. I. Synthesis of lithocholic acid sulfates and their identification in human bile. J. Lipid Res. 12:671-679, 1971.

h Palmer, R.H. Bile acids, liver injury, and liver disease. Arch. Intern. Med. 130:606-617, 1972.

i Palmer, R.H. Toxic effects of lithocholate on the liver and biliary tree. _In_ The Hepatobiliary System. Fundamental and Pathological Mechanism. W Taylor, ed. Plenum Press, New York, 1976, pp 227-240.

j Palmer, R.H. The gallbladder and bile composition (editorial). Dig. Dis. & Sci. 21:795-796, 1976.

k Palmer, R.H. Bile acid heterogeneity and the gastrointestinal epithelium: From diarrhea to colon cancer. J. Lab. Clin. Med. 94:655-660, 1979.

l Palmer, R.H. and Carey, M.C. Sounding Board. An optimistic view of the National Cooperative Gallstone Study. N. Engl. J. Med. 306:1171-1174, 1982.

m Palmer, R.H. and McSherry, C.K. Lithocholate metabolism in baboons fed chenodeoxycholate. J. Lab. Clin. Med. 99:533-538, 1982.

n Papp, J., Feher, T., Laszlo, P., Szam, I., Vass, A., and Wittman, I. Results of chenodeoxycholic acid treatment in cholelithiasis. 10. Int'l. Cong. Gastroenterol, Budapest, June, 1976 (abstract).

o Paraf, A., Coste, T., Rautureau, M., Rautureau, J., and Gouffier, E. Lithiase choledocienne et agenesie de la vesicule. Anomalies de la composition de la bile. Nouvelle Presse Medicale 3:2203-2204, 1973.

a Park, Y.H., Igimi, H., and Carey, M.C. Human cholesterol (ChM) gallstones dissolve as fast in simulated 'urso'-rich bile as in 'cheno'-rich bile. Gastroenterology 80:1248, 1981 (abstract).

b Parkin, D.M., Cussons, D.F., Rooney, P., O'Moore, R.R., Warwick, R.R.G., Percy-Robb, I.W., and Shearman, D.J.C. Evaluation of the "breath test" in the detection of bacterial colonisation of the upper gastrointestinal tract. Lancet 2:777-780, 1972.

c Parl, F. and Gutstein, W.H. Association of coronary artery endothelial injury with elevation of serum bile acids in the rat. Atheroscl. Proc. Int. Symp., 1974, pp 229-232.

d Parmentier, G. and Eyssen, H. Synthesis and characteristics of the specific monosulfates of chenodeoxycholate, deoxycholate, and their taurine or glycine conjugates. Steroids 30:583-590, 1977.

e Parmentier, G. and Eyssen, H. Thin-layer chromatography of bile salt sulphates. J. Chromatogr. 152:285-289, 1978.

f Parmentier, G., Janssen, G.A., Eggermont, E.A., and Eyssen, H.J. C_{27} bile acids in infants with coprostanic acidemia and occurrence of a 3a-, 7a-, 12a-trihydroxy-5b-C_{29} dicarboxylic bile acid as a major component in their serum. Europ. J. Biochem. 102:173-183, 1979.

g Parquet, M., Rey, C., Groussard, M., and Infante, R. Pharmacokinetics and metabolism of ^{14}C-ursodeoxycholic acid in the rat. Biochim. Biophys. Acta 665:299-305, 1981.

h Patel, D.C. and Higuchi, W.I. Mechanism of cholesterol gallstone dissolution. I. The determination of the binding of alkyl amines to bile micelles using dynamic membrane transport methods. J. Colloid Interface Sci. 74:201-210, 1980.

i Patton, J.S. and Carey, M.C. Inhibition of human pancreatic lipase-colipase activity by mixed bile salt-phospholipid micelles. Am. J. Phys. 241: G328-G336, 1981.

j Paumgartner, G. and Grabner, G. Das Verhalten konjugierter Gallensauren des Serums bei Erkrankungen der Leber. Acta Hepatosplen. 17:344-353, 1970.

k Paumgartner, G. Storungen des Gallensaurenstoffwechsels. Z. Gastroenterol. 11:121-130, 1973.

l Paumgartner, G., Sauter, K., Schwarz, H.P., and Herz, R. Hepatic excretory transport maximum for free and conjugated cholate in the rat. Effect of enzyme induction. In The Liver. Quantitative Aspects of Structure and Function. G Paumgartner and R Preisig, eds. S Karger Verlag, Basel, 1973, pp 337.

m Paumgartner, G., Sauter, K., Schwarz, H.P., and Herz, R. Hepatic excretory transport maximum for free and conjugated cholate in the rat. Effect of phenobarbital. Gastroenterology 64:161, 1973 (abstract).

a Paumgartner, G. and Schwarz, H.P. Elevation of free chenodeoxycholic acid in serum after therapeutic doses of the bile acid in man. Gastroenterology 65:563, 1973 (abstract).

b Paumgartner, G. Grundlagen und Ergebnisse der Pharmakotherapie des Cholesteringallensteinleidens. Therapeutische Umschau/Revue Therapeutique 31:852-858, 1974.

c Paumgartner, G. Pathophysiologishe Grundlagen der Gallensteinbildung. Leber Magen Darm 4:17, 1974.

d Paumgartner, G., Herz, R., Sauter, K., and Schwarz, H.P. Taurocholate excretion and bile formation in the isolated perfused rat liver. An in vitro - in vivo comparison. Naunyn-Schmiedebergs Arch. Pharm. 285:165, 1974.

e Paumgartner, G., Reichen, J., and Preisig, R. Evaluation of ^{14}C-taurocholate for estimation of hepatic blood flow in man. Digestion 10:373, 1974 (abstract).

f Paumgartner, G. Cholelitholyse. Grundlagen und Ergebnisse. Z. Gastroenterol. 13:295-299, 1975.

g Paumgartner, G. Medikamentose Cholelitholyse. Hepatologen argumentieren Pro und Contra. Indikation: Erhohtes Op-Risiko. Med. Tribune, Nr. 20, pp 49, 1975.

h Paumgartner, G. Pharmacokinetic aspects of chenodeoxycholic acid therapy. Hosp. Prac. 10:117-122, 1975.

i Paumgartner, G. Was ist gesichert in der internistischen Therapie des Gallensteinleidens? Internist 16:566-570, 1975.

j Paumgartner, G. and Reichen, J. Different pathways for hepatic uptake of taurocholate and indocyanine green. Experientia 31:306, 1975.

k Paumgartner, G., Reichen, J., von Bergmann, K., and Preisig, R. Elaboration of hepatocytic bile. Bull. N.Y. Acad. Med. 51:455-471, 1975.

l Paumgartner, G. and Reichen, J. Kinetics of hepatic uptake and excretion of organic anions. In The Hepatobiliary System. W Taylor, ed. Plenum Publishing Corp., New York, 1976, pp 287.

m Paumgartner, G. Die Gallensteinauflosung mit Chenodesoxylsaure in der Praxis. Therap. Umschau 34:767-771, 1977.

n Pearlman, B.J. and Schoenfield, L.J. Gallstones. The present and future of medical dissolution. Med. Clin. N. Am. 62:87-105, 1978.

o Pearlman, B.J., Bonorris, G., Phillips, M., Chung, A., Vimadalal, S., Marks, J., and Schoenfield, L. Cholesterol gallstone formation and prevention by chenodeoxycholic and ursodeoxycholic acids. Gastroenterology 77:634-641, 1979.

a Pearlman, B.J., Marks, J.W., Bonorris, G.G., and Schoenfield, L.J. Gallstone dissolution--A progress report. Clin. Gastroenterol. 8:123-140, 1979.

b Pedersen, L., Arnfred, T., and Hess Thaysen, E. Cholesterol kinetics in patients with cholesterol gallstones before and during chenodeoxycholic acid treatment. Scand. J. Gastroenterol. 9:787-791, 1974.

c Pedersen, L. Medicinsk behandlung af galdesten. Ugeskr. Laeg. 137:1569-1574, 1975.

d Pedersen, L. and Arnfred, T. Kinetics and pool size of chenodeoxycholic acid in cholesterol gallstone patients. Scand. J. Gastroenterol. 10:557-560, 1975.

e Pedersen, L. and Bremmelgaard, A. Biliary bile acid composition and hepatic morphology during chenodeoxycholic acid therapy for radiolucent gallstones. Scand. J. Gastroenterol. 10:34-35, 1975.

f Pedersen, L. and Bremmelgaard, A. Hepatic morphology and bile acid composition of bile and urine during chenodeoxycholic acid therapy for radiolucent gallstones. Scand. J. Gastroenterol. 11:385-389, 1976.

g Pedersen, L. Medical treatment of cholesterol gallstones. Ugeskr. Laeger. 141:527-528, 1979.

h Pelissier, E., Carayon, P., and Spitz, J.F. The dissolution of residual calculi in the common bile duct using chenodeoxycholic acid. Chirurgie 104:775-779, 1978.

i Pellizzari, E.D., O'Neil, F.S., Farmer, R.W., and Fabre, L.F. Identification of lithocholic and measurement of other bile acids in serum of healthy humans. Clin. Chem. 19:248-252, 1973.

j Percy-Robb, I.W. and Boyd, G.S. The synthesis of bile acids in perfused rat liver subjected to chronic biliary drainage. Biochem. J. 118:519-530, 1970.

k Percy-Robb, I.W., Telfer Brunton, W.A., Gould, J.C., Jalan, K.N., McManus, J.P.A., and Sircus, W. Composition and bile salt transforming capacity of the bacterial flora of ileal effluent in patients with ileostomies. Scand. J. Gastroenterol. 6:625-630, 1971.

l Percy-Robb, I.W. and Collee, J.G. Bile acids: A pH dependent antibacterial system in the gut? Brit. Med. J. 3:813-815, 1972.

m Percy-Robb, I.W. Cholesterol gallstones. Scot. Med. J. 18:157-165, 1973.

n Percy-Robb, I.W. and Boyd, G.S. The biosynthesis of bile acids. Scot. Med. J. 18:166-174, 1973.

o Percy-Robb, I.W. Bile acid synthesis: An alternative pathway leading to hepatotoxic compounds? Essays Med. Biochem. 1:59-80, 1977.

a Perman, E. Medical resolution of gallstones--the current situation. Lakartidnigen, 75:4237, 1978 (Letter to Editor).

b Perry, P.M., White, J., and Dowling, R.H. Bile acid absorption by jejunum and colon after ileal resection in the rat. Brit. J. Surg. 59:310, 1972 (abstract).

c Perry, W.F. The metabolism of cholesterol and its alteration by various factors. Manitoba Med. Rev. 48:382-384, 1968.

d Pertsemlidis, D., Kirchman, E.H., and Ahrens, E.H., Jr. Regulation of cholesterol metabolism in the dog. I. Effects of complete bile diversion and of cholesterol feeding on absorption, synthesis, accumulation and excretion rates measured during life. J. Clin. Invest. 52:2353-2367, 1973.

e Pertsemlidis, D., Kirchman, E.H., and Ahrens, E.H. Jr. Regulation of cholesterol metabolism in the dog. II. Effects of complete bile diversion and of cholesterol feeding on pool size of tissue cholesterol measured at autopsy. J. Clin. Invest. 52:2368-2378, 1973.

f Pertsemlidis, D., Panveliwalla, D., and Ahrens, E.H., Jr. Effects of clofibrate and of an estrogen-progestin combination on fasting biliary lipids and cholic acid kinetics in man. Gastroenterology 66:565-573, 1974.

g Peskin, G.W. The treatment of silent gallstones. Surg. Clin. N. Am. 53:1063-1069, 1973.

h Pessoa, V.C., Kim, K.S., and Ivy, A.C. Fat absorption in absence of bile and pancreatic juice. Am. J. Physiol. 174:209-218, 1953.

i Peters, H. and Keimes, A.M. Die Cholezystektomie als pradisponierender Faktor in der Genese des kolorektalen Karzinoms? Dtsch. med. Wschr. 104: 1581-1583, 1979.

j Pethica, B.A. and Schulman, J.H. Hemolytic and surface activity of sodium taurocholate. Nature 170:117-118, 1952.

k Petite, J.P. Le traitement de la lithiase biliaire par l'acide chenodesoxycholique. La Revue du Praticien 27:757-759, 1976.

l Phillips, G.B. The lipid composition of human bile. Biochim. Biophys. Acta 41:361, 1960.

m Phillips, M.J., Oda, M., Mak, E., Fisher, M.M., and Jeejeebhoy, K.N. Microfilament dysfunction as a possible cause of intrahepatic cholestasis. Gastroenterology 69:48-58, 1975.

n Phillips, M.J., Oda, M., Mak, E., Edwards, V., Yousef, I.M., and Fisher, M.M. The bile canalicular network in vitro. J. Ultrastructural Res. 57:163-167, 1976.

o Phillips, M.J., Funatsu, K., Oda, M., Edwards, V., and Mickle, D.A.G. Dissolution of human cholesterol gallstones in vitro with ethanol and ether. Lab. Invest. 39:488-504, 1978.

a Phillips, S.F. and Gaginella, T.S. Intestinal secretion as a mechanism in diarrheal disease. In Progress in Gastroenterology. GB Jerzy-Glass, ed. Grune and Stratton, Inc., New York, Vol III, 1977, pp 481-504.

b Phlippen, R., Herold, G., Oette, K., Friedmann, G., Hoeffken, W., Huebner, W., Adler, K., and Hirschmann, W.D. Aetioloie, pathogenese und therapie der cholesterin-gallensteine mit chenodesoxycholsaeure. In Aktuelle Probleme der Inneren Medizin. FK Shattauer Verlag, Stuttgart-New York, 1977, pp 299-342.

c Pimstone, N.R. and Mok, H.Y. Current status of medical treatment of gallstones. Surg. Clin. North Am. 61:865-874, 1981.

d Pirotte, J. Cholelithiasis treatment. I. Medical treatment. Rev. Med. Liege 33:602-606, 1978.

e Pitt, H.A. and Cameron, J.L. Sodium cholate dissolution of retained biliary stones: Mortality rate following intrahepatic infusion. Surgery 85:457-460, 1979.

f Plant, J.C.D., Percy, I., Bates, T., Gastard, J., Hita de Nercy, Y. Incidence of gallbladder disease in Canada, England and France. Lancet 2:249-251, 1973.

g du Plessis, D.J. and Jersky, J. The management of acute cholecystitis. Surg. Clin. N. Am. 53:1071-1077, 1973.

h Podda, M., Zuin, M., Dioquardi, M.L., Festorazzi, S., and Dioguardi, N. A combination of cheno- and ursodeoxycholic acid is more effective than either alone in reducing bile cholesterol saturation. Gastroenterology 78:1316, 1978 (abstract).

i Podda, M., Zuin, M., Dioguardi, M., and Lesma, S. Comparison of effects of cheno- and ursodeoxycholic acid and their combination on biliary lipids in obese patients with gallstones. Gastroenterology 80:1344, 1981 (abstract).

j Podda, M., Zuin, M., Carulli, N., Ponz de Leon, M., and Dioguardi, M.L. Gallstone dissolution after 6 months of ursodeoxycholic acid (UDCA): Effectiveness of different doses. J. Int. Med. Res. 10:59-63, 1982.

k Podesta, M.T., McGuffie, C.A., Murphy, G.M., and Dowling, R.H. Faecal bile acid (BA) excretion in patients with cholelithiasis before and during chenodeoxycholic (CDCA) and ursodeoxycholic (UDCA) acid therapy. Gut 19:A991, 1978 (abstract).

l Podesta, M.T., Murphy, G.M., Sladen, G.E., and Dowling, R.H. Sulphated faecal bile acid excretion--an underestimated factor. Clin. Sci. Mol. Med. 54:32p-33p, 1978 (abstract).

m Podesta, M.T., Murphy, G.M., Sladen, G.E., Breuer, N.F., and Dowling, R.H. Fecal bile acid excretion in diarrhea: effect of sulfated and non-sulfated bile acids on colonic structure and function. In Biological Effects of Bile Acids. G Paumgartner, A Stiehl, W Gerok, eds. MTP Press, Lancaster, 1979, pp 245-256.

a Podesta, M.T., Murphy, G.M., and Dowling, R.H. Measurement of faecal bile acid sulphates. J. Chromatogr. 182:293-300, 1980.

b Poley, J.R., Dower, J.C., Owen, C.A., Jr., and Stickler, G.B. Bile acids in infants and children. J. Lab. Clin. Med 63:838-846, 1964.

c Poley, J.R. Fat digestion and absorption in lipase and bile acid deficiency. In Lipid Absorption: Biochemical and Clinical Aspects. K Rommel, H Goebell, R Bohmer, eds. Medical and Technical Publishing, Co. Ltd., Lancaster, 1976, pp 151-202.

d Poley, J.R. and Hofmann, A.F. Role of fat maldigestion in pathogenesis of steatorrhea in ileal resection. Fat digestion after two sequential test meals with and without cholestyramine. Gastroenterology 71:38-44, 1976.

e Poliakova, E.D., Vasileva, L.E., Denisenko, T.V., Dizhe, E.B., Klimova, T.A., Petrova, L.A., and Klimov, A.N. Biosynthesis of cholic and chenodeoxycholic acids from (1-^{14}C) acetyl-CoA and (2-^{14}C) malonyl-CoA in a reconstituted system from the rat liver. Biokhimiia 46:462-472, 1981.

f Polli, E., Inter-Hospital Clinical Research Group (GRRC). The effect of ursodeoxycholic acid (UDCA) on "dyspepsia" in patients with gallstones or other biliary tract anomalies. Curr. Therap. Res. 26:230-233, 1979.

g Polli, E.E., Bianchi, P.A., Conte, D., and Sironi, L. Treatment of radiolucent gallstones with CDCA or UDCA: A multicenter trial. Digestion 22: 185-191, 1981.

h Polonovski, M. and Bourrillon, R. Etude sur la composition des biles dans la serie animale. Bull. Soc. Chim. Biol. 34:703-711, 1952.

i Polonovski, M. and Bourrillon, R. Les Phospholipides de la Bile. Bull. Soc. Chim. Biol. 34:712-719, 1952.

j Polter, D.E., Boyle, J.D., Miller, L.G., and Finegold, S.M. Anaerobic bacteria as cause of the blind loop syndrome: A case with observations on response to antibacterial agents. Gastroenterology 54:1148-1154, 1968.

k Pomare, E.W. and Heaton, K.W. Increased bacterial degradation of bile salts in cholecystectomized subject. Gut 13:321-327, 1972.

l Pomare, E.W. and Heaton, K.W. Alteration of bile salt metabolism by dietary fibre (bran). Brit. Med. J. 4:262-264, 1973.

m Pomare, E.W. and Heaton, K.W. Bile salt metabolism in patients with gallstones in functioning gallbladders. Gut 14:885-890, 1973.

n Pomare, E.W. and Heaton, K.W. The effect of cholecystectomy on bile salt metabolism. Gut 14:753-762, 1973.

o Pomare, E.W. and Low-Beer, T.S. Measurement and validation of human bile salt pool size and synthesis. Clin. Chim. Acta 57:239-248, 1974.

a Pomare, E.W. and Low-Beer, T.S. Selective suppression of chenodeoxycholate synthesis by cholate metabolites in man. Clin. Sci. Mol. Med. 48:315-321, 1975.

b Pomare, E.W., Low-Beer, T.S., and Heaton, K.W. The effect of wheat-bran on bile salt metabolism and bile composition. In Advances in Bile Acid Research. S Matern, J Hackenschmidt, P Back, and W Gerok, eds. F.K. Schattauer Verlag, Stuttgart-New York, 1975, pp 355-360.

c Pomare, E.W., Heaton, K.W., Low-Beer, T.S., and Espiner, H.J. The effect of wheat bran upon bile salt metabolism and upon the lipid composition of bile in gallstone patients. Am. J. Dig. Dis. 21:521-526, 1976.

d Poncelet, P.R. and Thompson, A.G. Role of infected bile in spasm of the sphincter of Oddi. Am. J. Surg. 126:387-391, 1973.

e Ponz de Leon, M., Carulli, N., Loria, P., Iori, R., and Zironi, F. The effect of chenodeoxycholic acid (CDCA) on cholesterol absorption. Gastroenterology 77:223-230, 1979.

f Ponz de Leon, M., Carulli, N., Zironi, F., Loria, P., and Iori, R. Cholesterol absorption during bile acid feeding in man: The effect of urso-deoxycholic acid (UDCA) and cholic acid (CA). Gut 20:A930, 1979 (abstract).

g Ponz de Leon, M. and Carulli, N. How does bile acid feeding regulate cholesterol entry into bile? Gastroenterology 78:425-426, 1980.

h Ponz de Leon, M., Carulli, N., Iori, R., Loria, P., Smerieri, A., and Zironi, F. Medical treatment of radiolucent gallstones with chenodeoxycholic acid (CDCA): Follow-up report at four years. Ital. J. Gastroenterol. 12:17-22, 1980.

i Ponz de Leon, M., Carulli, N., Loria, P., Iori, R., and Zironi, F. Cholesterol absorption during bile acid feeding. Effect of ursodeoxycholic acid (UDCA) administration. Gastroenterology 78:214-219, 1980.

j Ponz de Leon, M., Carulli, N., Loria, P., Romano, G., and Zironi, F. Effect of chenodeoxycholic acid (CDCA) and ursodeoxycholic acid (UDCA) on cholesterol absorption in man. Ital. J. Gastroenterol. 12:222, 1980.

k Ponz de Leon, M., Loria, P., Carulli, N., Murphy, G., and Dowling, R.H. Intestinal solubilization, absorption, pharmacokinetics and bioavailability of chenodeoxycholic acid. Europ. J. Clin. Invest. 10:261-271, 1980.

l Ponz de Leon, M. and Carulli, N. The influence of bile acid pool composition on the regulation of cholesterol absorption. In Bile Acids and Lipids. G Paumgartner, A Stiehl, and W Gerok, eds. MTP Press, Lancaster, 1981, pp 133-140.

m Ponz de Leon, M., Carulli, N., Loria, P., Iori, R., Romani, M., and Piccagli, I. Effect of deoxycholic (DCA) and cholic acid (CA) pool expansion on dietary cholesterol absorption and bile saturation in man. Ital. J. Gastroenterol. 13:293-294, 1981 (abstract).

a Pope, J.L., Parkinson, T.M., and Olson, J.A. Action of bile salts on the metabolism and transport of water-soluble nutrients by perfused rat jejunum in vitro. Biochim. Biophys. Acta 130:218-232, 1966.

b Popper, H. and Schaffner, F. Pathophysiology of cholestasis. Human Path. 1:1-24, 1970.

c Popper, H. Gallensauren und Cholestase. Leber, Magen, Darm 2:205-207, 1972.

d Porter, H.P. and Saunders, D.R. Isolation of the aqueous phase of human intestinal content during the digestion of a fatty meal. Gastroenterology 60:997-1007, 1971.

e Porter, H.P., Saunders, D.R., Tytgat, G., Brunser, O., and Rubin, C.E. Fat absorption in bile fistula man: A morphological and biochemical study. Gastroenterology 60:1008-1019, 1971.

f Porterfield, G., Cheung, L.Y., and Berenson, M. Detection of occult gallbladder disease by duodenal drainage. Am. J. Surg. 134:702-704, 1977.

g Portman, O.W. and Mann, G.V. The disposition of taurine-S^{35}- and taurocholate-S^{35} in the rat: Dietary influence. J. Biol. Chem. 213:733-734, 1955.

h Portman, O.W. Further studies of the intestinal degradation products of cholic acid-24-C^{14} in rats: Formation of deoxycholic acid. Arch. Biochem. Biophys. 78:125-137, 1958.

i Portman, O.W. and Murphy, P. Bile acid-lipoprotein relationships using cholic acid-24-C^{14}. Am. J. Physiol. 195:189-193, 1958.

j Portman, O.W. and Murphy, P. Excretion of bile acids and b-hydroxy sterols by rats. Arch. Biochem. Biophys. 76:367-376, 1958.

k Portman, O.W. Nutritional influences on the metabolism of bile acids. Am. J. Clin. Nutr. 8:462, 1960.

l Portman, O.W. and Bruno, D. Various natural and modified bile acids in cholesterol metabolism. J. Nutr. 73:329, 1961.

m Portman, O.W. Importance of diet, species, and intestinal flora in bile acid metabolism. Fed. Proc. 21:896-902, 1962.

n Portman, O.W. and Shah, S. The determination of concentrations of bile acids in peripheral, portal and hepatic blood of Cebus monkeys. Arch. Biochem. Biophys. 96:516, 1962 (abstract).

o Portman, O.W., Shah, S., Antonis, A., and Jorgensen, B. Alterations of bile salts by bacteria. Proc. Soc. Exptl. Biol. Med. 109:959, 1962.

p Portman, O., Osuga, T., and Tanaka, N. Biliary lipids and cholesterol gallstone formation. Adv. Lipid Res. 13:135-193, 1975.

a Portman, O., Alexander, M., Tanaka, N., and Osuga, T. Role of diet in normal biliary physiology and gallstone formation. In Primates in Nutritional Research, Academic Press, New York, 1979, pp 140-180.

b Portman, O., Alexander, M., Tanaka, N., and Osuga, T. Relationships between cholesterol gallstones, biliary function, and plasma lipoproteins in Squirrel monkeys. Oregon Regional Primate Research Center publication no. 1078.

c Poulsen, H. and Christoffersen, P. Abnormal bile duct epithelium in liver biopsies with histological signs of viral hepatitis. Acta Path. Microbiol. Scand. 76:383-390, 1969.

d Poupon, O., Poupon, R., Grosdemouge, M.L., Dumont, M., and Erlinger, S. Influence of bile acids upon biliary cholesterol and phospholipid secretion in the dog. Europ. J. Clin. Invest. 6:279-284, 1976.

e Poupon, R., Poupon, R., Dumont, M., and Erlinger, S. Hepatic storage and biliary transport maximum of taurocholate and taurochenodeoxycholate in the dog. Europ. J. Clin. Invest. 6:431-437, 1976.

f Poupon, R.E., Poupon, R.Y., Duval, M., LeQuernec, L., and Erlinger, S. Chronic administration of chenodeoxycholic acid increases cholesterol saturation in bile in the dog. Europ. J. Clin. Invest. 9:103-105, 1979.

g Poupon, R.Y., et al. Acides biliares seriques et disparition de l'acide cholique au cours des maladies du foie d'origine aloolique. Gastroenterol. Clin. Biol. 2:475-480, 1978.

h Powell, G.K., Jones, L.A., and Richardson, J. A new syndrome of bile acid deficiency - A possible synthetic defect. J. Pediat. 83:758-766, 1973.

i Pradalier, A., Dry, J., and Luce, H. Essai de prevention de la migraine commune par l'acide chenodesoxycholique. La Nouv. Presse Med. 10:180, 1981 (abstract).

j Prakongpan, S., Higuchi, W.I., Kwan, K.H., and Molokhia, A.M. Dissolution rate studies of cholesterol monohydrate in bile acid-lecithin solutions using the rotating disk method. J. Pharm. Sci. 65:685, 1976.

k Prandi, D., Erlinger, S., Glasinovic, J.C., and Dumont, M. Canalicular bile production in man. Europ. J. Clin. Invest. 5:1-6, 1975.

l Prange, I., Christensen, F., and Dam, H. Alimentary production of gallstones in hamsters. J. Nutr. Sci. 3:59-78, 1962-1963.

m Prange, I. and Dam, H. Alimentary production of gallstones in hamsters. 23. Influence of hydrogenated palm oil and hydrogenated palm oil in mixture with sunflower seed oil on the ratio between lipid-soluble phosphorus and cholesterol in the bladder bile. Z. Ernahr. 10:303-307, 1971.

a Prange, I., Sondergaard, E., and Dam, H. Alimentary production of gallstones in hamsters. 26. The influence of orally ingested lithocholic, cholic, dehydrocholic and deoxycholic acids on gallstone production compared with the influence of chenodeoxycholic acid. Z. Ernahr. 12:92-107, 1973.

b Preisig, R., Cooper, H.L., and Wheeler, H.O. The relationship between taurocholate secretion rate and bile production in the unanesthetized dog during cholinergic blockade and during secretin administration. J. Clin. Invest. 41:1152-1162, 1962.

c Preisig, R., Halter, F., and Bircher, J. Neue Aspekte in der Behandlung von Cholezysto- und Choledocholithiasis. Schweiz. med. Wschr. 111:297-302, 1981.

d Prentice, R.T.W. Dissolution of gallstones. Lancet 2:1230, 1981 (letter).

e Pribam, B.O.C. Method for dissolution of common duct stones remaining after operation. Surgery 22:806-817, 1947.

f Pribam, B.O.C. Ether treatment of retained postoperative biliary tree stones. Acta Chir. Scand. 116:437, 1959.

g Pries, J.M., Sherman, C.A., Williams, G.C., and Hanson, R.F. The fractional hepatic extraction of cholic acid conjugates in the conscious dog. Gastroenterology 73:1240, 1977 (abstract).

h Pries, J.M., Sherman, C.A., Williams, G.C., and Hanson, R.F. Hepatic extraction of bile salts in conscious dog. Am. J. Physiol. 236:E191-E197, 1979.

i Priestly, B.G., Cote, M.G., and Plaa, G.L. Biochemical and morphological parameters of taurolithocholate-induced cholestasis. Canad. J. Physiol. Pharmacol. 49:1078-1091, 1971.

j Probstein, J.G. and Eckert, C.T. Injection of ether into the biliary tract as treatment for choledocholithiasis. Arch. Surg. 35:258, 1937.

k Quarfordt, S.H. and Greenfield, M.F. Estimation of cholesterol and bile acid turnover in man by kinetic analysis. J. Clin. Invest. 52:1937-1945, 1973.

l Quarfordt, S.H., Oelschlaeger, H., Krigbaum, W.R., Jakoi, L., and Davis, R. Effect of biliary obstruction on canine plasma and biliary lipids. Lipids 8:522-530, 1973.

m Quintao, E., Grundy, S.M., and Ahrens, E.H., Jr. Effects of dietary cholesterol on the regulation of total body cholesterol in man. J. Lipid Res. 12:233-247, 1971.

n Rachmilewitz, D. and Saunders, D.R. Metabolism of chenodeoxycholate by intestinal mucosa. Gastroenterology 71:82-86, 1976.

a Raedsch, R. and Stiehl, A. Zunehmende Sulfatierungen der Lithocholsaure nach Chenodesoxycholsaurebehandlung. 80. Tagung der Dtsch. Ges. Inn. Med., Wiesbaden, April, 1974 (abstract).

b Raedsch, R., Hofmann, A.F., and Tserng, K-Y. Separation of individual sulfated bile acid conjugates as calcium complexes using reversed-phase partition thin-layer chromatography. J. Lipid Res. 20:796-800, 1979.

c Raedsch, R., Stiehl, A., and Cyzgan, P. Ursodeoxycholic acid and gallstone calcification. Lancet 2:1296, 1981 (Letter to editor).

d Raedsch, R., Stiehl, A., Czygan, P., Gotz, R., Manner, Ch., Walker, S., and Kommerell, B. Increased glycine conjugation of biliary bile acids during treatment of gallstone patients with chenodeoxycholic acid or ursodeoxycholic acid: effects on biliary cholesterol saturation. In Bile Acids and Lipids. G Paumgartner, A Stiehl, and W Gerok, eds. MTP Press, Lancaster, 1981, pp 195-202.

e Raedsch, R., Stiehl, A., Gotz, R., Walker, S., and Kommerell, B. Kinetics of cholesterol gallstone dissolution by glycocheno-, glycoursodeoxycholic acid, and mixtures of both in vitro. Z. Gastroenterol. 19:159-163, 1981.

f Raha, P.K., Sengupta, K.P., and Aikat, B.K. Chronic cholecystitis and cholelithiasis: An experimental study. Indian J. Med. Res. 59:873-879, 1971.

g Rahban, S., Bonorris, G.G., Marks, J.W., Chung, A., and Schoenfield, L.J. The effect of dihydroxy bile acids on intestinal secretion, cyclic nucleotides, and Na^+,K^+ ATPase. Am. J. Med. Sci. 279:141-146, 1980.

h Raicht, R.F., Cohen, B.I., and Mosbach, E.H. Effects of sodium taurochenodeoxycholate and sodium taurocholate on cholesterol absorption in the rat. Gastroenterology 67:1155-1161, 1974.

i Raicht, R.F., Cohen, B.I., Eliav, B., Mosbach, E., and Zimmon, D. Effect of a hydrocholeretic agent (zanchol) on sterol metabolism in rats. Gastroenterology 72:507-509, 1977.

j Raicht, R.F., Cohen, B.I., Sarwal, A., and Takahashi, M. Ursodeoxycholic acid. Effects on sterol metabolism in rats. Biochim. Biophys. Acta 531:1-8, 1978.

k Rajagopalan, N. and Lindenbaum, S. The binding of Ca^{2+} to taurine- and glycine-conjugated bile salt micelles. Biochim. Biophys. Acta 711:66-74, 1982.

l Ranajit, P. and Balaram, P. A fluorescent probe study of the solubilization of cholesterol by bile salt-phospholipid micelles. BBRC 81:850-857, 1978.

m Rask-Madsen, J., Kamper, J., and Krag, E. The influence of bile acids on epithelial transport mechanisms illustrated by ileal perfusion in a patient with congenital chloridorrhea. Scand. J. Gastroenterol. 10:31-32, 1975.

a Rask-Madsen, J., Kamper, J., Oddsson, E., and Krag, E. Congenital chloridorrhoea. A question of reversed brush border processes and varying junctional tightness? Scand. J. Gastroenterol. 11:377, 1976.

b Rauen, H.M., Schriewer, H., Gebauer, B., Abu Tair, M., Ruther, N., and The, L.G. Die hepatotoxische Wirkung von Desoxycholat. Ein Modell der multivariaten Analyse experimentaller Leberschadigungen. Arzneimittel-Forschung 23:127-133, 1973.

c Rautureau, J. La lithiase biliaire. Mecanismes physiopathologiques. Nouv. Presse Med. 1:1553-1555, 1972.

d Rautureau, J., Rautureau, M., and Coste, T. Acid chenodeoxycholique Donnees biologiques. M.C.D. 4(Suppl 1):7-11, 1975.

e Rautureau, J. Medical treatment of biliary lithiasis with chendeoxycholic acid. Nouv. Presse Med. 6:20-21, 1977.

f Rautureau, J. Calculi recurrence after stopping chenic acid treatment. Med. Chir. Dig. 7:352-353, 1978.

g Rautureau, M. and Rautureau, J. Les acides et les sels biliaires. Arch. Fran. Mal. App. Dig. 60:445-462, 1971.

h Rautureau, M., Coste, Th., Rautureau, J., Paraf, A., and Gouffier, E. Lithiase biliaire et court circuit intestinal. Dosages des acides biliaires dans la bile, le sang peripherique et le sang portal. Arch. Fran. Mal. App. Dig. 63:401-406, 1974.

i Realini, S., Reiner, M., and Frigerio, G. Le traitment des troubles dyspeptiques de la lithiase et de la dyscinesie biliaires avec l'acide ursodesoxycholique. Schweiz. Med. Wschr. 110:879-880, 1980.

j Reddy, B.S., Watanabe, K., Weisburger, J.H., and Wynder, E.L. Promoting effect of bile acids in colon carcinogenesis in germ-free and conventional F344 rats. Cancer Research 37:3238-3242, 1977.

k Reddy, B.S. and Wynder, E.L. Metabolic epidemiology of colon cancer. Fecal bile acids and neutral sterols in colon cancer patients and patients with adenomatous polyps. Cancer 39:2533-2539, 1977.

l Reddy, B.S. and Watanabe, K. Effect of cholesterol metabolites and promoting effect of lithocholic acid in colon carcinogenesis in germ-free and conventional F344 rats. Cancer Res. 39:1521-1524, 1979.

m Reddy, B.S. Diet and excretion of bile acids. Cancer Res. 41:3766-3768, 1981.

n Redgrave, T.G. The absorption of micellar lipid into the lymph of unanaesthetised rats. Quart. J. Exptl. Phys. 52:130, 1967.

o Redinger, R.N. and Small, D.M. Bile composition, bile salt metabolism and gallstones. Arch. Intern. Med. 130:618-630, 1972.

a Redinger, R.N., Hermann, A.H., and Small, D.M. Primate biliary physiology X. Effects of diet and fasting on biliary lipid secretion and relative composition and bile salt metabolism in the Rhesus monkey. Gastroenterology 64:610-621, 1973 (Letter to Editor).

b Redinger, R.N. and Small, D.M. Primate biliary physiology. VIII. The effects of phenobarbital upon bile salt synthesis and pool size, biliary lipid secretion and bile composition. J. Clin. Invest. 52:161-172, 1973.

c Redinger, R.N., Strasberg, S.M., and Small, D.M. Effects of acute biliary obstruction on biliary lipid metabolism in the monkey. Am. J. Physiol. 226:676-683, 1974.

d Redinger, R.N. Cholelithiasis. Review of advances in research. Postgrad. Med. 65:56-62, 1979.

e Redinger, R.N. The effects of phenobarbital on biliary lipid metabolism in cholesterol gallstone subjects. Lipids 14:277-284, 1979.

f Rees, W. and Rhodes, J. Bile reflux in gastro-oesophageal disease. Clin. Gastroenterol. 6:179-200, 1977.

g Reichen, J. and Paumgartner, G. Kinetics of taurocholate uptake by the perfused rat liver. Gastroenterology 68:132-136, 1975.

h Reichen, J., Messerli, J., and Paumgartner, G. Decreased Na^+ -K^+-ATPase activity in canalicular plasma membranes of cholestatic rat liver. Experientia 32:760, 1976 (abstract).

i Reichen, J. and Paumgartner, G. Decreased canalicular Na^+ -K^+-ATPase activity in taurolithocholate-induced cholestasis in the rat. Digestion 14:542, 1976 (abstract).

j Reichen, J. and Paumgartner, G. Uptake of bile acids by perfused rat liver. Am. J. Physiol. 231:734-742, 1976.

k Reichen, J., Preisig, R., and Paumgartner, G. Influence of chemical structure on hepatocellular uptake of bile acids. In Bile Acid Metabolism in Health and Disease. G Paumgartner and A Stiehl, eds. MTP Press, Ltd., Lancaster, 1977, pp 113-123.

l Reichen, J. and Paumgartner, G. Inhibition of hepatic Na^+, K^+-adenosinetriphosphatase in taurolithocholate-induced cholestasis in the rat. Experientia 35:1186-1188, 1979.

m Reid, J.M., Fullmer, S.D., Pettigrew, K.D., Burch, T.A., Bennett, P.H., Miller, M., and Whedon, G.D. Nutrient intake of Pima Indian women: Relationships to diabetes mellitus and gallbladder disease. Am. J. Clin. Nutr. 24:1281-1289, 1971.

n Reinhold, J.G. and Wilson, D.R. The acid-base composition of hepatic bile. III. The effects of sodium cholate and sodium dehydrocholate (decholin). Am. J. Physiol. 107:400-405, 1934.

a Reiser, R. Serum cholesterol levels and faecal bile acids as altered by the development of intestinal flora in previously germ-free swine. Fed. Proc. 30:348, 1971.

b Reiss-Husson, F. and Luzzati, V. Phase transitions in lipids in relation to the structure of membranes. Adv. Biol. Med. Phys. 11:87-107, 1967.

c Reuben, A. and Dowling, R.H. Does obesity complicate chenodeoxycholic acid (CDCA) threatment of gallstones. Gut 19:A452, 1978.

d Reuben, A., Murphy, G.M., and Dowling, R.H. Factors influencing the bioavailability of chenodeoxycholic acid. Clin. Sci. & Mol. Med. 54:15p, 1978 (abstract).

e Reunanen, A. Treatment of gallstones by dissolution. Duodecim. 89:1357-1359, 1973.

f Rewbridge, A.G. The disappearance of gallstone shadows following the prolonged administration of bile salts. Surgery 1:395-400, 1937.

g Reynier, M., Sireix, R., Calba, A., and Mariaud, J.F. Action des acids cholaniques et du cholesterol sur l'activite de l'isoenzyme-L-phenylalanine-sensible de la phosphatase alcaline serique. Clin. Chim. Acta 46:311-319, 1973.

h Reynier, M.O., Marteau, C.H., Vigne, J.L., Mule, A., Crotte, C., and Gerolami, A. Action of three bile acids on hepatic and intestinal cholesterogenesis in the rat. Lipids 12:254-257, 1977.

i Reynier, M.O., Montet, J-C., Crotte, C., Marteau, C., and Gerolami, A. Cholesterol absorption from mixed micelles. In vitro effects of taurocholate (TC), taurochenodeoxycholate (TCDC) and tauroursodeoxycholate (TUDC). VI Internat'l Bile Acid Meeting, Freiburg, 1980, pp 85 (abstract).

j Reynier, M.O, Montet, J.C., Crotte, C., Marteau, C., and Gerolami, A. Intestinal cholesterol uptake from mixed micelles. In vitro effects of taurocholate, taurochenodeoxycholate and tauroursodeoxycholate. Biochim. Biophys. Acta 664:616-619, 1981.

k Reynier, M.O., Montet, J.C., Gerolami, A., Marteau, C., Crotte, C., Montet, A.M., and Mathieu, S. Comparative effects of cholic, chenodeoxycholic and ursodeoxycholic acids on micellar solubilization and intestinal absorption of cholesterol. J. Lipid Res. 22:467-473, 1981.

l Rhodes, J., Barnardo, D.E., Phillips, S.F., Rovelstad, R.A., and Hofmann, A.F. Increased reflux of bile into the stomach in patients with gastric ulcer. Gastroenterology 57:241-252, 1969.

m Rice, P.L., Stanley, M.M., Greenlee, H.B., Gacke, D., and Murphy, J. Studies of bile acid kinetics from percutaneously aspirated gallbladder bile in the dog with subcutaneous cholecystopexy. Clin. Res. 24:434A, 1976 (abstract).

a Rich, A. and Blow, D.M. Formation of a helical steroid complex. Nature 182:423-426, 1958.

b Richardson, J.D., Southfield, F.D., Proudfoot, W.H., and Benenson, A.S. Epidemiology of gallbladder disease in an Appalachian community. Health Service Reports 88:241-246, 1973.

c Riemann, J.F. Internist therapy of cholelithiasis. Fortschr. Med. 99: 755-760, 1981.

d Ripatti, P.O. and Sidorov, V.S. Quantitative composition of vertebrate bile acids in relation to the nature of their nutrition. Dokl. Akad. Nauk. USSR 212:770-773, 1973 (Russ).

e Robins, S.J. and Fasulo, J. Mechanism of lithogenic bile production: Studies in the hamster fed an essential fatty acid-deficient diet. Gastroenterology 65:104-114, 1973.

f Roda, A., Aldini, R., Festi, D., Mazzella, G., Sama, C., Roda, E., and Barbara, L. Diurnal variations of serum levels of conjugated primary bile acids in normal and hepatobiliary patients. Rendic. Gastroenterol. 9:234, 1977 (abstract).

g Roda, A., Roda, E., Festi, D., Sama, C., Mazzella, G., Aldini, R., and Barbara, L. A radioimmunoassay of primary bile acid conjugates in human serum. La Riccerca Clin. Lab. 7:163-178, 1977.

h Roda, A., Bazzoli, F., Petronelli, A., Aldini, R., Festi, D., and Frabboni, R. Intestinal cholesterol absorption during CDCA and UDCA administration in man. VI Internat'l Bile Acid Meeting, Freiburg, 1980, pp 128 (abstract).

i Roda, A., Roda, E., Sama, C., Festi, D., Aldini, R., Morselli, A.M., Mazzella, G., and Barbara, L. Serum primary bile acids in Gilbert's syndrome. Gastroenterology 82:77-83, 1982.

j Roda, E., Festi, D., Roda, A., Sama, C., Aldini, R., and Mazzella, G. Results of chenic acid therapy in patients with cholesterol calculi. Min. Med. 68:3027-3029, 1977.

k Roda, E., Roda, E., Aldini, R., Festi, D., Mazzella, G., Sama, C., and Barbara, L. Development, validation and application of a single-tube radioimmunoassay for cholic and chenodeoxycholic conjugated bile acids in human serum. Clin. Chem. 23:2107-2113, 1977.

l Roda, E., Aldini, R., Mazzella, G., Roda, A., Sama, C., Festi, D., and Barbara, L. Enterohepatic circulation of bile acids after cholecystectomy. Gut 19:640-649, a978.

m Roda, E., Roda, A., Sama, C., Festi, D., Mazzella, G., Aldini, R., and Barbara, L. Effect of ursodeoxycholic acid adminstration on biliary lipid composition and bile acid kinetics in cholesterol gallstone patients. Am. J. Dig. Dis. 24:123-128, 1979.

a Roda, E., Mazzella, G., Roda, A., Aldini, R., Sama, C., Festi, D., Morselli, A., and Barbara, L. Lithocholic acid metabolism before and after chenodeoxycholic acid therapy in gallstone patients. Ital. J. Gastroenterol. 12:171-176, 1980.

b Roda, E., Mazzella, G., Roda, A., Morselli, A., Mastroroberto, L., Rossi, R., Petronelli, A., and Barbara, L. Bile lipid secretion rate during ursodeoxycholic acid treatment. VII International Symposium on Drugs Affecting Lipid Metabolism, 1980.

c Roda, E., Mazzella, G., Roda, A., Bazzoli, F., Messale, E., Morselli, A.M., Festi, D., Aldini, R., and Barbara, L. Effect of chenodeoxycholic acid and ursodeoxycholic acid administration on biliary lipid secretion in normal weight and obese gallstone patients. In Bile Acids and Lipids. G Paumgartner, A Stiehl, W Gerok, eds. MTP Press, Lancaster, 1981, pp 189-193.

d Rodgers, J.B., O'Brien, R.J., and Balint, J.A. The absorption and subsequent utilization of lecithin by the rat jejunum. Am. J. Dig. Dis. 20:208-213, 1975.

e Roepke, R.R. and Mason, H.L. Micelle formation in aqueous solutions of bile salts. J. Biol. Chem. 133:103-108, 1940.

f Roller, R.J. and Kern, F., Jr. Minimal bile acid malabsorption and normal bile acid breath tests in cystic fibrosis and acquired pancreatic insufficiency. Gastroenterology 72:661-665, 1977.

g Ros, E., Small, D., and Carey, M. Effects of chlorpromazine hydrochloride on bile salt synthesis, bile formation and biliary lipid secretion in the Rhesus monkey: a model for chlorpromazine-induced cholestasis. Europ. J. Clin. Invest. 9:29-41, 1979.

h Rosato, E.F. and Rosato, F.E. Chenodeoxycholic acid: Problem of small stones. N. Engl. J. Med. 290:404-405, 1974 (Letter to Editor).

i Rose, G., Blackburn, H., Keys, A., Taylor, H.L., Kannel, W.B., Paul, O., Reid, D.D., and Stamler, J. Colon cancer and blood-cholesterol. Lancet 1:181-183, 1974.

j Roslyn, J., DenBesten, L., Thompson, J., and Cohen, K. Chronic cholelithiasis and decreased bile salt pool size. Cause or effect? Am. J. Surg. 139:119-124, 1980.

k Ross, J.K. and Leklem, J.E. The effect of dietary citrus pectin on the excretion of human fecal neutral and acid steroids and the activity of 7a-dehydroxylase and b-glucuronidase. Am. J. Clin. Nutr. 34:2068-2077, 1981.

l Ross, P.E., Pennington, C.R., and Bouchier, I.A.D. Gas-liquid chromatographic assay of serum bile acids. Anal. Biochem. 80:458-465, 1977.

m Rotstein, O.D., Kay, R.M., Wayman, M., and Strasberg, S.M. Prevention of cholesterol gallstones by lignin and lactulose in the hamster. Gastroenterology 81:1098-1103, 1981.

a Roullet-Audy, J.C. and Guivarch, M. Therapeutic indications in biliary calculi. Med. Chir. Dig. 7:361-365, 1978.

b Rowe, G.G. Control of tenesmus and diarrhea by cholestyramine administration. Am. J. Med. Sci. 255:84-88, 1968.

c Roze, C. Pharmacologie de l'acide chenodesoxycholique chez l'homme. Therapie 32:393-400, 1977.

d Ruben, ATh. and van Berge-Henegouwen, G.P. A simple reverse-phase high pressure liquid chromatographic determination of conjugated bile acids in serum and bile using a novel radial compression separation system. Clin. Chim. Acta 119:41-50, 1982.

e Rubulis, A., Basantani, G.K., Flood, M.S., and Faloon, W.W. Fecal lipid, bile acid and sterol following ileojejunostomy: Excretory patterns and influence of metronidazole. Gastroenterology 68:976, 1975 (abstract).

f Rudman, D. and Kendall, F.E. Bile acid content of human serum. I. Serum bile acids in patients with hepatic disease. J. Clin. Invest. 36:530-537, 1957.

g Rudman, D. and Kendall, F.E. Bile acid content of human serum. II. The binding of cholanic acids by human plasma proteins. J. Clin. Invest. 36:538-542, 1957.

h Ruppin, D.C. and Dowling, R.H. Is recurrence inevitable after gallstone dissolution by bile-acid treatment? Lancet 1:181-185, 1982.

i Ruppin, D.C. and Dowling, R.H. Is recurrence inevitable on withdrawing treatment after complete dissolution with chenodeoxycholic (CDC) and ursodeoxycholic (UDC) acids? Gut 22:432A, 1981 (abstract).

j Russell, R.I. Clinical aspects of alterations in bile acid metabolism. The wrong bile acids in the wrong place. Scot. Med. J. 18:146-151, 1973.

k Russell, R.I., Allan, J.G., Gerskowitch, V.P., and Cochran, K.M. The effect of conjugated and unconjugated bile acids on water and electrolyte absorption in the human jejunum. Clin. Sci. Mol. Med. 45:301-311, 1973.

l Sachatello, C.R., Hedgecock, H. Jr., and Armstrong, A. What can experimental colorectal cancer tell us about colorectal cancer in man? Dis. Colon Rectum 23:80-85, 1980.

m Sackett, D.L. Laboratory screening: A critique. Fed. Proc. 34:2157-2165, 1975.

n Sacquet, E.C., van Hajenoort, Y., Riottot, M., and Leprince, C. Action of microbial flora of the digestive tract on the metabolism of bile acids in the rat. Biochim. Biophys. Acta 380:52-65, 1975.

o Sacquet, E.C., Raibaud, P.M., Mejean, C., Riottot, M.J., Leprince, C., and Leglise, P.C. Bacterial formation of w-muricholic acid in rats. Appl. & Envtl. Microbiol. 37:1127-1131, 1979.

a Safrany, L. Duodenoscopic sphincterotomy and gallstone removal. Gastroenterology 72:338-343, 1977.

b Saint Clair, R.W., Henderson, G.R., Heaster, V., Wagner, W.D., Bond, M.G., and McMahan, M.R. Influence of dietary fat and an oral contraceptive on plasma lipids, high density lipoproteins, gallstones, and atherosclerosis in African green monkeys. Atherosclerosis 37:103-121, 1980.

c Salen, G., Ahrens, E.H., Jr., and Grundy, S.M. The metabolism of b-sitosterol in man. J. Clin. Invest. 49:952-967, 1970.

d Salen, G. and Polito, A. Biosynthesis of 5a-cholestan-3b-ol in cerebrotendinous xanthomatosis. J. Clin. Invest. 51:134-140, 1972.

e Salen, G., Dyrszka, H., Chen, T., Saltzman, W.H., and Mosbach, E.H. Toxicity of chenodeoxycholic acid in Rhesus monkeys. Lancet 2:1517-1518, 1974.

f Salen, G., Tint, G.S., Eliav, B., Deering, N., and Mosbach, E.H. Increased formation of ursodeoxycholic acid in patients treated with chenodeoxycholic acid. J. Clin. Invest. 53:612-621, 1974.

g Salen, G., Dyrszka, H., Chen, T., Saltzman, W.H., and Mosbach, E.H. Prevention of chenodeoxycholic acid toxicity with Lincomycin. Lancet 1:1082, 1975 (Letter to Editor).

h Salen, G., Meriwether, T.W., and Nicolau, G. Chenodeoxycholic acid inhibits increased cholesterol and cholestanol synthesis in patients with cerebrotendinous xanthomatosis. Biochem. Med. 14:57-64, 1975.

i Salen, G., Nicolau, G., Shefer, S., and Mosbach, E.H. Hepatic cholesterol metabolism in patients with gallstones. Gastroenterology 69:676-684, 1975.

j Salen, G., Shefer, S., Zaki, F.G., and Mosbach, E.H. Inborn errors of bile acid synthesis. Clin. Gastroenterol. 6:91-101, 1977.

k Salen, G., Fedorowski, T., Colalillo, A., Tint, G.S., and Mosbach, E.H. The metabolism of ursodeoxycholic acid in man. In Bile Acid Metabolism in Health and Disease. G Paumgartner, A Stiehl, eds. MTP Press, Lancaster, 1979, pp 167-172.

l Salen, G., Shefer, S., Mosbach, E., Hauser, S., Cohen, B., and Nicolau, G. Metabolism of potential precursors of chenodeoxycholic acid in cerebrotendinous xanthomatosis. J. Lipid Res. 20:22-30, 1979.

m Salen, G., Colalillo, A., Verga, D., Bagan, E., Tint, G., and Shefer, S. Effect of high and low doses of ursodeoxycholic acid on gallstone dissolution in humans. Gastroenterology 78:1412-1418, 1980.

n Salen, G., Tint, G.S., Verga, D., and Shefer, S. The metabolism of 7-ketolithocholic acid in man. In Bile Acid and Lipids. G Paumgartner, A Stiehl, and W Gerok, eds. MTP Press, Lancaster, 1981, pp 97-101.

a Sali, A. and Iser, J. The non-operative management of gallstones. Aust. N. Z. J. Surg. 48:484-488, 1978.

b Sallee, V.L. Apparent monomer activity of saturated fatty acids in micellar bile salt solutions measured by a polyethylene partitioning system. J. Lipid Res. 15:56-64, 1974.

c Salvioli, G., Lugli, R., Salati, R., Valeria Beldelli, M. Gli Acidi Biliari nel siero e nelle urine in soggetti con colestasi. Il Fegato 20:387-402, 1974.

d Salvioli, G. and Salati, R. Faecal bile acid loss and bile acid pool size during short-term treatment with ursodeoxycholic acid and chenodeoxycholic acid in patients with radiolucent gallstones. Gut 20:698-704, 1979.

e Salvioli, G., Salati, R., and Fratalocchi, A. Eliminazione fecale e pool degli acidi billiari in corso di somministrazione di acido chenico (CDCA) e ursodesossicolico (UDCA). Ital. J. Gastroenterol. 2(Supple.):49, 1979.

f Salvioli, G., Salati, R., Fratalocchi, A., and Lugli, R. Ursodeoxycholic acid therapy for radiolucent gallstone dissolution. Curr. Therap. Res. 26:995-1004, 1979.

g Salvioli, G. and Carey, M.C. In vitro perfusion system to study membrane dissolution by bile salts: Differential detergent effects of taurocheno deoxycholate (UCDC) and tauroursodeoxycholate (TUDC) on lecithin and cholesterol 'secretion'. 16th Meeting of the EASL, Lisbon, 1981 (abstract).

h Salvioli, G., Igimi, H., and Carey, M. Crystalline cholesterol monohydrate (ChM) dissolves in 'urso'-rich bile by both liquid crystalline and micellar mechanisms: A phase equilibria explanation and possible clinical relevance. Gastroenterology 80:1268, 1981 (abstract).

i Salvioli, G., Igimi, H., and Carey, M.C. During gallstone dissolution with ursodeoxycholic acid (UDC) liquid crystals cooperate with micelles in the solubilization of cholesterol monohydrate (ChM). Ital. J. Gastroenterol. 13:281, 1981 (abstract).

j Sama, C. and LaRusso, N.F. Effect of deoxycholic, chenodeoxycholic, and cholic acids on intestinal absorption of cholesterol in humans. Mayo Clin. Proc. 57:44-50, 1982.

k Sama, C., LaRusso, N.F., Lopez del Pino, V., and Thistle, J. Effects of acute bile acid administration on biliary lipid secretion in healthy volunteers. Gastroenterology 82:515-525, 1982

l Sampliner, R.E., Bennett, P.H., Comess, L.J., Rose, F.A., and Burch, T.A. Gallbladder disease in Pima Indians. Demonstration of high prevalence and early onset by cholecystography. N. Engl. J. Med. 283:1358-1364, 1970.

m Samuel, P., Saypol, E., Meilman, E., Mosbach, E.H., and Chafizadeh, M. Absorption of bile acids from the large bowel in man. J. Clin. Invest. 47:2070-2078, 1968.

a Samuel, P. Perl, W., Holtzman, C.M., Rochman, N.D., and Lieberman, S. Long-term kinetics of serum and xanthoma cholesterol radioactivity in patients with hypercholesterolemia. J. Clin. Invest 51:266-278, 1972.

b Samuel, P., Holtzman, C.M., Meilman, E., and Sekowski, I. Effect of neomycin and other antibiotics on serum cholesterol levels and on 7a-dehydroxylation of bile acids by the fecal bacterial flora in man. Circ. Res. 33:393-402, 1973.

c Samuel, P. and Lieberman, S. Improved estimation of body masses and turnover of cholesterol by computerized input-output analysis. J. Lipid Res. 14:189-196, 1973.

d Samuel, P., Schussheim, A., Lieberman, S., and Don, E.C. Relation of serum cholesterol to in vitro 7a-dehydroxylation of primary bile acids by fecal bacteria in infants and children. Pediatrics 54:222-228, 1974.

e Samuels, A.D. and Palmer, R.H. Conversion of chenodeoxycholic acid to cholic acid in humans with obstructive jaundice. Gastroenterology 64:168, 1973 (abstract).

f Samuelson, K. Radioimmunoassay compared to an enzymatic method for serum bile acid determination. Scand. J. Clin. Lab. Invest. 40:289-291, 1980.

g Samuelson, K. and Eklund, A. Determination of urinary cholic and cheno deoxycholic acid conjugates with radioimmunoassay. Scand. J. Clin. Lab. Invest. 40:555-561, 1980.

h Samuelsson, B. The metabolism of 7-ketolithocholic acid-24-^{14}C in the rat. Acta Chem. Scand. 13:236, 1959.

i Samuelsson, B. On the metabolism of chenodeoxycholic acid in the rat. Acta Chem. Scand. 13:976, 1959.

j Samuelsson, B. On the metabolism of ursodeoxycholic acid in the rat. Acta Chem. Scand. 13:970, 1959.

k Samuelsson, B. Metabolism of 3a,7b,12a-trihydroxycholanic acid in the rat. Acta Chem. Scand. 14:21, 1960.

l Samuelsson, B. Bile acids and steroids. On the mechanism of the biological formation of deoxycholic acid from cholic acid. J. Biol. Chem. 235:361-366, 1960.

m Sanchez, H.M. A comparison of the metal composition of cholesterol (CS) and pigment (PS) gallstones and surrounding biles. Gastroenterology 68:1003, 1975 (abstract).

n Sarfeh, I.J., Beeler, D.A., Treble, D.H., and Balint, J.A. Studies of the hepatic excretory defects in essential fatty acid deficiency. Their possible relationship to the genesis of cholesterol gallstones. J. Clin. Invest. 53:423-430, 1974.

a Sarles, H., Crotte, C., Gerolami, A., Mule, A., Domingo, N., and Hauton, J. Influence of cholestyramine, bile salt, and cholesterol feeding on the lipid composition of hepatic bile in man. Scand. J. Gastroenterol. 5:603-608, 1970.

b Sarles, H., Hauton, J., Planche, N.E., Lafont, H., and Gerolami, A. Diet, cholesterol gallstones, and composition of the bile. Am. J. Dig. Dis. 15:251-260, 1970.

c Sarles, H., Crotte, C., Gerolami, A., Mule, A., Domingo, N., and Hauton, J. The influence of calorie intake and of dietary protein on the bile lipids. Scand. J. Gastroenterol. 6:189-191, 1971.

d Sarles, H., Gerolami, A., and Bord, A. Diet and cholesterol gallstones. Digestion 17:128-134, 1978.

e Sarva, R.P., Fromm, H., Carlson, G.L., Mendelow, L., and Ceryak, S. Intracolonic conversion in man of chenodeoxycholic acid (CDC) to ursodeoxycholic acid (UDC) with and without formation of 7-ketolithocholic acid (KLC) as an intermediate. Gastroenterology 78:1252, 1980 (abstract).

f Sarva, R.P., Fromm, H., Farivar, S., Sembrat, R.F., Mendelow, H., Shinozuka, H., and Wolfson, S.K. Comparison of the effects between ursodeoxycholic and chenodeoxycholic acid on liver function and structure and on bile acid composition in the Rhesus monkey. Gastroenterology 79:629-636, 1980.

g Sarva, R., Farivar, S., Fromm, H., and Poller, W. Study of the sensitivity and specificity of computerized tomography in the detection of calcified gallstones which appear radiolucent by conventional roentgenography. Gastrointest. Radiol. 6:165-167, 1981.

h Sarva, R.P., Farivar, S., Fromm, H., Bazzoli, F., Wald, A., and Amin, P. Comparative sensitivity of eight and 24-hour bile acid breath tests and Schilling test in ileopathies. Am. J. Gastroenterol. 76:432-437, 1981.

i Sarwal, A.N., Cohen, B.I., Raicht, R.F., Takahashi, M., and Fazzini, E. Effects of dietary administration of chenodeoxycholic acid on N-methyl-N-nitrosourea-induced colon cancer in rats. Biochim. Biophys. Acta 574: 423-432, 1979.

j Sasson, L. Dissolution and flushing technics for removal of retained common duct stones. Am. J. Gastroenterol. 51:354-409, 1969.

k Sauer, H.D., deHeer, K., and Mitschke, H. Chenodeoxycholic acid therapy and colorectal carcinoma--an experimental approach. Z. Gastroenterol. 17:236-243, 1979.

l Sauerbruch, T. Pharmakotherapie von Cholesteringallensteinen. Med. Mo. Pharm. 4:263-268, 1981.

m Saunders, D.R. Insignificance of the enterobiliary circulation of lecithin in man. Gastroenterology 59:848-852, 1970.

a Sawada, H., Kinoshita, S., Yoshida, T., and Taguchi, H. Microbial production of chenodeoxycholic acid precursor, 12-ketochenodeoxycholic acid, from dehydrocholic acid. Europ. J. Appl. Microbiol. Biotechnol. 10:107-112, 1980.

b Schaefer, R.A., Javitt, N.B., Finlayson, N.D.C., and Prince, A.M. Serum chenodeoxycholate levels in hepatitisB-antigen carriers. Gastroenterology 66:865, 1974 (abstract).

c Schaffner, F. and Javitt, N.B. Morphologic changes in hamster liver during intrahepatic cholestasis induced by taurolithocholate. Lab. Invest. 15:1783-1792, 1966.

d Schaffner, F., Bacchin, P.G., Hutterer, F., Scharnbeck, H.H., Sarkozi, L.L., Denk, H., and Popper, H. Mechanism of cholestasis. IV. Structural and biochemical changes in the liver and serum in rats after bile duct ligation. Gastroenterology 60:888-897, 1971.

e Schalm, S.W. Serum levels of chenodeoxycholic acid in health and nonhepatic disease. Acta Gastroenterol. Belg. 40:406-407, 1977.

f Schalm, S.W., van Berge-Henegouwen, G.P., Hofmann, A.F., and Turcotte, J. Radioimmunoassay of serum bile acids for conjugates of chenodeoxycholic acid. Development, validation, and preliminary application. Gastroenterology 73:285-290, 1977.

g Schalm, S.W. and van Berge Henegouwen, G.P. Behandling van Galsteendragers met Chenodesoxycholzuur. Ned. T. Geneesk. 122:266-270, 1978.

h Schalm, S.W., LaRusso, N.F., Hofmann, A.F., Hoffman, N.E., van Berge Henegouwen, G.P., and Korman, M.G. Diurnal serum levels of primary conjugated bile acids. Assessment by specific radioimmunoassays of cholic and chenodeoxycholic acid. Gut 19:1-9, 1978.

i Scharschmidt, B.F., Waggoner, J.G., and Berk, P.D. Hepatic organic anion uptake in the rat. J. Clin. Invest. 56:1280-1292, 1975.

j Scharschmidt, B.F. and Schmid, R. The micellar sink. A quantitative assessment of the association or organic anions with mixed micelles and other macromolecular aggregates in rat bile. J. Clin. Invest. 62:1122-1132, 1978.

k Scharschmidt, B.F., Keeffe, E.B., Vessey, D.A., Blankenship, N.M., and Ockner, R.K. In vitro effect of bile salts on rat liver plasma membrane, lipid fluidity, and ATPase activity. Hepatology 1:137-145, 1981

l Scharschmidt, B.F. and Stephens, J.E. Transport of sodium, chloride, and taurocholate by cultured rat hepatocytes. Proc. Natl. Acad. Sci. USA 78:986-990, 1981.

m Scheig, R. Hepatic metabolism of medium chain fatty acids. In Medium Chain Triglycerides. JR Senior, ed. University of Pennsylvania Press, 1968, pp 39-50.

a Schein, C.J., Hurwitt, E.S., and Rosenblatt, M.A. The significance of calculus size in determining the indication for elective cholecystectomy. Gastroenterology 29:377-380, 1955.

b Schenk, J., Koch, H., Stolte, M., and Schmack, B. Tissue compatability of the gallstone solubilizer Capmul 8210 - A study in cats. Gastroenterology 76:1237, 1979 (abstract).

c Schenk, J., Dobronte, Z., Koch, H., and Stolte, M. Studies on tissue compatibility of d-limonene as a dissolving agent of cholesterol gallstones. Z. Gastroenterol. 18:389-394, 1980.

d Schenk, J., Schmack, B., Riemann, J.F., and Rosch, W. Treatment of chole docholithiasis using the transpapillary perfusion technique. Endoscopy 12:224-227, 1980.

e Schenk, J., Schmack, B., Rosch, W., Riemann, J.F., Koch, H., and Demling, L. Spulbehandlung von Choledochussteinen mit Octanoat (Capmul 8210). Dtsch. med. Wschr. 105:917-921, 1980.

f Schentke, K.U. Clinical and internal medicine therapy of biliary tract disease. Z. Gesamte Inn. Med. 35:642-646, 1980.

g von Schentke, U., Jaross, W., and Trubsbach, A. Lipide der Blasengalle bei Lebergesunden, Leberkranken und Gallensteintragern. Dtsch. Z. Verdau.- u. Stoffwechselkr. 32:303-310, 1972.

h Schersten, T., Gottfries, A., and Nilsson, S. Human bile phospholipids in normal conditions and in acute cholecystitis. Eur. Soc. Clin. Invest., 1968 (abstract).

i Schersten, T., Nilsson, S., and Cahlin, E. Current concepts on the pathogenesis of human gallstones. Scand. J. Gastroenterol. 5:473-478, 1970.

j Schersten, T. Bile acid conjugation. In Metabolic Conjugation and Metabolic Hydrolysis, Vol 2. Fichman, ed. Academic Press, New York-London, 1971, pp 75-121.

k Schersten, T., Nilsson, S., Cahlin, E., Filipson, M., and Brodin-Persson, G. Relationship between the biliary excretion of bile acids and excretion of water, lecithin and cholesterol in man. Europ. J. Clin. Invest. 1:242-247, 1971.

l Schersten, T. Bile acids as a determining factor for synthesis and excretion of human bile lecithin. Helv. Med. Acta 37:161-168, 1973.

m Schersten, T. Formation of lithogenic bile in man. Digestion 9:540-553, 1973.

n Schersten, T., Cahlin, E., Jonsson, J., Lindblad, L., and Nilsson, S.W. Supersaturated bile: Is it due to a metabolic disorder or to an impaired gallbladder? Scand. J. Gastroenterol. 9:501-506, 1974.

a Schersten, T., Lindblad, L., and Lundholm, K. The influence of cholic and chenic acid on the bile flow and the biliary secretion of lecithin and cholesterol in man. Second Int'l. Gstaad Symp., Sept., 1975, pp 275-286.

b Schersten, T. Medical treatment of gallstones. Scand. J. Gastroenterol. 13:129-131, 1978 (Review).

c Schersten, T. and Lindblad, L. Biliary cholesterol output during ursodeoxycholic acid secretion in man. In Biological Effects of Bile Acids, G Paumgartner, A Stiehl, W Gerok, eds. MTP Press, Ltd., Lancaster, 1979, pp 53-60.

d Schiff, E.R., Small, N.C., and Dietschy, J.M. Characterization of the kinetics of the passive and active transport mechanisms for bile acid absorption in the small intestine and colon of the rat. J. Clin. Invest. 51:1351-1362, 1972.

e Schiff, E.R., Parker, I.T., and Dick, R.D. The effect of phenobarbital on bile acid kinetics in man. Gastroenterology 67:828, 1974 (abstract).

f Schiff, L., Carey, J.B., and Dietschy, J.M. Bile Salt Metabolism. Chas. C. Thomas, Springfield, 1969, pp 306.

g Schiff, M. Gallenbildung, abhangig von der Aufsaugung der Gallenstoffe. Phlueger Arch. Ges. Physiol. 3:598-613, 1870.

h Schlierf, G., Stiehl, A., Heuck, C.C., Lang, P.D., Oster, P., and Schellenberg, B. Does chenodeoxycholic acid have a lipid lowering effect in primary hyperlipoproteinemia? Europ. J. Clin. Pharmacol. 10:147-149, 1976.

i Schlierf, G., Schellenberg, B., Stiehl, A., and Oster, P. Biliary cholesterol saturation and weight reduction--effect of fasting and low calorie diet. Digestion 21:44-49, 1981.

j Schluter, K.J., Petersen, K-G., and Kerp, L. Einfluss von Mono-, Di- und Trihydroxygallensauren auf die Insulinrezeptorbildung. Z. Gastroenterol. XIX (9), 1981 (abstract).

k Schmack, B. Clinical significance of bile acids. Fortsch. Med. 97:690-693, 1979.

l Schmack, B., Schenk, J., Riemann, J., Koch, H., and Rosch, W. Dissolution of biliary-duct stones with mono-octanoin. Lancet 2:423-424, 1979 (letter).

m Schmidt, H.D. and Rothmund, M. Cholecystectomy or drug litholysis of biliary calculi? Surgical viewpoint. Dtsch. med. Wschr. 104:606-607, 1979.

n Schmidt, L.H. and Hughes, H.B. Studies on bile metabolism. I. The fate of cholic acid in the guinea pig. J. Biol. Chem. 143:771-783, 1942.

o Schoenfield, L.J. Bile acid composition of gallstones from man. J. Lab. Clin. Med. 68:186-192, 1966.

a Schoenfield, L.J. and Sjovall, J. Bile acids and cholesterol in guinea pigs with induced gallstones. Am. J. Physiol. 211:1069-1074, 1966.

b Schoenfield, L.J. and Sjovall, J. Identification of bile acid and neutral sterols in guinea pig bile. Acta Chem. Scand. 20:1297-1303, 1966.

c Schoenfield, L.J., Sjovall, J., and Sjovall, K. Bile acid composition of gallstones from man. J. Lab. Clin. Med. 68:186-194, 1966.

d Schoenfield, L.J., Sjovall, J. and Perman, E. Bile acids on the skin of patients with pruritic hepatobiliary disease. Nature 213:93-94, 1967.

e Schoenfield, L.J. The relationship of bile acids to pruritus in hepatobiliary disease. In Bile Salt Metabolism. L Schiff, ed. C.C. Thomas, Springfield, 1969, pp 257-265.

f Schoenfield, L.J. Genesis and treatment of gallstones. Min. Med. 54:626, 1971 (Editorial).

g Schoenfield, L.J. Animal models of gallstone formation. Gastroenterology 63:189-191, 1972 (Editorial).

h Schoenfield, L.J. Diseases of the gallbladder and biliary tract. Tice's Prac. Int. Med. VII:1-58, 1973.

i Schoenfield, L.J., Bonorris, G.G., and Ganz, P. Induced alterations in the rate-limiting enzymes of hepatic cholesterol and bile acid synthesis in the hamster. J. Lab. Clin. Med. 82:858-868, 1973.

j Schoenfield, L.J., Danzinger, R.G., Hofmann, A.F., and Thistle, J.L. Effect of chenodeoxycholic acid on bile composition, bile acid kinetics and gallstones. In The Liver. Quantitative Aspects of Structure and Function. Karger, Basel, 1973, pp 174-178.

k Schoenfield, L.J. Clinical aspects of the chenodeoxycholic acid trial. Hosp. Prac. 9:53-57, 1974.

l Schoenfield, L.J. Clinical trends and topics: Medical therapy for gallstones. Gastroenterology 67:725-729, 1974.

m Schoenfield, L.J., Bonorris, G.G., Coyne, M.J., and Goldstein, L.I. Hepatic HMG-CoA reductase and 7a-hydroxylase activities during gallstone dissolution. In Advances in Bile Acid Research. S Matern, J Hackenschmidt, P Back, and W Gerok, eds. F.K. Schattauer Verlag, Stuttgart-New York, 1975, pp 311-313.

n Schoenfield, L.J. and Coyne, M.J. Cholesterol gallstones, 1975. Viewpoints on Digestive Diseases 7(1), 1975.

a Schoenfield, L.J., Coyne, M.J., Conley, D.R., Chung, A., and Bonorris, G.G. Inhibition of bile acid stimulation of colonic secretion and adenylate cyclase. In The Liver. Quantitative Aspects of Structure and Function. Editio Cantor, Aulendorf, 1976, pp 413-418.

b Schoenfield, L.J., Goldstein, L.I., Panish, J., Shore, J.M. Gallstones. West. J. Med. 124:299-315, 1976.

c Schoenfield, L.J. Stone dissolution and the National Cooperative Gallstone Study. Am. J. Dig. Dis. 22:1115-1116, 1977.

d Schoenfield, L.J., Coyne, M.J., Bonorris, G.G., Key, P.H., and Marks, J.W. Chenodeoxycholic acid for the dissolution of cholesterol gallstones. In Liver and Bile, L Bianchi, ed. Univ. Park Press, Baltimore, 1977, pp 297-308.

e Schoenfield, L.J. The disappearing gallstone and the National Cooperative Gallstone Study. JAMA 239:1138-1144, 1978 (Editorial).

f Schoenfield, L.J. and Associates. Gallstones--1977. Am. J. Dig. Dis. 23:737-751, 1978.

g Schoenfield, L.J. Chenodeoxycholic acid: Uses and limitations. Hosp. Prac. 14:57-65, 1979.

h Schoenfield, L.J., Lachin, J.M., the NCGS Steering Committee, and the NCGS Group: National Cooperative Gallstone Study: A controlled trial of the efficacy and safety of chenodeoxycholic acid for dissolution of gallstones. Annals Intern. Med. 95:257-282, 1981.

i Schoenfield, L.J. Medical dissolution of gallstones. In Alternativas de tratamiento en padecimientos del aparato digestivo. Asociacion Mexicana de Gastroenterologiea, 1981, pp 93-98.

j Scholmerich, J., Schmidt, K., Kremer, B., Becher, M.S., and Gerok, W. Different effect of taurolithocholate and chenodeoxycholate on structure and function of isolated hepatocytes. Klin. Wschr. 59:655-668, 1981.

k Schreiber, J., Erb., W., and Boehle, E. Analysis of fecal bile acids. Verh. Dtsch. Ges. Inn. Med. 75:920-923, 1969.

l Schriewer, H., Badde, R., Roth, G., and Rauen, H.M. Die Pharmakokinetik der antihepatotoxischen Wirkung des Silymarins bei der Leberschadigung der Ratte durch CCl_4 und Desoxycholat. Arzneimittel-Forschung 23:157-158, 1973.

m Schriewer, H., von Bassewitz, D.B., and Rauen, H.M. Lipidmetabolstorung der Leber durch parenteral verabreichtes Desoxycholat bei der Ratte. Klin. Wschr. 51:39-40, 1973.

n Schwaier, A. Tupiais (tree shrews)--a new animal model for gallstone research. Res. Exp. Med. 176:15-24, 1979.

a Schwartz, C.C., Vlahcevic, Z.R., Halloran, L.G., Gregory, D.H., Meek, J.B., and Swell, L. Evidence for the existence of definitive hepatic cholesterol precursor compartments for bile acids and biliary cholesterol in man. Gastroenterology 69:1379-1382, 1975.

b Schwartz, C.C., Cohen, B.I., Vlahcevic, Z.R., Gregory, D.H., Halloran, L.G., Kuramoto, T., Mosbach, E.H., and Swell, L. Quantitative aspects of the conversion of 5b-cholestane intermediates to bile acids in man. J. Biol. Chem. 251:6308-6314, 1976.

c Schwartz, C.C., Berman, M., Vlahcevic, Z.R., Halloran, L.G., Gregory, D.H., and Swell, L. Multicompartmental analysis of cholesterol metabolism in man. J. Clin. Invest. 61:408-423, 1978.

d Schwartz, C.C., Almond, H.R., Vlahcevic, Z.R., and Swell, L. Bile acid metabolism in cirrhosis. V. Determination of biliary lipid secretion rates in patients with advanced cirrhosis. Gastroenterology 77:1177-1182, 1979.

e Schwartz, H.P. and Paumgartner, G. Elevation of serum bile acids following therapeutic doses of chenodeoxycholic acid in man. Digestion 8:431, 1973 (abstract).

f Schwartz, H.P., Paumgartner, G., and Preisig, R. Diagnostiche Bedeutung der Serumgallensauren. Schwz. med. Wschr. 105:533-535, 1975.

g Schwarz, L.R., Burr, R., Schwenk, M., Pfaff, E., and Greim, H. Uptake of taurocholic acid into isolated rat liver cells. Europ. J. Biochem. 55:617-623, 1975.

h Schwenk, M., Hofmann, A., Carlson, G., Carter, J., Couston, F., and Greim, H. Bile acid conjugation in the chimpanzee: Effective sulfation of lithocholic acid. Arch. Toxicol. 40:109-118, 1978.

i Scopinaro, N., Civalleri, D., Mortola, G., Anfossi, A., Gianetta, E., and Berti Riboli, E. Mono-octanoin T-tube infusion for the treatment of cholesterol retained bile duct stones. Ital. J. Gastroenterol. 12:353, 1980 (abstract).

j Scott, V.F., Roth, H.P., Bellon, E.M., and Neiderhiser, D.H. Effect of regular emptying of the gallbladder on gallstone formation in the rabbit. Gastroenterology 63:851-855, 1972.

k Sedaghat, A. and Grundy, S. Cholesterol crystals and the formation of cholesterol gallstones. N. Engl. J. Med. 302:1274-1277, 1980.

l Segiet, R. Auflosung eines intrahepatischen Gallengangkonkrementes durch orale Chenodesoxycholsaurebehandlung. Med. Welt 30:658-660, 1979.

m Sehlin, R.C., Cussler, E.L., and Evans, D.F. Diffusion in bile and its implications on detergency. Biochim. Biophys. Acta 388:385-396, 1975.

n Seifert, E. Cholelithiasis: Indications for cholecystectomy, papillotomy and gallstone dissolution. Leber Magen Darm 7:324-327, 1977.

a Selye, H. Prevention by catatoxic steroids of lithocholic acid-induced biliary concrements in the rat. Proc. Soc. Exptl. Biol. Med. 141:555-558, 1972.

b Semb, B.K.H., Norderval, Y., and Halvorsen, J.F. The non-operative removal of retained common duct stones after biliary surgery. Acta Chir. Scand. 140:469, 1974.

c Semple, P.F. and Russell, R.I. Role of bile acids in the pathogenesis of aspirin-induced gastric mucosal hemorrhage in rats. Gastroenterology 68:67-70, 1975.

d Senior, J.R., Budz, D.M., and Isselbacher, K.J. Demonstration of an intestinal monoglyceride lipase: An enzyme with a possible role in the intracellular completion of fat digestion. J. Clin. Invest. 42:187-195, 1963.

e Senior, J.R. Medium Chain Triglycerides. University of Pennsylvania Press, 1968, 300 pp.

f Setchell, K.D.R., Lawson, A.M., Blackstock, E.J., and Murphy, G.M. Diurnal changes in serum unconjugated bile acids in normal man. Gut 23:637-642, 1982.

g Sewell, R., Hoffman, N.E., Smallwood, R., and Cockbain, S. Bile acid structure and bile formation: A comparison of hydroxy and keto bile acids. Am. J. Physiol. 239:G10-G17, 1980.

h Shaffer, E.A., Braasch, J.W., and Small, D.M. Bile composition at and after surgery in normal persons and patients with gallstones. Influence of cholecystectomy. N. Engl. J. Med. 287:1317-1322, 1972.

i Shaffer, E.A. and Beaudoin, M. Cholesterol gallstones. Formation and medical treatment. Union Med. Can. 103:2061-2069, 1974.

j Shaffer, E.A., Beaudoin, M., Small, D.M., O'Brien, J., and Williams, L. Relationship between gallbladder function and the enterohepatic circulation of bile salts during fasting. Gastroenterology 66:775, 1974 (abstract).

k Shaffer, E.A. Gallstones: Current concepts of pathogenesis and medical dissolution. Can. J. Surg. 23:517-532, 1980.

l Shaffer, E.A., McOrmond, P., and Duggan, H. Quantitative cholescintigraphy: Assessment of gallbladder filling and emptying and duodenogastric reflux. Gastroenterology 79:899-906, 1980.

m Shankland, W. The equilibrium and structure of lecithin-cholate mixed micelles. Chem. Phys. Lipids 4:109-130, 1970.

n Shankland, W. The ionic behavior of fatty acids solubilized by bile salts. J. Colloid Interface Sci. 34:9-25, 1970.

o Shapero, T.F., Lee, V., Wilson, R.S., Rosen, I.E., and Fisher, M.M. A problem in the evaluation of gallstone dissolution. Gastroenterology 80:1348, 1981 (abstract).

a Shapiro, D.J. and Rodwell, V.W. Diurnal variation and cholesterol regulation of hepatic HMG-CoA reductase activity. Biochem. Biophys. Res. Comm. 37:867-872, 1969.

b Shapiro, S. The pill, thromboembolism, and gallbladder disease. Lancet 2:567, 1973 (Letter to Editor).

c Sharp, H., Carey, J., Peller, J., et al. Lithocholic acid in meconium. Pediat. Res. 2:293, 1968.

d Sharp, H.L. Primary and secondary bile acids in meconium. Pediat. Res. 5:274-279, 1971.

e Sharp, H.L. and Mirkin, B.L. Effect of phenobarbital on hyperbilirubinemia, bile acid metabolism, and microsomal enzyme activity in chronic intrahepatic cholestasis of childhood. J. Pediat. 81:116-126, 1972.

f Sharp, K.W. and Gadacz, T.R. Rate of gallstone dissolution with monooctanoin compared to gallstone composition. Gastroenterology 80:1282, 1981 (abstract).

g Shaw, R. and Elliott, W.H. Bile acids. LV. 2,2-Dimethoxypropane: An esterifying agent preferred to diazomethane for chenodeoxycholic acid. J. Lipid Res. 19:783-787, 1978.

h Shefer, S., Hauser, S., and Mosbach, E.H. 7a-Hydroxylation of cholestanol by rat liver microsomes. J. Lipid Res. 9:328-333, 1968.

i Shefer, S., Hauser, S., Bekersky, I., and Mosbach, E.H. Feedback regulation of bile acid biosynthesis in the rat. J. Lipid Res. 10:646-655, 1969.

j Shefer, S., Hauser, S., Bekersky, I., and Mosbach, E.H. Biochemical site of regulation of bile acid biosynthesis in the rat. J. Lipid Res. 11:404-411, 1970.

k Shefer, S., Hauser, S., Lapar, V., and Mosbach, E.H. HMG-CoA reductase of intestinal mucosa and liver of the rat. J. Lipid Res. 13:402-412, 1972.

l Shefer, S., Hauser, S., and Mosbach, E.H. Stimulation of cholesterol 7a-hydroxylase by phenobarbital in two strains of rats. J. Lipid Res. 13:69-70, 1972.

m Shefer, S., Hauser, S., Lapar, V., and Mosbach, E.H. Regulatory effects of dietary sterols and bile acids on rat intestinal HMG-CoA reductase. J. Lipid Res. 14:400-405, 1973.

n Shefer, S., Hauser, S., Lapar, V., and Mosbach, E.H. Regulatory effects of sterols and bile acids on hepatic 3-hydroxy-3-methylglutaryl CoA reductase and cholesterol 7a-hydroxylase in the rat. J. Lipid Res. 14:573-580, 1973.

o Shefer, S., Nicolau, G., and Mosbach, E.H. Isotope derivative assay of microsomal cholesterol 7a-hydroxylase. J. Lipid Res. 17:92-96, 1975.

a Shefer, S., Salen, G., Fedorowski, T., Dyrszka, H., and Mosbach, E.H. Inhibition of cholesterol biosynthesis by chenodeoxycholic acid in the rhesus monkey. J. Steroid Biochem. 6:1563-1564, 1975.

b Shefer, S., Cheng, F.W., Batta, A.K., Dayal, B., Tint, G.S., and Salen, G. Biosynthesis of chenodeoxycholic acid in man. Sterospecific side chain hydroxylations of 5b-cholestane-3a,7a-diol. J. Clin. Invest. 62:539-545, 1978.

c Shefer, S., Cheng, F.W., Batta, A.K., Dayal, B., Tint, G.S., Salen, G., and Mosbach, E. Stereospecific side chain hydroxylations in the biosynthesis of chenodeoxycholic acid. J. Biol. Chem. 253:6386-6392, 1978.

d Shefer, S., Salen, G., Hauser, S., Dayal, B., and Batta, A.K. Metabolism of iso-bile acids in the rat. J. Biol. Chem. 257:1401-1406, 1982.

e Sherman, C.A. Bile acid biosynthesis: The metabolism of 7a-hydroxy-4-cholestan-3-one in the bile fistula rat. Gastroenterology 68:1092, 1974 (abstract).

f Sherr, H.P., Sasaki, Y., Newman, A., Banwell, J.G., Wagner, H.N., Jr., and Hendrix, T.R. Detection of bacterial deconjugation of bile salts by a convenient breath-analysis technic. N. Engl. J. Med. 285:656-661, 1971.

g Sherr, H.P., Nair, P.P., Banwell, J.G., White, J.J., and Lockwood, D.H. Bile acid metabolism and hepatic disease following small bowel bypass for obesity. Am. J. Clin. Nutr. 27:1369-1379, 1974.

h Shimada, K., Bricknell, K.S., and Finegold, S.M. Deconjugation of bile acids by intestinal bacteria: Review of literature and additional studies. J. Inf. Dis. 119:273-281, 1969.

i Shimada, K., Sutter, V.L., and Finegold, S.M. Effect of bile acid deoxycholate on gram-negative anaerobic bacteria. Appl. Microbiol. 20:737-741, 1970.

j Shimoda, S.S., O'Brien, T.K., and Saunders, D.R. Fat absorption after infusing bile salts into the human small intestine. Gastroenterology 67:7-18, 1974.

k Shin, Y.C. Some observations on the morphological evidence for the mechanism of the bile secretion. Acta Anat. 100:499-511, 1978.

l Shindo, K. and Fukushima, K. Deconjugation of bile acids by human intestinal bacteria. Gastroenterol. Jpn. 11:167-174, 1976.

m Shiner, M. Effect of bile acids on the small intestinal mucosa in man and rats: A light and electron microscope study. In Bile Salt Metabolism. Schiff, Carey, and Dietschy, eds. Thomas, Springfield, 1969, pp 41-55.

n Shinoda, K., Nakagawa, T., Tamamushi, B., et al. Colloidal Surfactants, Some Physical Chemical Properties. Academic Press, New York, 1963.

a Shinozaki, K. and Nakagawa, S. Sulfated bile acid in urine of patients with hepatobiliary disease. Lipids 8:47-49, 1973.

b Shinozaki, K. Pharmacokinetic study of oral ursodeoxycholic acid tolerance test. Acta Hepatol. Japon. 20:782-794, 1979.

c Shirakawa, Y. Hepatic bile production and bile acid metabolism after relief of biliary obstruction. J. Japan Surg. Soc. 82:633-646, 1981.

d Shoda, M. Uber die Ursodesoxycholsaure aus Barengallen und ihre physiologische Wirkung. J. Biochem. 7:505-517, 1927.

e Shridi, F.A., Chitranukroh, A., Pourfarzaneh, M., Billing, B.H., and Ekeke, G. A direct fluoroimmunoassay for conjugated chenodeoxycholic acid using antibody coupling to magnetisable particles. Ann. Clin. Biochem. 17:188-191, 1980.

f Sickinger, K. Die Behandlung der Chologenen diarrhoe und steatorrhoe des enteralen Gallensaure-verlustsyndroms mit Cholestyramin und mittelkettigen Triglyceriden. Dtsch. med. Wschr. 94:1151-1157, 1969.

g Sickinger, K. Medikamentose Auflosung von Gallensteinen. Indikationsfeld: rontgennegative multiple kleine Kondremente. Arztl. Praxis Nr. 95:3843, 1975.

h Siegfried, C.M., Doisy, E.A., Jr., and Elliott, W.H. Bile acids. XLIV. Quantitation of bile acids from the bile fistula rat given (4-^{14}C) cholesterol. Biochim. Biophys. Acta 380:66-75, 1975.

i Sierra Ruiz, E. Resultados terapeuticos en la litiasis biliar con un nuevo coleretico, trimetoxi-chalcona (1314 CB), asociado a espasmoliticos oddianos. Rev. Esp. Enf. Ap. Dig. 32:907-918, 1970.

j Signer, E., Murphy, G.M., Edkins, S., and Anderson, C.M. The role of bile salts in the fat malabsorption of premature infants. Arch. Dis. Childh. 49:174-180, 1974.

k Sigstad, H. Drug dissolution of biliary calculi. Tidsskr. Nor Laegeforen 99:227-228, 1979.

l Silen, W. and Forte, T.G. Effects of bile salts on amphibian gastric mucosa. Am. J. Physiol. 228:637-644, 1975.

m Simmonds, W.J., Hofmann, A.F., and Theodor, E. Absorption of cholesterol from a micellar solution: Intestinal perfusion studies in man. J. Clin. Invest. 46:874-890, 1967.

n Simmonds, W.J. Effect of bile salts on the rate of fat absorption. Am. J. Clin. Nutr. 22:266-272, 1969.

o Simmonds, W.J., Korman, M.G., Go, V.L.W., and Hofmann, A.F. Radioimmunoassay of conjugated cholyl bile acids in serum. Gastroenterology 65:705-711, 1973.

a Simmonds, W.J. Absorption of lipids. In Gastrointestinal Physiology. MTP International Review of Science. ED Jacobson and LL Shanbour, eds. University Park Press, Baltimore, 1974, pp 343-376.

b Simmons, F. and Bouchier, I.A.D. Intraluminal bile salt concentrations and fat digestion after cholecystectomy. S. African Med. J. 46:2089-2092, 1972.

c Simmons, F., Ross, A.P.J., and Bouchier, I.A.D. Alterations in hepatic bile composition after cholecystectomy. Gastroenterology 63:466-471, 1972.

d Simon, B., Czygan, P., Stiehl, A., and Kather, H. Human colonic adenylate cyclase: Effects of bile acids. Europ. J. Clin. Invest. 8:321-323, 1978.

e Singer, S.S., Federspiel, M.J., Green, J., Lewis, W.G., Martin, V., Witt, K.R., and Tappel, J. Enzymatic sulfation of steroids. XV. Studies differentiating between rat liver androgen, estrogen, bile acid, glucocorticoid and phenol sulfotransferases. Biochim. Biophys. Acta 700:110-117, 1982.

f Siperstein, M.D. Regulation of cholesterol synthesis in normal and malignant tissues. In Current Topics in Cellular Regulation. BL Horecker and ER Stadtman, eds. Vol 2, Academic Press, New York, 1970, pp 74-76.

g Sjodahl, R. and Tagesson, C. On the mediation of inflammatory reaction in the human gallbladder epithelium. Scand. J. Gastroenterol. 11:321-328, 1976.

h Sjodahl, R., Tagesson, C. and Wetterfors, J. On the pathogenesis of acute cholecystitis. Surg. Gyn. & Obst. 146:199-202, 1978.

i Sjovall, J. Dietary glycine and taurine on bile acid conjugation in man. Proc. Soc. Exptl. Biol. Med. 100:676, 1959.

j Sjovall, J. The occurrence of 7b-hydroxylated bile acids in human bile. Acta Chem. Scand. 13:711-716, 1959.

k Sjovall, J. On the concentration of bile acids in the human intestine during absorption. Acta Physiol. Scand. 46:339, 1959.

l Sjovall, J. Bile acids in man under normal and pathological conditions. Bile acids and steroids 73. Clin. Chim. Acta 5:33-42, 1960.

m Sjovall, J. and Sjovall, K. Serum bile acid levels in pregnancy with pruritus. Clin. Chim. Acta 13:207-211, 1966.

n Sladen, G.E. and Harries, J.T. Studies on the effects of unconjugated dihydroxy bile salts on rat small intestinal function in vivo. Biochem. Biophys. Acta 288:443-456, 1972.

o Smadja, M. and Bauer, P. La lithiase du choledoque du suject age. La Revue de Medicine 20:1973-1977, 1981.

a Small, D.M. and Bourges, M.C. Lyotropic paracrystalline phases obtained with ternary and quaternary systems of amphiphilic substances in water: Studies on aqueous systems of lecithin, bile salts and cholesterol. Molecular Crystals 1:541-561, 1966.

b Small, D.M., Bourges, M.C., and Dervichian, D.G. The biophysics of lipidic associations. I. The ternary systems lecithin-bile salt-water. Biochim. Biophys. Acta 125:563, 1966.

c Small, D.M., Bourges, M.C., and Dervichian, D.G. Ternary and quaternary aqueous systems containing bile salt, lecithin and cholesterol. Nature 211:816-818, 1966.

d Small, D.M. Phase equilibria and structure of dry and hydrated egg lecithin. J. Lipid Res. 8:551-557, 1967.

e Small, D.M. Physicochemical studies of cholesterol gallstone formation. Gastroenterology 52:607-610, 1967.

f Small, D.M. A classification of biologic lipids based upon their interaction in aqueous systems. J. Am. Oil Chemists' Soc. 45:108-119, 1968.

g Small, D.M. Gallstones. N. Engl. J. Med. 279:588-593, 1968.

h Small, D.M. Size and structure of bile salt, micelles: Influence of structure, concentration, counterion concentration, pH and temperature. In Molecular Association in Biological and Regulated Systems. RF Gould, ed. Adv. Chem. Ser. 84:31-52, 1968.

i Small, D.M. Liquid crystals in biological systems: Bile secretion and gallstone formation. Molec. Crystals Liquid Crystals 8:209-214, 1969.

j Small, D.M. and Admirand, W.H. Solubility of bile salts. Nature 221:265-267, 1969.

k Small, D.M. The formation of gallstones. Adv. Intern. Med. 16:243-264, 1970.

l Small, D.M., Penkett, S.A., and Chapman, D. Studies on simple and mixed bile salt micelles by nuclear magnetic resonance spectroscopy. Biochim. Biophys. Acta 176:178-189, 1969.

m Small, D.M. Surface and bulk interactions of lipids and water with a classification of biologically active lipids based on these interactions. Fed. Proc. 291:1320-1326, 1970.

n Small, D.M. and Rapo, S. Source of abnormal bile in patients with cholesterol gallstones. N. Engl. J. Med. 283:53-57, 1970.

o Small, D.M. Gallstones, 1971. Viewpoints on Digestive Diseases 3, May, 1971.

a Small, D.M. The physical chemistry of the cholanic acids. In The Bile Acids, Chemistry, Physiology and Metabolism. PP Nair and D Kritchevsky, eds. Plenum Publishing Co., New York, 1971, pp 249-356.

b Small, D.M. Prestone gallstone disease - Is therapy safe? N. Engl. J. Med. 284:214-216, 1971 (Editorial).

c Small, D.M. Gallstones: Diagnosis and treatment. Postgrad. Med. 51:187-193, 1972.

d Small, D.M., Dowling, R.H., and Redinger, R.N. The enterohepatic circulation of bile salts. Arch. Intern. Med. 130:552-573, 1972.

e Small, D.M., Shaffer, E.A., and Braasch, J.W. Bile composition at and after surgery in normals, pigment stone patients and cholesterol stone patients. In Bile Acids in Human Disease. P Back and W Gerok, eds. FK Shattauer Verlag, Stuttgart-New York, 1972, pp 175-178.

f Small, D.M. Advantages of a varied and individualized approach. In Controversies in Internal Medicine. FJ Ingelfinger, RV Ebert, M Finland, and AS Relman, eds. Saunders, Philadelphia, 1974, vol II, pp 545-559.

g Small, D.M., Beaudoin, M., Shaffer, E., O'Brien, J., and Williams, L. The gallbladder and the enterohepatic circulation. In Advances in Bile Acid Research. S Matern, J Hackenschmidt, P Back, and W Gerok, eds. F.K. Schattauer Verlag, Stuttgart-New York, 1975, pp 293-298.

h Small, D.M. The etiology and pathogenesis of cholesterol gallstone disease. Adv. Surg. 10:63-85, 1976.

i Small, D.M. The formation and treatment of gallstones. In Diseases of the Liver. Shiff, ed. Lippincott Company, Philadelphia, 1976, pp 146-162.

j Small, D.M. Symposium of Gallstones. In Advances in Surgery, WP Longmire, Jr., ed. Year Book Medical Publishers, Inc., New York, 1976, pp 61-85.

k Small, D.M. Nucleation and growth of cholesterol gallstones. Med. Chir. Dig. 9:619-635, 1980.

l Smallwood, R.A., Jablonski, P., and Watts, J.McK. Intermittent secretion of abnormal bile in patients with cholesterol gallstones. Brit. Med. J. 4:263-266, 1972.

m Smallwood, R.A., Lester, R., Piasecki, G.J., Klein, P.D., Greco, R., and Jackson, B.T. Fetal bile salt metabolism. II. Hepatic excretion of endogenous bile salt and of a taurocholate load. J. Clin. Invest. 51:1388-1397, 1972.

n Smallwood, R.A., Jablonski, P., and Watts, J.McK. Bile acid synthesis in the developing sheep liver. Clin. Sci. Mol. Med. 45:403-406, 1973.

a Smallwood, R.A. and Hoffman, N.E. Bile acid structure and biliary secretion of cholesterol and phospholipid in the cat. Gastroenterology 71:1064-1066, 1976.

b Smith, D.C., Crook, J.N., McAllister, R.A., and MacKay, C. The comparison of gallbladder bile in patients with gallstones and in patients with duodenal ulcer before and after vagotomy. Brit. J. Surg. 59:306, 1972 (abstract).

c Smith, D.C., McAllister, R.A., and Mackay, C. The effect of cholecystectomy on the composition of bile in gallstone patients. Brit. J. Surg. 60:899, 1973 (abstract).

d Smith, L.H. and Hofmann, A.F. Acquired hyperoxaluria, urolithiasis, and intestinal disease: A new digestive disorder. Gastroenterology 66:1257-1261, 1974 (Editorial).

e Smythe, A., Mangnall, D., and Johnson, A.G. A simple method for the separation of bile acid groups by ion-exchange chromatography. Anal. Biochem. 118:65-69, 1981.

f Sobotka, H. Physiological Chemistry of the Bile. Baltimore, Williams and Wilkins, 1937, pp 2.

g Sobotka, H. The Chemistry of the Steroids. The Williams & Wilkins Company, Baltimore, 1938, 202 pp.

h Soderlund, C.H. Medical resolution of gallstones: No alternative to surgical treatment. Lakartidningen 76:399-400, 1979.

i Sodhi, H.S., Kudchodkar, B.J., and Horlick, L. Determinants of increased fecal excretion of cholesterol and its metabolites in response to hypocholesterolemic agents. Circulation 46:276, 1972 (abstract).

j Sodhi, H.S. and Kudchodkar, B.J. Catabolism of cholesterol in hypercholesterolemia and its relationship to plasma triglycerides. Clin. Chim. Acta 46:161-171, 1973.

k Sohrabi, A., Max, M.H., and Hershey, C.D. Cholate sodium infusion for retained common bile duct stones. Arch. Surg. 11:1169-1172, 1979.

l Solis-Herruzo, J.A. Papel de la bilis en la genesis de la malabsorpcion de los enfermos con hepatopatias cronicas. Rev. Clin. Esp. 125:301-312, 1972.

m Solis-Herruzo, J.A. Patogenia y tratamiento medico de la litiasis biliar. La medicina, hoy 220:41-46, 1976.

n Solis-Herruzo, J.A. Treatment of biliary calculi of cholesterol with chenodeoxycholic acid. Rev. Clin. Esp. 145:411-418, 1977.

o Solis-Herruzo, J.A. and Rodriguez Agullo, J.L. Mechanismo de la formacion de calculos biliares de colesterol. I. Fisiopatologia de la formacion de calculos. Rev. Clin. Esp. 147:447-452, 1977.

a Solis-Herruzo, J.A. and Rodriguez Agullo, J.L. Mechanismo de la formacion de calculos biliares de colesterol. II. Causas de bilis litogenica. Rev. Clin. Esp. 147:453-460, 1977.

b Solomons, N.W., Schoeller, D.A., Wagonfeld, J.B., Ott, D., Rosenberg, I.H., and Klein, P.D. Application of a stable isotope (^{13}C) labeled glycocholate breath test to diagnosis of bacterial overgrowth and ileal dysfunction. J. Lab. Clin. Med. 90:431-439, 1977.

c Soloway, R.D., Thistle, J.L., and Schoenfield, L.J. Hepatic lipid secretion and cholelithiasis. Am. J. Dig. Dis. 16:437-454, 1971.

d Soloway, R.D., Clark, M.L., Powell, K.M., Senior, J.R., and Brooks, F.P. Effects of secretin and bile salt infusions on canine bile composition and flow. Am. J. Physiol. 222:681-686, 1972.

e Soloway, R.D., Hofmann, A.F., Thomas, P.J., Schoenfield, L.J., and Klein, P.D. Triketocholanoic (dehydrocholic) acid. Hepatic metabolism and effect on bile flow and biliary lipid secretion in man. J. Clin. Invest. 52:715-724, 1973.

f Soloway, R.D., Powell, K.M., Senior, J.R., and Brooks, F.P. Interrelationship of bile salts, phospholipids, and cholesterol in bile during manipulation of the enterohepatic circulation in the conscious dog. Gastroenterology 64:1156-1162, 1973.

g Soloway, R.D. Gallstone disease. In Gastrointestinal Pathophysiology. FP Brooks, ed. Oxford University Press, New York, 1974, pp 172.

h Soloway, R.D. and Schoenfield, L.J. Effects of meals and interruption of the enterohepatic circulation on flow, lipid composition, and cholesterol saturation of bile in man after cholecystectomy. Am. J. Dig. Dis. 20:99-109, 1975.

i Soloway, R.D., Trotman, B.W., and Ostrow, J.D. Pigment gallstones. Progress in Hepatology. Gastroenterology 72:167-182, 1977.

j von Sonnenberg, A., Leuschner, U., and Leuschner, M. Erwartungskosten bie der konservativen und chirurgischen Behandlung der unkomplizierten Cholezystolithiasis. Z. Gastroenterol. 20:66-77, 1982.

k Sonnenshein, M., Siegel, J.H., Rosenthal, W.S., Sable, R., and Balthazar, E. Recurrent choledocholithiasis following cholecystectomy, sphincterotomy and choledochoduodenostomy: successful treatment with chenodeoxycholic acid. Am. J. Med. 69:163-166, 1980.

l Sorensen, T.I.A. and Krag, E. Fat digestion after jejunoileal bypass operation for obesity. Scand. J. Gastroenterol. 11:491, 1976.

m Sorensen, T.I.A., Bruusgaard, A., Andersen, A.N., and Andersen, B. Serum levels and clearance of bile acids are unaffected by jejunoileal bypass with 3:1 or 1:3 jejunoileal ratio. Scand. J. Gastroent. 16:705-711, 1981.

a Spanner, G.O. and Bauman, L. The behavior of cholesterol and other bile constituents in sodium solutions of bile salts. J. Biol. Chem. 98:181-183, 1932.

b Sperber, I. Secretion of organic anions in the formation of urine and bile. Pharm. Rev. 11:109, 1951.

c Spitzer, H.L., Kyriakides, E.C., and Balint, J.A. Biliary phospholipids in various species. Nature 204:288, 1965 (Letter to Editor).

d Spritz, N., Ahrens, E.H., Jr., and Grundy, S. Sterol balance in man as plasma cholesterol concentrations are altered by exchanges of dietary fats. J. Clin. Invest. 44:1482-1493, 1965.

e Stadler, G.A. Pathogenesis of gallstones, effectiveness and indications of medical treatment. Ther. Umsch. 34:866-868, 1977.

f Stahl, E. and Arnesjo, B. Taurocholate metabolism in man. Scand. J. Gastroenterol. 7:559-566, 1972.

g Standaert, L.O. Oplossen van galstenen. Tijdschr. Gastroenterol. 15:155-158, 1972.

h Standaert, L.O. Le point sur les modifications de la composition de la bile. Lille Med. 18:279-283, 1973.

i Stanley, M.M. and Nemchausky, B. Fecal ^{14}C bile acid excretion in normal subjects and patients with steroid-wasting syndromes secondary to ileal dysfunction. J. Lab. Clin. Med. 70:627-639, 1967.

j Stanley, M.M. Steroid-wasting enteropathy: Clinical picture, bile salt absorption and fecal excretion, and therapy. In Bile Salt Metabolism. L Schiff, JB Carey, and JM Dietschy, eds. C. C. Thomas, Springfield, 1969, pp 266-283.

k Stanley, M.M. Quantification of intestinal functions during fasting: Estimations of bile salt turnover, fecal calcium and nitrogen excretions. Metabolism 19:865-875, 1970.

l Stanley, M.M., Gacke, D., and Murphy, J. Effect of colestipol on fecal excretion of cholate in man. Clin. Res. 21:869, 1973 (abstract).

m Stanley, M.M., Paul, D., Gacke, D., and Murphy, J. Effects of cholestyramine, metamucil, and cellulose on fecal bile salt excretion in man. Gastroenterology 65:889-894, 1973.

n Starkey, B.J. and Marks, V. Determination of total bile acids in serum. A comparison of a radioimmunoassay with an enzymatic-fluorimetric method. Clin. Chim. Acta 119:165-177, 1982.

o Stein, W.D. The Movement of Molecules Across Cell Membranes. Academic Press, New York, 1969, 369 pp.

a Stellwag, E. and Hylemon, P. Purification and characterization of bile salt hydrolase from bacteroids fragilis subsp. fragilis. Biochim. Biophys. Acta 452:165-176, 1976.

b Stellwag, E.J. and Hylemon, P.B. 7a-Dehydroxylation of cholic acid and chenodeoxycholic acid by Clostridium leptum. J. Lipid Res. 20:325-333, 1979.

c Stempel, J.M. and Duane, W.C. Biliary lipids and bile acid pool size after vagotomy in man: Evidence against a predisposition to gallstones. Gastroenterology 75:608-611, 1978.

d Stephan, Z., Armstrong, M., and Hayes, K. Bile lipid alterations in taurine-depleted monkeys. Amer. J. Clin. Nutr. 34:204-210, 1981.

e Stiehl, A. Gallensauren und Gallensaurensulfate in der Haut von Patienten mit Cholestase. 28. Tagung Dtsch. Ges. Verdau. Stoffwechselkr. Erlangen, Sept., 1973 (abstract).

f Stiehl, A. Bildung und Auflosung von Gallensteinen. G. Kurs praktische Gastroenterol., Erlangen, Nov., 1974 (abstract).

g Stiehl, A. Bile salt sulphates in cholestasis. Europ. J. Clin. Invest. 4:59-63, 1974.

h Stiehl, A. Sulfation of bile salts: A new metabolic pathway. Digestion 11:406-413, 1974.

i Stiehl, A., Czygan, P., and Raedsch, R. Sulphation of lithocholate in patients during chenodeoxycholate treatment. A protective mechanism. In Advances in Bile Acid Research. S Matern, J Hackenschmidt, P Back, and W Gerok, eds. F.K. Schattauer Verlag, Stuttgart-New York, 1974, pp 347-350.

j Stiehl, A. Bildung und Auflosung von Gallensteinen. In Gallenblase - Pankreas. Boecker, ed. Thieme, Stuttgart, 1975, pp 28-32.

k Stiehl, A. Die Sulfatierung der Gallensauren. Ein neuer und quantitativ wichtiger Stoffwechselweg. Fortsch. Med. 93:1092-1093, 1975.

l Stiehl, A. Lithogene Galle und Cholelithiasis. Entstehung von Cholesterin-Gallensteinen und Behandlung mit Chenodeoxycholsaure. Fortschr. Med. 93:343-344, 1975.

m Stiehl, A. Veranderungen des Gallensaurestoffwechsels wahrend der Behandlung mit Chenodesoxycholsaure. Z. Gastroenterol. 13:300-301, 1975.

n Stiehl, A., Earnest, D.L., and Admirand, W.H. Sulfation and renal excretion of bile salts in patients with cirrhosis of the liver. Gastroenterology 68:534-544, 1975.

o Stiehl, A., Kommerell, B., Regula, M., and Raedsch, R. Zur Behandlung von Patienten mit Cholesteringallensteinen mit Chenodesoxycholsaure: Veranderungen im Gallensaurenstoff wechsel. Inn. Med. 2:13-18, 1975.

a Stiehl, A., Raedsch, R., and Kommerell, B. Increased sulfation of lithocholate in patient with cholesterol gallstones during chenodeoxycholate treatment. Digestion 12:105-110, 1975.

b Stiehl, A., Raedsch, R., Regula, M., and Kommerell, B. Elevated serum transaminase following chenodeoxycholate treatment. Correlation to chenodeoxycholate dose and chenodeoxycholate concentration in the serum. 10th Meeting of EASL. Digestion 12:4-6, 1975.

c Stiehl, A., Raedsch, R., Regula, M., and Kommerell, B. Treatment of patients with cholesterol gallstones with chenodeoxycholic acid: Alterations in the bile salt metabolism. Inn. Med. 2:13-18, 1975.

d Stiehl, A., Regula, M., and Kommerell, B. Transaminasenhohungen nach Chenodesoxycholsaurebehandlung Abhangigkeit von Chenodesoxycholsauredosis und Chenodesoxycholsaurekonzentration im Serum. 81. Tagung Dtsch. Ges. Inn. Med., Wiesbaden, April, 1975, 401:278 (abstract).

e Stiehl, A., Ast, E., Czygan, P., Frohling, W., and Kommerell, B. Elevated transaminases following treatment of patients with cholesterol gallstones with chenodeoxycholic acid. Inn. Med. 3:75-80, 1976.

f Stiehl, A., Ast, E., Czygan, P., Frohling, W., and Kommerell, B. Serumtransaminasen und Gallensaurenkonzentrationen im Serum von Patienten mit Gallensteinen wahrend der Behandlung mit Chenodesoxycholsaure. Z. Gastroenterol. 14:40-41, 1976.

g Stiehl, A., Ast, E., Czygan, P., and Liersch, M. Formation, metabolism and excretion of bile salt sulfates in man. In The Hepatobiliary System. W Taylor, ed. Plenum Publishing Corp., New York, 1976, pp 453-465.

h Stiehl, A. Disturbances of bile acid metabolism in cholestasis. Clin. Gastroenterol. 6:45-67, 1977.

i Stiehl, A., Czygan, P., Frohling, W., and Kommerell, B. Changes in biliary bile acid composition and cholesterol saturation of bile in patients with cholesterol gallstones following treatment with ursodeoxycholic acid. Verh. Dtsch. Ges. Inn. Med. 83:501-502, 1977.

j Stiehl, A., Ast, E., Czygan, P., Frohling, W., Raedsch, R., and Kommerell, B. Pool size, synthesis, and turnover of sulfated and nonsulfated cholic acid and chenodeoxycholic acid in patients with cirrhosis of the liver. Gastroenterology 74:572-577, 1978.

k Stiehl, A., Czygan, P., Kommerell, B., Weis, H.J., and Holtermuller, K.H. Ursodeoxycholic acid versus chenodeoxycholic acid. Gastroenterology, 75:1016-1020, 1978.

a Stiehl, A., Raedsch, R., Czygan, P., Gotz, R., Manner, C.H., Walker, S., and Kommerell, B. Effects of biliary bile acid composition on biliary cholesterol saturation in gallstone patients treated with chenodeoxycholic and/or ursodeoxycholic acid. Gastroenterology 79:1192-1198, 1980.

b Stiehl, A. Neue Aspekte der konservativen Gallensteinbehandlung: Theorie und Praxis. Schweiz. med. Wschr. 111:1630-1631, 1981.

c Stiehl, A. Die konservative Behandlung der Cholelithiasis. Media 2:554-557, 1981.

d Stiehl, A. Effects of chenodeoxycholic acid and ursodeoxycholic acid on bile acid and biliary lipid metabolism in patients with radiolucent gallstones. Correlation with efficacy and toxicity. In Bile Acids and Lipids. G Paumgartner, A Stiehl, and W Gerok, eds. MTP Press, Lancaster, 1981, pp 309-317.

e Stiehl, A., Raedsch, R., Walker, S., Gotz, R., Czygan, P., and Kommerell, B. Taurin- und Glycin-Konjugation sulfatierter und glucuronidierter Gallensauren bein Patienten mit alkaholischer Leberzirrhose und Cholestase. Z. Gastroenterol. XIX (9), 1981 (abstract).

f Stock, S. Gallstones under attack. New Scientist, December 29, 1972.

g Stolk, A. Induction of hepatic cirrhosis in Iguana iguana by 3-monohydroxycholanic treatment. Experientia 16:507, 1960.

h Stolk, A. Induction of hepatic cirrhosis in the axoloth by 3-monohydroxycholanic treatment. Naturwiss 48:671, 1961.

i Strange, R.C., Nimmo, I.A., and Percy-Robb, I.W. Binding of bile acids by 100,000 g supernatants from rat liver. Biochem. J. 162:659-664, 1977.

j Strange, R.C., Beckett, G.J., and Percy-Robb, I.W. Nuclear and cytosolic distrubution of conjugated cholic acid and radiolabelled glycocholic acid in rat liver. Biochem. J. 178:71-78, 1979.

k Strange, R.C., Chapman, B.T., Johnston, J.D., Nimmon, I.A., and Percy-Robb, I.W. Partitioning of bile acids into subcellular organelles and the in vivo distribution of bile acids in rat liver. Biochim. Biophys. Acta 573:535-545, 1979.

l Strange, R.C., Nimmo, I.A., and Percy-Robb, I.W. Studies in the rat on the hepatic subcellular distribution and biliary excretion of lithocholic acid. Biochim. Biophys. Acta 588:70-80, 1979.

m Strange, R.C. Hepatic bile salt transport. Biochem. Soc. Trans. Biochem. Rev. 9:170-174, 1981.

n Strasberg, S.M., Dorn, B.C., Redinger, R.N., Small, D.M., and Egdahl, R.H. Effects of alteration of biliary pressure on bile composition - A method for study. Primate biliary physiology. Gastroenterology 61:357-362, 1971.

a Strasberg, S.M., Ilson, R.G., and Siminovitch, K.A. Bile production in fasted and fed primates. Ann. Surg. 180:356-363, 1974.

b Strasberg, S.M. and Ilson, R.G. The effect of bile acid synthesis on cholesterol secretion into the bile. Ann. Surg. 181:458-465, 1975.

c Strasberg, S.M., Ilson, R.G., Simonovitch, K.A., Brenner, D., and Palaheimo, J.E. Analysis of the components of bile flow in the rhesus monkey. Am. J. Physiol. 228:115-121, 1975.

d Strasberg, S.M., Petrunka, C.N., and Ilson, R.G. The contribution of the extrahepatic bile ducts to bile formation. Canad. J. Physiol. Pharmacol. 54:757-763, 1976.

e Strasberg, S.M., Petrunka, C.N., and Ilson, R.G. Effect of bile acid synthesis rate on cholesterol secretion rate in the steady state. Gastroenterology 71:1067-1070, 1976.

f Strasberg, S.M., Petrunka, C.N., and Ilson, R.G. Unilateral hepatic duct obstruction in the primate. Surgery 81:91-99, 1977.

g Strasberg, S.M., Kay, R.M., Ilson, R.G., Petrunka, C.N., and Paloheimo, J.E. Taurolithocholic acid and chlorpromazine cholestasis in the rhesus monkey. Can. J. Physiol. Pharmacol. 57:1138-1147, 1979.

h von Stremmel, W. Zur medikamentosen auflosung von Gallensteinen mit Chenodesoxycholsaure. Z. Allgemeinmed. 29:1504-1507, 1976.

i von Stremmel, W. Can gallstones be dissolved by drugs? Med. Klin. 75:42-45, 1980.

j Stremmel, W. Prophylaxis of gallstone formation. Zentralbl. Chir. 105: 162-166, 1980.

k Strohmeyer, G. Auflosung von Gallensteinen. Der Internist 13:342-343, 1972.

l Sturdevant, R.A.L., Dayton, S., and Pearce, M.L. Increased prevalence of gallstones in men ingesting a serum cholesterol lowering diet. N. Engl. J. Med. 288:24-27, 1973.

m Sturdevant, R.A.L. Medical treatment of gallstones. Scand. Med. J. 68:76-78, 1975.

n Sturman, J.A., Hepner, G.W., Hofmann, A.F., and Thomas, P.J. Metabolism of ^{35}S taurine in man. J. Nutr. 105:1206-1214, 1975.

o Su, C.C., Park, J.Y., Higuchi, W.I., Alkan, M.H., Corrigan, O.I., Hofmann, A.F., and Danzinger, R.G. Mesophase formation during in vitro cholesterol gallstone dissolution: a specific effect of ursodeoxycholic acid. J. Pharm. Sci. 70:713-715, 1981.

a Subbiah, M.T.R., Kuksis, A., and Mookerjea, S. Secretion of bile salts by intact and isolated rat livers. Canad. J. Biochem. 47:847-854, 1969.

b Subbiah, M.T.R. Cholestanol and chenodeoxycholic acid: Metabolites of injected cholesterol-4-^{14}C in pigeon bile. Experientia 29:404-405, 1973.

c Subbiah, M.T.R. and Buscaglia, M.D. Studies concerning the hypercholesterolemia of pregnancy: Cholesterol catabolism and excretion during late pregnancy in the rat. Res. Comm. Chem. Path. Pharm. 13:529-539, 1976.

d Sue, S.O., Taub, M., Pearlman, B.J., Marks, J.W., Bonorris, G.G., and Schoenfield, L.J. Treatment of choledocholithiasis with oral chenodeoxycholic acid. Surgery 90:32-34, 1981.

e Sugata, F. and Shimizu, M. Retrospective studies on gallstone disappearance. Jap. J. Gastroenterol. 71:70-80, 1974.

f Sugata, F., Kobayashi, a., Yamamura, M., and Shimizu, M. Five year follow-up study on UDCA therapy for cholelithiasis with special reference to recurrence. XI Internat'l Congress of Gastroenterology, Hamburg, 1980, E34.11 (abstract).

g Summerfield, J.A. Medical treatment of gallstones. Brit. J. Hosp. Med. 21:482-489, 1979.

h Suzuki, N., Nagashima, H., Matsushiro, T., Saitoh, T., Nakamura, N., Hatanaka, T., Kobayashi, N., Nakamura, Y., and Sato, T. Role of sulfated glycoproteins in the gallstone formation. Gastroenterol. Jpn. 9:214, 1974 (abstract).

i Svanvik, J. and Jansson, R. An experimental method for studying in vivo gallbladder absorption. Gastroenterology 72:634-638, 1977.

j Swell, L., Bell, C.C., Jr., and Entenman, C. Bile acids and lipid metabolism. III. Influence of bile acids on phospholipids in liver and bile of the isolated perfused dog liver. Biochim. Biophys. Acta 164:278-284, 1968.

k Swell, L., Entenman, C., Leong, C.F., and Holloway, R.J. Bile acids and lipid metabolism. IV. Influence of bile acids on biliary and liver organelle phospholipids and cholesterol. Am. J. Physiol. 215:1390-1396, 1968.

l Swell, L., Bell, C.C., Jr., and Vlahcevic, Z.R. Relationship of bile acid pool size to biliary lipid excretion and the formation of lithogenic bile in man. Gastroenterology 61:716-722, 1971.

m Swell, L., Bell, C.C., Jr., Gregory, D.H., and Vlahcevic, Z.R. The cholesterol saturation index of human bile. Am. J. Dig. Dis. 19:261-265, 1974.

n Swell, L., Gregory, D.H., and Vlahcevic, Z.R. Current concepts of the pathogenesis of cholesterol gallstones. Med. Clin. N. Am. 58:1449-1471,1974.

a Swell, L., Schwartz, C.C., Halloran, L.G., and Vlahcevic, Z.R. Rapid feedback inhibition of endogenous cholic and chenodeoxycholic acid synthesis by exogenous chenodeoxycholic acid in man. Biochem. Biophys. Res. Comm. 64:1083-1089, 1975.

b Swell, L., Gustafsson, J., Schwartz, C.C., Halloran, L.G., Danielsson, H., and Vlahcevic, Z.R. An in vivo evaluation of the quantitative significance of several potential pathways to cholic and chenodeoxycholic acids from cholesterol in man. J. Lipid Res. 21:455-466, 1980.

c Swell, L., Gustafsson, J., Danielsson, H., Schwartz, C.C., Halloran, L.G., and Vlahcevic, Z.R. Bile acid synthesis in humans. Cancer Res. 41:3757-3758, 1981.

d Switz, D.M., Hislop, I.G., and Hofmann, A.F. Factors influencing the absorption of bile acids by the human jejunum. Gastroenterology 58:999, 1970 (abstract).

e Szalatnay, Z., Mohr, P., and Akovbiantz, A. Zur nichtchirurgischen Behandlung postoperativ retinierter Hepato-Choledochussteine. Schw. med. Wschr. 106:876-880, 1976.

f Szczepanik, P.A., Hachey, D.L., Thistle, J.L., Hofmann, A.F., and Klein, P.D. Sensitive complete quantitation of biliary bile acids by mass spectrometry in gallstone patients undergoing chenotherapy. Gastroenterology 69:869, 1975 (abstract).

g Szczpanik, P.A., Hachey, D.L., and Klein, P.D. Evaluation of Poly-S-179 as a stationary phase for the gas-liquid chromatography/mass spectrometry of bile acid methyl ester acetates. J. Lipid Res. 19:280-283, 1978.

h Tabaqchali, S. and Booth, C.C. Jejunal bacteriology and bile-salt metabolism in patients with intestinal malabsorption. Lancet 2:12-15, 1966.

i Tabaqchali, S., Hatzioannou, J., and Booth, C.C. Bile salt deconjugation and steatorrhea in patients with the stagnant loop syndrome. Lancet 2:12-16, 1968.

j Tabaqchali, S. The pathophysiological role of small intestinal bacterial flora. Scand. J. Gastroenterol. 6(Suppl.):139-163, 1970.

k Takabayashi, A., Watkins, J., Soloway, R., Rios-Dalenz, J., and Henson, D. Glycolithocholic acid is greatly increased in stones from patients with carcinoma of the gallbladder. Gastroenterology 79:1058, 1980 (abstract).

l Takagi, T. and Takeda, M. Chenodeoxycholic acid-induced diarrhea in rats. Effects of atropine and codeine. Arch. Int. Pharmacodyn. Ther. 240:328-339, 1979.

m Takahashi, H., Tozuka, K., Miyashita, T., and Miyamoto, K. Chronic toxicity studies of ursodeoxycholic acid orally administered for six months in Wistar male rat. Kiso to Rinsho (Clinical Report) 9:3209-3222, 1975.

a Takahashi, H., Tozuka, K., Miyashita, T., and Miyamoto, K. Toxicity studies of ursodeoxycholic acid orally administered for three months in Wister male rat. Kiso to Rinsho (Clinical Report) 9:3203-3208, 1975.

b Takahashi, H., Tozuka, K., Miyashita, T., Usui, K., and Miyamoto, K. Influence of ursodeoxycholic acid administered during pregnancy on the development of foetus and postnatal growth in rats and mice. Kiso to Rinsho (Clinical Report) 9:3223-3242, 1975.

c Takahashi, H., Tozuka, K., Miyashita, T., Usui, K., and Miyamoto, K. Subacute toxicity studies of intraperitoneally administered ursodeoxycholic acid in Wistar rat. Kiso to Rinsho (Clinical Report) 9:3183-3202, 1975.

d Takahashi, H., Tozuka, K., Miyashita, T., Usui, K., and Miyamoto, K. Subacute toxicity studies of orally administered ursodeoxycholic acid in Wistar rat. Kiso to Rinsho (Clinical Report) 9:3167-3181, 1975.

e Takasawa, Y., Suzuki, N., Takahashi, W., and Uematsu, I. A fundamental study on the dissolution and disintegration of calcium bilirubinate stone. Japanese J. Gastroenterol. 79:836-844, 1982.

f Takeda, K. Disintegration effects of sodium hexametaphosphate on the structure of human gallstones with special reference to soft x-ray findings. Fukuoka Acta Med. 40:404-426, 1970.

g Tamesue, N. and Juniper, K., Jr. Concentrations of bile salts at the critical micellar concentration of human gallbladder bile. Gastroenterology 52:473-479, 1967.

h Tamesue, N., Inoue, T., and Juniper, K., Jr. Solubility of cholesterol in bile salt-lecithin model systems. Am. J. Dig. Dis. 18:670-678, 1974.

i Tanaka, N., Portman, O.W., and Osuga, T. Effect of type of dietary fat, cholesterol, and chenodeoxycholic acid in gallstone formation, bile acid kinetics, and plasma lipids in squirrel monkeys. J. Nutr. 106:1123-1134, 1976.

j Tanaka, N. and Portman, O. Effect of type of dietary fat and cholesterol on cholesterol absorption rate in Squirrel monkeys. J. Nutr. 107:814-821, 1977.

k Tanaka, N., Osuga, T., Torii, M., Oda, T., and Mashige, F. Clinical significance of determination of serum bile acid in liver diseases. Acta Hepatol. Japonica 22:785-802, 1981.

l Tangedahl, T.N. Dissolution of gallstones--when and how? Surg. Clin. North Am. 59:797-809, 1979.

a Tangedahl, T.N., Thistle, J.L., Hofmann, A.F., and Matseshe, J.W. Effect of b-sitosterol alone or in combination with chenic acid on cholesterol saturation of bile and cholesterol absorption in gallstones patients. Gastroenterology 76:1341-1346, 1979.

b Tangedahl, T.N., Hofmann, A.F., and Kottke, B.A. Biliary lipid secretion in hypercholesterolemia. J. Lipid Res. 20:125-133, 1979.

c Tanikawa, K. and Maeyama, T. Treatment of gallstones with ursodeoxycholic acid--lipid and bile composition in bile. Nippon Shokakibyo Gakkai Zasshi 75:1196-1203, 1978.

d Tanimura, H. and Hikasa, Y. Cholelithiasis - Cholesterol stone. Jap. J. Clin. Med. 30:234-241, 1972.

e Tanimura, H. and Hikasa, Y. The etiology and pathophysiology of cholelithiasis. Gastroent. Japonica 10:90, 1975 (abstract).

f Tanimura, H. and Takenaka, M. Experimental studies on dissolution of cholesterol gallstones in hamsters with chenodeoxycholic acid. Arch. Jap. Chir. 44:3-20, 1975.

g Tanimura, H. and Hikasa, Y. Diurnal rhythm of lithogenic bile and treatment with chenodeoxycholic acid. Nippon Geka Hokan 47:474-482, 1978.

h Tanimura, H., Shioda, R., Nagase, M., Takenaka, M., Kobayashi, N., Setoyama, M., Kamata, T., Mukaihara, S., Maruyama, K., Kato, H., Miki, K., and Hikasa, Y. Initiating factors in the formation of cholesterol gallstones. Arch. Jpn. Chir. 47:427-445, 1978.

i Tao, J.C., Cussler, E.L., and Evans, D.F. Accelerating gallstone dissolution. Proc. Natl. Acad. Sci. 10:3917, 1974.

j Tappeiner, A.J.F.H. Ueber die Aufsaugung der Gallsauren alkalien im Dunndarme. Wien. Akad. Sitzber. 77:281-304, 1878.

k Tarpila, S., Miettinen, T.A., and Metsaranta, L. Effects of bran on serum cholesterol, feacal mass, fat, bile acids and neutral sterols, and biliary lipids in patients with diverticular disease of the colon. Gut 19:137-145, 1978.

l Tashiro, A. Oral ursodeoxycholic acid tolerance test for patients with hepatobiliary disease. Acta Hepatol. Jap. 20:369-375, 1979.

m Tateyama, T. and Matsushiro, T. Bile acid composition affecting cholesterol dissolution rate: A use of multiple regression analysis. Tohoku J. exp. Med. 133:467-475, 1981.

a Tateyama, T., Nezu, Y., Tsutsumi, J., Katayama, K., Fujisawa, K., and Matsushiro, T. Studies on biotransformation of chenodeoxycholic acid in man: Effects of chenodeoxycholic acid ingestion on the bile acid kinetics and on the cholesterol dissolution. Proc 12th Symp on Drug Metabolism and Action, Kanazawa, 1981 (abstract).

b Tatsumura, T., Sato, H., Yamamoto, K., and Ueyama, T. Ursodeoxycholic acid prevents gastrointestinal disorders caused by anticancer drugs. Jpn. J. Surg. 11:84-89, 1981.

c Taub, M., Bonorris, G., Chung, A., Coyne, M.J., and Schoenfield, L.J. Effect of propanol on bile acid- and cholera enterotoxin-stimulated cAMP and secretion in rabbit intestine. Gastroenterology 72:101-105, 1977.

d Taub, M., Coyne, M., Bonorris, G., Chung, A., Coyne, B., and Schoenfield, L. Inhibition by propranolol of bile acid- and PGE_1-stimulated cAMP and intestinal secretion. Am. J. Gastroenterol. 70:129-135, 1978.

e Taylor, I., Basu, P., Hammond, P., Darby, C., and Flynn, M. Effect of bile acid perfusion on colonic motor function in patients with the irritable colon syndrome. Gut 21:843-847, 1980.

f Taylor, W., Ellis, W.R., and Bell, G.D. The effect of cholesterol feeding on gallbladder bile acids of the rabbit. Biochem. J. 198:639-643, 1981.

g Teem, M.V. and Phillips, S.F. Dihydroxy bile acids inhibit water absorption by the hamster jejunum in vivo. J. Lab. Clin. Med. 76:876-877, 1970.

h Teem, M.V. and Phillips, S.F. Perfusion of the hamster jejunum with conjugated and unconjugated bile acids: Inhibition of water absorption and effects on morphology. Gastroenterology 62:261-267, 1972.

i Tenneson, M.E., Owen, R.W., and Mason, A.N. The anaerobic side-chain cleavage of bile acids by _Escherichia coli_ isolated from human faeces. Biochem. Soc. Trans. 5:1758-1760, 1977.

j Tenneson, M.E., Baty, J.D., Bilton, R.F., and Mason, A.N. The degradation of chenodeoxycholic acid by Pseudomonas Spp. N.C.I.B. 10590. J. Steroid Biochem. 10:311-316, 1979.

k Teplick, S.K., Pavlides, C.A., Goodman, L.R., and Babayan, V.K. In vitro dissolution of gallstones: comparison of monooctanoin, sodium dehydrocholate, heparin, and saline. Am. J. Roentgen. 138:271-273, 1982.

l Tera, H. Stratification of human gallbladder bile in vivo. Acta Chir. Scand. Suppl. 256:1-85, 1960.

m Testa, R., Bocchini, R., Dellepiane, F., Mansi, C., and Celle, G. Postprandial serum bile acids after ursodeoxycholic acid. Preliminary results in healthy subjects, in patients with ileal resection and patients with liver disease. Ital. J. Gastroenterol. 12:339, 1980 (abstract).

n Teufel, H. Cholesterinsteine. Z. Allgemeinmed. 52:328, 1976.

a Hess Thaysen, E. and Pedersen, L. Diarrhoea associated with idiopathic bile acid malabsorption. Fact or fantasy? Dan. Med. Bull. 20:174-177, 1973.

b Hess Thaysen, E. Diagnostic value of the ^{14}C-cholylglycine breath test. Clin. Gastroenterol. 6:227-245, 1977.

c Theodor, E., Spritz, N., and Sleisenger, M.H. Metabolism of intravenously injected isotopic cholic acid in viral hepatitis. Gastroenterology 55:183-190, 1968.

d Thiele, H. Dissolution of gallstones left in the common bile duct. Langenbecks Arch. Cir. 344:123-129, 1977.

e Thistle, J.L. and Schoenfield, L.J. Induced alterations of bile composition in humans with cholelithiasis. J. Lab. Clin. Med. 74:1020-1021, 1969 (abstract).

f Thistle, J.L., Eckhert, K.L., Nensel, R.E., Nobrega, F.T., Poehling, G.G., Reimer, M., and Schoenfield, L.J. Prevalence of gallbladder disease among Chippewa Indians. Mayo Clin. Proc. 46:603-608, 1971.

g Thistle, J.L. and Schoenfield, L.J. Induced alterations in composition of bile of persons having cholelithiasis. Gastroenterology 61:488-496, 1971.

h Thistle, J.L. and Schoenfield, L.J. Lithogenic bile among young Indian women. Lithogenic potential decreased with chenodeoxycholic acid. N. Engl. J. Med. 284:177-181, 1971.

i Thistle, J.L. Cholesterol gallstone dissolution. Current status. Arch. Surg. 107:831-832, 1973.

j Thistle, J.L. Gallstones: Pathophysiology and dissolution. Postgrad. Med. 53:65-71, 1973.

k Thistle, J.L. and Hofmann, A.F. Dissolution of cholesterol gallstones by chenodeoxycholic acid: Current status of the Mayo Clinic therapeutic trial. Biol. Gastroenterol. 6:170, 1973.

l Thistle, J.L. and Hofmann, A.F. Efficacy and specificity of chenodeoxycholic acid therapy for dissolving gallstones. N. Engl. J. Med. 289:655-659, 1973.

m Thistle, J.L. and Hofmann, A.F. Medical therapy of gallstones: Ethical aspects. N. Engl. J. Med. 289:1372, 1973 (Letter to Editor).

n Thistle, J.L. and Hofmann, A.F. Chenodeoxycholic acid: Problem of small stones. N. Engl. J. Med. 290:404-405, 1974 (Letter to Editor).

o Thistle, J.L., Yu, P.Y.S., Hofmann, A.F., and Ott, B.J. Prompt return of bile to supersaturated state followed by gallstone recurrence after discontinuance of chenodeoxycholic acid therapy. Gastroenterology 66:789, 1974 (abstract).

a Thistle, J.L., Hofmann, A.F., Ott, B.J., and Yu, P.Y.S. Gallstone dissolution with chenodeoxycholic acid, 1969-1976. Gastroenterology 70:943, 1976 (abstract).

b Thistle, J.L. Effetto dell'acido chenico sulla composizione lipidica biliare e sul metabolismo degli acidi biliari nei pazienti litiasici. Min. Med. 68:3019-3021, 1977.

c Thistle, J.L., Carlson, G.L., Hofmann, A.F., and Babayan, V.K. Medium chain glycerides rapidly dissolve cholesterol gallstones in vitro. Gastroenterology 72:1141, 1977 (abstract).

d Thistle, J.L., Hofmann, A.F., Yu, P.Y.S., and Ott, B.J. Effect of varying doses of chenodeoxycholic acid on bile lipid and biliary bile acid composition in gallstone patients: A dose response study. Am. J. Dig. Dis. 22:1-6, 1977.

e Thistle, J.L. Therapy of gallstones. Ration. Drug Therap. 12:1-5, 1978.

f Thistle, J.L., Carlson, G.L., LaRusso, N.F., and Hofmann, A.F. Effective dissolution of biliary duct stones by intraductal infusion of mono-octanoin. Gastroenterology 74:1103, 1978 (abstract).

g Thistle, J.L., Hofmann, A.F., Ott, B.J., and Stephens, D.H. Chenotherapy for gallstones. I. Efficacy and safety. JAMA 239:1138-1144, 1978.

h Thistle, J.L., Carlson, G.L., Hofmann, A.F., LaRusso, N.F., MacCarty, R.L., Flynn, G.L., Higuchi, W.I., and Babayan, V.K. Monooctanoin, a dissolution agent for retained cholesterol bile duct stones: physical properties and clinical application. Gastroenterology 78:1016-1022, 1980.

i Thistle, J.L. Gallstone dissolution: 1981 Update. Mayo Clin. Proc. 56:336, 1981 (Clinical Brief).

j Thistle, J.L. Medical management of gallstones. Prac. Gastroenterol. 5:31-38, 1981.

k Thistle, J.L. Treatment of bile duct stones. In Bile Acids and Lipids. G Paumgartner, A Stiehl, and W Gerok, eds. MTP Press, Lancaster, 1981, pp 351-356.

l Thistle, J.L., LaRusso, N.F., Hofmann, A.F., Turcotte, J., Carlson, G.L., and Ott, B.J. Differing effects of ursodeoxycholic or chenodeoxycholic acid on biliary cholesterol saturation and bile acid metabolism in man: A dose response study. Dig. Dis. & Sci. 12:161-168, 1982.

m Thjodleifsson, B., Barnes, S., Chitranukroh, A., Billing, B.H., and Sherlock, S. Cholyl-^{14}C-glycine clearance and serum bile acid concentration for the detection of liver disease. Digestion 14:553-554, 1976 (abstract).

n Thomas, P.J.. Hsia, S.L., Matschiner, J.T., Doisy, E.A., Jr., Elliott, W.H., Thayer, S.A., and Doisy, E.A. XIX. Metabolism of lithocholic acid-24-^{14}C in the rat. J. Biol. Chem. 239:102-105, 1964.

a Thomas, P.J. and Hsia, S.L. XXI. Metabolism of 3a,6b-dihydroxy-5b-cholanoic acid-24-^{14}C-6a-^{3}H in the rat. J. Biol. Chem. 240:1059-1063, 1965.

b Thomas, P.J. and Hofmann, A.F. A simple calculation of the lithogenic index: Expressing biliary lipid composition on rectangular coordinates. Gastroenterology 65:698-700, 1973 (Letter to Editor).

c Thompson, G.R., MacMahon, M., and Claes, P. Precipitation of neomycin compounds of fatty acid and cholesterol from mixed micellar solutions. Europ. J. Clin. Invest. 1:40-47, 1970.

d Thompson, W.G. Cholestyramine. Canad. Med. Assn. J. 104:305-309, 1971.

e Thomson, A.B.R. and Cleland, L. Intestinal cholesterol uptake from phospholipid vesicles and from simple and mixed micelles. Lipids 16:881-887, 1981.

f Thornell, E., Kral, J.G., Jansson, R., and Svanvik, J. Inhibition of prostaglandin synthesis as a treatment for biliary pain. Lancet 1:584, 1979 (Preliminary Communication).

g Thornton, J.R., Emmett, P.M., and Heaton, K.W. Effects of refined and unrefined carbohydrate diets on bile cholesterol saturation and bile acid metabolism. Gut 22:A886, 1981 (abstract).

h Thudichum, J. A Treatise on Gall-Stones: Their Chemistry, Pathology, and Treatment. John Churchill and Sons, London, 1863, 323 pp.

i Thureborn, E. Human hepatic bile. Acta Chir. Scand. 303(Suppl.):7-63, 1962.

j Thurston, O.G., McDougall, R.M. and Walker, K. The effect of prosthetic gallstones on total bile acid pool size in dogs. Surg. Gyn. & Obst. 146: 911-913, 1978.

k Tilvis, R.S., Aro, J., Strandberg, T.E., Lempinen, M., and Miettinen, T.A. Lipid composition of bile acid gallbladder mucosa in patients with acalculous cholesterolosis. Gastroenterology 82:607-615, 1982.

l Tint, G.S., Salen, G., Colallilo, A., Graber, D., Verga, D., Speck, J., and Shefer, S. Ursodeoxycholic acid: A clinical trial of a safe and effective agent for dissolving cholesterol gallstones. Gastroenterology 80:1304, 1981 (abstract).

m Tobiasson, P. and Forkman, A. Serum bile acids in acute hepatitis. Scand. J. Gastroenterol. 16:145-149, 1981.

n Tobiasson, P., Fryden, A., and Tagesson, C. Serum bile acids after test meals and oral load of chenodeoxycholic acid. Scand. J. Gastroenterol. 16: 763-767, 1981.

o Togo, M. Cholesterol gallstone formation in hamsters correlated with histological findings in livers and gallbladders. Arch. Jap. Chir. 38:565-580, 1969.

a Tohma, M., Nakata, Y., Yamada, H., Kurosawa, T., Makino, I., and Nakagawa, S. Quantitative determination of ursodeoxycholic acid and its deuterated derivative in human bile by gas chromatography-mass fragmentography. Chem. Pharm. Bull. 29:137-145, 1981.

b Tokyo Cooperative Gallstone Study Group. Efficacy and indications of ursodeoxycholic acid treatment for dissolving gallstones. Gastroenterology 78:542-548, 1980.

c Tokyo Tanabe. Literature. Urso. Brand of ursodeoxycholic acid. Tokyo Tanabe, Co., Ltd., Japan.

d Tompkins, R.K., Burke, L.G., Zollinger, R.M., and Cornwell, D.G. Relationship of biliary phospholipid and cholesterol concentrations to the occurrence and dissolution of human gallstones. Ann. Surg. 172:936-945, 1970.

e Tompkins, R.K., Kraft, A.R., and Zollinger, R.M. Alterations in biliary phospholipid/cholesterol ratios following vagotomy. Surg. Forum 21:396-397, 1970.

f Tompkins, R.K. Current status of investigations into the etiology of gallstones. Am. J. Surg. 122:1-2, 1971.

g Tompkins, R.K., Kraft, A.R., Zimmerman, E., Lichtenstein, J.E., and Zollinger, R.M. Clinical and biochemical evidence of increased gallstone formation after complete vagotomy. Surgery 71:196-200, 1972.

h Tompkins, R.K. Comments on chenotherapy of cholesterol cholelithiasis. Am. J. Surg. 127:501-502, 1974 (Editorial).

i Tondury, G.D. The treatment of dyspeptic disturbances with ursodeoxycholic acid. Praxis 70:969-973, 1981.

j Toor, E.W., Evans, D.F., and Cussler, E.L. The nucleation of cholesterol monohydrate crystals in model bile solutions. In Gallstones. MM Fisher, CA Goresky, EA Shaffer, and SM Strasberg. Plenum Press, New York, 1979, pp 169-181.

k Toouli, J., Jablonski, P., and Watts, J. Dissolution of stones in the common bile duct with bile-salt solutions. Aust. N. Z. J. Surg. 44: 336-340, 1974.

l Toouli, J., Jablonski, P., and Watts, J.McK. Gallstone dissolution in man using cholic acid and lecithin. Lancet 2:1124-1126, 1975.

m Toouli, J., Williamson, B.W., Gooszen, H., and Blumgart, L.H. In vitro dissolution of human gallstones: The efficacy of heparinized solutions. Brit. J. Surg. 66:770-771, 1979.

n Toouli, J., Jablonski, P., and Watts, J. Treatment of gallstones by chenodeoxycholic acid. Med. J. Aust. 1:478-479, 1980.

a Toouli, J., Jablonski, P., and Watts, J.M. Treatment of gallstones by chenodeoxycholic acid. Med. J. Aust. 1:478-479, 1980.

b Toshaki, O. Study on the dissolution of gallstones with ursodeoxycholic acid: A double-blind trial. Advances in Med. 101:922-936, 1977.

c Touchstone, J.C., Levitt, R.E., Soloway, R.D., and Levin, S.S. Separation of conjugated dihydroxy bile acids by thin-layer chromatography. J. Chromatogr. 178:566-570, 1979.

d Touchstone, J., Levitt, R., Levin, S., and Soloway, R. Separation of conjugated bile acids by reverse phase thin layer chromatography. Lipids 15:386-387, 1980.

e Tournut, R. Pathogeny and medical treatment of cholelithiasis. Rev. Med. Toulouse 11:51-59, 1975.

f Toyoshima, S., Fujita, H., Sato, R., and Kashima, M. Reproduction studies of ursodeoxycholic acid in rats. IV. Perinatal and postnatal study. Pharmacometrics 15:1141-1155, 1978.

g Toyoshima, S., Fujita, H., Sato, R., Kashima, M., and Sato, S. Reproduction studies of ursodeoxycholic acid in rats. I. Fertility study. Pharmacometrics 15:923-930, 1978.

h Toyoshima, S., Fujita, H., Sato, R., Kashima, M., and Sato, S. Teratogenicity study of ursodeoxycholic acid in rabbits. Pharmacometrics 15:1133-1140, 1978.

i Toyoshima, S. Fujita, H., Sakurai, T., Sato, R., and Kashima, K. Reproduction studies of ursodeoxycholic acid in rats. II. Teratogenicity study. Pharmacometrics 15:931-945, 1978.

j Treble, D.H., Frumkin, S., Balint, J.A., and Beeler, D.A. The entry of choline into lecithin, in vivo, by base exchange. Biochim. Biophys. Acta 202:163, 1970.

k Trias, X., Strebel, H.M., Paumgartner, G., and Wiesmann, U. Toxic effects of bile and bile acids on cultured human fibroblasts. Digestion 12(4-6), 1975.

l Trimmer, E. Drop in gallstone surgery soon. Med. News, January 14, 1974.

m Trotman, B.W. and Soloway, R.D. Comparison of gallbladder bile and stone composition from women with and without heterozygous hemoglobinopathy. Gastroenterology 64:811, 1973 (abstract).

n Trotman, B.W. and Soloway, R.D. Influence of age, race or sex on pigment and cholesterol gallstone incidence. Gastroenterology 65:573, 1973 (abstract).

a Trotman, B.W. and Soloway, R.D. The influence of age, sex and race on gallstone and gallbladder bile composition. Gastroenterology 64:811, 1973 (abstract).

b Trotman, B.W., Ostrow, J.D., Soloway, R.D., Cheong, E.B., and Longyear, R.B. Pigment vs cholesterol cholelithiasis: Comparison of stone and bile composition. Am. J. Dig. Dis. 19:585-590, 1974.

c Trotman, B.W., Petrella, E., Soloway, R.D., Sanchez, H., Morris, T., III, and Miller W.T. Evaluation of radiographic lucency or opaqueness of gallstones as a means of identifying cholesterol or pigment stones. Correlation of radiopaqueness with mineral content. Gastroenterology 66:791, 1974 (abstract).

d Trotman, B.W., Morris, T.A., III, Cheney, H.M., Ostrow, J.D., Soloway, R.D., Sanchez, H.M., and Conn, H.O. Two types of pigment gallstones (PS) formed in cirrhotic and noncirrhotic patients: Analysis and comparison. Gastroenterology 68:872, 1975 (abstract).

e Trotman, B.W., Petrella, E.J., Soloway, R.D., Sanchez, H., Morris, T.A., III, and Miller, W.T. Evaluation of radiographic lucency or opaqueness of gallstones as a means of identifying cholesterol or pigment stones. Correlation of lucency or opaqueness with calcium and mineral. Gastroenterology 68:1563-1566, 1975.

f Trotman, B.W. and Soloway, R.D. Pigment vs cholesterol cholelithiasis. Clinical and epidemiologic aspects. Am. J. Dig. Dis. 20:735-740, 1975.

g Trotman, B.W., Soloway, R.D., and Cheong, E. Bile acid conjugation in man and woman with and without gallstones. Gastroenterology 71:932, 1976 (abstract).

h Trotman, B.W., Morris, T., Sanchez, H., Soloway, R., and Ostrow, D. Pigment versus cholesterol cholelithiasis: Identification and quantification by infrared spectroscopy. Gastroenterology 72:495-498, 1977.

i Trotman, B., Morris, T., Cheney, H., Ostrow, D., Sanchez, H., Soloway, R., and Conn, H. Pigment gallstone composition in cirrhotic and noncirrhotic subjects. Am. J. Dig. Dis. 23:872-876, 1978.

j Trulzsch, D., Greim, H., Czygan, P., Hutterer, F., Schaffner, F., Popper, H., Cooper, D.Y., and Rosenthal, O. Cytochrome P-450 in 7*a*-hydroxylation of taurodeoxycholic acid. Biochemistry 12:76-79, 1972.

k Trulzsch, D., Roboz, J., Greim, H., Czygan, P., Rudick, J., Hutterer, F., Schaffner, F., and Popper, H. Hydroxylation of taurolithocholate and taurodeoxycholate by human liver microsomes. *In* Bile Acids in Human Diseases. P Back and W Gerok, eds. FK Schattauer Verlag, Stuttgart, 1972, pp 71-72.

l Trulzsch, D., Roboz, J., Greim, H., Czygan, P., Rudick, J., Hutterer, F., Schaffner, F., and Popper, H. Hydroxylation of taurolithocholate by isolated human liver microsomes. I. Identification of metabolic product. Biochem. Med. 9:158-166, 1974.

a Truswell, A.S., McVeigh, S., Michell, W.D., and Bronte-Stewart, B. Effect in man of feeding taurine on bile acid conjugation and serum cholesterol levels. J. Atheroscl. Res. 5:526-532, 1965.

b Tserng, K-Y. and Klein, P.D. Synthesis of sulfate esters of lithocholic acid, glycolithocholic acid, and taurolithocholic acid with sulfur trioxide-triethylamine. J. Lipid Res. 18:491-495, 1977.

c Tserng, K-Y. A convenient synthesis of 3-keto bile acids by selective oxidation of bile acids with silver carbonate - celite. J. Lipid Res. 19: 501-504, 1978.

d Tserng, K-Y. and Klein, P.D. Bile acid sulfates: II. Synthesis of 3-monosulfates of bile acids and their conjugates. Lipids 13:479-486, 1978.

e Tserng, K-Y. and Klein, P.D. Bile acid sulfates. III. Synthesis of 7- and 12-monosulfates of bile acids and their conjugates using a sulfur trioxide-triethylamine complex. Steroids 33:167-182, 1979.

f Tsuchiya, Y. Oral gallstone dissolution therapy of asymptomatic gallstones and their indication for surgery. Gastroenterol. Jpn. 14:633-634, 1979.

g Tuerck, D.G. and Comer, T.P. The pill, thromboembolism, and gallbladder disease. Lancet 2:317-318, 1973 (Letter to Editor).

h Turjman, N. and Nair, P.P. Nature of tissue-bound lithocholic acid and its implications in the role of bile acids in carcinogenesis. Cancer Res. 2:3761-3763, 1981.

i Turley, S.D. and Dietschy, J.M. Re-evaluation of the 3a-hydroxysteroid dehydrogenase assay for total bile acids in bile. J. Lipid Res. 19: 924-928, 1978.

j Turley, S.D. and Dietschy, J.M. Effect of clofibrate, cholestyramine, zanchol, probucol, and AOMA feeding on hepatic and intestinal cholesterol metabolism and on biliary lipid secretion in the rat. J. Cardiovasc. Pharm. 2:281-297, 1980.

k Turnberg, L.A. and Grahame, G. Bile salt secretion in cirrhosis of the liver. Gut 11:126-133, 1970.

l Tyor, M.P., Garbutt, J.T., and Lack, L. Metabolism and transport of bile salts in the intestine. Am. J. Med. 51:614, 1971.

m Tyor, M.P. The treatment of gallstones with chenodeoxycholic acid. N. C. Med. J. 39:37-38, 1978.

n Uchida, K., Takeuchi, N., and Yamamura, Y. Effect of glucose administration and cholesterol and bile acid metabolism in rats. Lipids 10:473-477, 1975.

o Uchida, K., Nomura, Y., Kadowaki, M., Takase, H., Takano, K., and Takeuchi, N. Age-related changes in cholesterol and bile acid metabolism in rats. J. Lipid Res. 19:544-552, 1978.

a Uchida, K., Nomura, Y., Kadowaki, M., Takase, H., and Takeuchi, N. Disturbance of cholesterol and bile acid metabolism in spontaneously hypersensitive rats (SHR). J. Biochem. 84:1113-1118, 1978.

b Uchida, K., Takase, H., Kadowaki, M., Nomura, Y., Matsubara, T., and Takeuchi, N. Altered bile acid metabolism in alloxan diabetic rats. Jpn. J. Pharm. 29:553-562, 1979.

c Uchida, K., Nomura, Y., and Takeuchi, N. Effects of cholic acid, chenodeoxycholic acid, and their related bile acids in cholesterol, phospholipid, and bile acid levels in serum, liver, bile and feces of rats. J. Biochem. 87:187-194, 1980.

d Ullrich, I.H., Lai, H-Y., Vona, L., Reid, R.L., and Albrink, M.J. Alterations of fecal steroid composition induced by changes in dietary fiber consumption. Am. J. Clin. Nutr. 34:2054-2060, 1981.

e Ulmenid Roche. Zur Auflosung von Cholesteringallensteinen. Roche, 1977.

f Update: Chenodeoxycholic acid and gallstones. JAMA 245:2378-2379 and 2383-2384, 1981.

g Uribe, M., Uscanga, L., Farca, S., Sanjurjo, J.L., LaGarriga, J., and Ortiz, J.H. Dissolution of cholesterol ductal stones in the biliary tree with medium-chain glycerides. Dig. Dis. Sci. 26:636-640, 1981.

h Vahouny, G.V. and Kay, R. Working group III: Lipid metabolites and intestinal flora. Summary, conclusion, and recommendations. Cancer Res. 41:3781-3782, 1981.

i Vaisrub, S. Cholesterol cholelitholysis. JAMA 228:874-875, 1974 (Editorial).

j Valdivieso, V. and Severin, M.C. Efecto de diferentes acidos biliares sobre la secrecion de lipidos biliares en la rata. Rev. Med. Chile 103:657-659, 1975.

k Valdivieso, V., Palma, R., Wunkhaus, R., Antezana, C., Severin, C., and Contreras, A. Effect of aging on biliary lipid composition and bile acid metabolism in normal Chilean women. Gastroenterology 74:871-874, 1978.

l Valdivieso, V., Palma, R., Nervi, F., Covarrubias, C., Severin, C., and Antezana, C. Secretion of biliary lipids in young Chilean women with cholesterol gallstones. Gut 20:997-1000, 1979.

m Vassilakis, J.S. and Nicolopoulos, N. Dissolution of gallstones following thyroxine administration. A case report. Hepato-Gastroenterol. 28:60-61, 1981.

n Velasco, M. and Csendes, J. Treatment of retained common duct stones with intraductal infusion of mono-octanoin. Med. Chile 108:1021-1023, 1980.

a Verkade, P.E. and Meerburg, W. The solubility of some normal saturated fatty acids in an aqueous sodium glycocholate solution. Rec. Trav. Chim. Pays. 74:263-270, 1955.

b Verzar, F. Absorption from the Intestine. Longmans, Green and Co., London, 1936, 294 pp.

c Vessey, D.A. The biochemical basis for the conjugation of bile acids with either glycine or taurine. Biochem. J. 174:621-626, 1978.

d Villa, L., Ideo, G., Agostoni, A., and Diogardi, N. Further studies on liver metabolism in subjects with gallbladder cholesterol stones. Acta Med. Scand. 175:691-695, 1964.

e Villalonga, E.F., Benitez, J.H., and Ramos, E.F. Encuesta sobre la alimentacion que han hecho los enfermos de litiasis biliar. Rev. Clin. Esp. 147:61-65, 1977.

f Viveros, J.G., Villalobos, J.J., and Wolpert, E. Litiasis biliar en enfermos con cirrhosis del higado. Rev. Invest. Clin. 27:269-273, 1975.

g Vlahcevic, Z.R., Bell, C.C., Jr., Buhac, I., Farrar, J.T., and Swell, L. Diminished bile acid pool size in patients with gallstones. Gastroenterology 59:165-173, 1970.

h Vlahcevic, Z.R., Bell, C.C., Jr., and Swell, L. Significance of the liver in the production of lithogenic bile in man. Gastroenterology 59:62-69, 1970.

i Vlahcevic, Z.R., Buhac, I., Bell, C.C., Jr., and Swell, L. Abnormal metabolism of secondary bile acids in patients with cirrhosis. Gut 11:420-422, 1970.

j Vlahcevic, Z.R., Bell, C.C., Jr., Juttijudata, P., and Swell, L. Bile-rich duodenal fluid as an indicator of biliary lipid composition and its applicability to detection of lithogenic bile. Am. J. Dig. Dis. 16:797-802, 1971.

k Vlahcevic, Z.R., Buhac, I., Farrar, J.T., Bell, C.C., Jr., and Swell, L. Bile acid metabolism in patients with cirrhosis. I. Kinetic aspects of cholic acid metabolism. Gastroenterology 60:491-498, 1971.

l Vlahcevic, Z.R., Miller, J.R., Farrar, J.T., and Swell, L. Kinetics and pool size of primary bile acids in man. Gastroenterology 61:85-90, 1971.

m Vlahcevic, Z.R., Bell, C.C., Jr., Gregory, D.H., Buker, G., Juttijudata, P., and Swell, L. Relationship of bile acid pool size to the formation of lithogenic bile in female Indians of the Southwest. Gastroenterology 62:73-83, 1972.

n Vlahcevic, Z.R., Juttijudata, P., Bell, C.C., Jr., and Swell, L. Bile acid metabolism in patients with cirrhosis. II. Cholic and chenodeoxycholic acid metabolism. Gastroenterology 62:1174-1181, 1972.

a Vlahcevic, Z.R., Yoshida, T., Juttijudata, P., Bell, C.C., Jr., and Swell, L. Bile acid metabolism in cirrhosis. III. Biliary lipid secretion in patients with cirrhosis and its relevance to gallstone formation. Gastroenterology 64:298-303, 1973.

b Vlahcevic, Z.R., Gregory, D.H., and Swell, L. Characterization of factors responsible for abnormal metabolism of deoxycholic acid in patients with alcoholic cirrhosis. In Advances in Bile Acid Research. S Matern, J Hackenschmidt, P Back, and W Gerok, eds. F.K. Schattauer Verlag, Stuttgart, 1974, pp 383-389.

c Vlahcevic, Z.R., Yoshida, T., and Swell, L. Characterization of the abnormality of deoxycholic acid metabolism in cirrhotic patients. Gastroenterology 66:897, 1974 (abstract).

d Vlahcevic, Z.R., Gregory, D.H., and Swell, L. Phenobarbital and cholesterol gallstone dissolution. Am. J. Dig. Dis. 21:429-433, 1976.

e Vlahcevic, Z.R., Prugh, M.F., Gregory, D.H., and Swell, L. Disturbances of bile acid metabolism in parenchymal liver cell disease. Clin. Gastroenterol. 6:25-43, 1977.

f Vlahcevic, Z.R., Schwartz, C.C., Gustaffson, J., Halloran, L.G., Danielsson, H., and Swell, L. Biosynthesis of bile acids in man. J. Biol. Chem. 255:2925-2933, 1980.

g Vochten, R. and Joos, P. Formation of micelles par des acides biliaires en milieu aqueux. J. Chim. Phys. 67:1372-1379, 1970.

h Voigt, W., Thomas, P.J., and Hsia, S.L. Enzymic studies of bile acid metabolism. I. 6 -Hydroxylation of chenodeoxycholic acid and taurochenodeoxycholic acids by microsomal preparations of rat liver. J. Biol. Chem. 243:3493-3499, 1968.

i Voigt, W., Fernandez, E.P., and Hsia, S.L. P-450 level and taurochenodeoxycholate 6 -hydroxylase system of rat liver microsomes. Proc. Soc. Exptl. Biol. Med. 133:1158-1161, 1970.

j Vold, R.D. and McBain, J.W. The solubility curve of sodium deoxycholate in water. J. Am. Chem. Soc. 63:1296-1298, 1941.

k Volpi, C., Ciravegna, G., Canepa, A., De Conca, D., Celle, G., Dodero, M., and Frigerio, G. A cross-over double blind trial comparing the effects of ursodeoxycholic acid (UDCA) and chenodeoxycholic acid (CDCA) on bowel habit in man. Curr. Therap. Res. 26:225-229, 1979.

l Vonk, R.J. Pharmacokinetics of indocyanine green during bile salt infusion. Digestion 10:326-327, 1974 (abstract).

m Vonk, R.J., Danhof, M., Coenraads, T., van Doorn, A.B.D., Keulemans, K., Scaf, A.H.J., and Meijer, D.K.J. Influence of bile salts on hepatic transport of dibromosulphthalein. Am. J. Physiol. 237:E524-E534, 1979.

a Vosseler, M.G. Chemische Hepatitis durch Chenodesoxycholsaure: Eine Frage der Dosierung. (Verlaufsbioptische Studie am Hund). Inauguraldissertation (Bibliothek Dr. Falk), 1976.

b Vuaridel, D., Borel, G.A., and Bron, B. Indications for medical dissolution of biliary lithiasis and value of the determination of the lithogenic index. Schweiz. med. Wschr. 110:877-879, 1980.

c Wachtel, N., Emerman, S., and Javitt, N.B. Metabolism of cholest-5-ene-3b, 26-diol in the rat and hamster. J. Biol. Chem. 243:5207-5212, 1968.

d van Waes, L. Etude: Clinique concernant l'emploi de l'acide chenodeoxycholique dans le traitement de la cholelithiase. Conference, Tielt, Belgium, Dec., 1974 (abstract).

e van Waes, L. and Demeulenaere, L. Behandeling van Galstenen met Cheninezuur. Tijdschr. voor Genessk. 24:1143-1145, 1974.

f van Waes, L., de Weert, M., Schurges, M., Beeckman, P., Barbier, F., and Demeulenaere, L. Behandeling van Galstenen met Cheninezuur. Actuele stand van een prospectieve Studie. Tijdschr. Gastroenterol. 17:287-295, 1974.

g van Waes, L., de Weert, M., Schurges, M., Barbier, F., and Demeulenaere, L. Traitement de la lithiase vesiculaire par l'acide chenique. Resultats preliminaires. M.C.D. 4(Suppl 1):19-22, 1975.

h van Waes, L., de Weert, M., Schurges, M., Beeckman, P., Barbier, F., and Demeulenaere, L. Traitement de la lithiase biliaire par l'acide chenique. Acta Gastro-Ent. Belg. 38:24-33, 1975.

i van Waes, L., Nachtegaele, P., Demeulenaere, L. Traitment de la lithiase biliare par l'acide chenodesoxycholique. Indications, facteurs de succes, resultats. Clin. Rev. Med. 20:1171-1179, 1979.

j Wagner, C.I., Trotman, B.W., and Soloway, R.D. Kinetic analysis of biliary lipid excretion in man and dog. J. Clin. Invest. 57:473-477, 1976.

k Wagner, C.I., Trotman, B.W., and Soloway, R.D. Biliary lipid excretion in patients with pigment gallstones. (A comparison with cholesterol gallstone patients.) Am. J. Dig. Dis. 23:85-88, 1978.

l Walker, J.W. The removal of gallstones by ether solution. Lancet 1:874, 1891.

m Walker, S., Raedsch, R., Stiehl, A., Gotz, R., and Kommerell, B. Resorption von freier, Glycin und Taurin konjugierter und sulfatierter Chenodesoxycholsaure im Kolon der Ratte. Z. Gastroenterol. XIX (9), 1981 (abstract).

n Walshe, E.L. and Ivy, A.C. Observations and the etiology of gallstones. Ann. Intern. Med. 4:134-144, 1930.

a Walters, W. and Wesson, H.R. Fragmentation and expulsion of a common duct stone into the duodenum by using ether and amyl nitrate. Surg. Gyn. & Obst. 65:695-697, 1937.

b Wanitschke, R., Nell, G., and Rummel, W. The influence of deoxycholate on the unidirectional sodium-fluxes in rat colon in vitro. Arch. Pharmacol. 277:R87, 1973 (abstract).

c Wanitschke, R. and Ammon, H.V. Effects of dihydroxy bile acids and hydroxy fatty acids on the absorption of oleic acid in the human jejunum. J. Clin. Invest. 61:178-186, 1978.

d Watanabe, H. Effect of 17a-ethinylestradiol on biliary excretion of bile acids. Biochim. Biophys. Acta 399:79-84, 1975.

e Watari, N., Torizawa, K., Kanai, M., Sato, T., and Yokoi, K. The protective effect of ursodeoxycholic acid for the pancreatic injury caused by alloxan administration. J. Clin. Elec. Micr. 8:477-478, 1975 (abstract).

f Watari, N., Torizawa, K., and Kanai, M. Ultrastructural studies on the preventive effect of ursodeoxycholic acid in possible alloxan-induced pancreatic injury. J. Clin. Electron Microscopy 9:69-81, 1976.

g Watari, N., Mabuchi, Y., and Hotta, Y. Electron microscopical observations on the curative effect of ursodeoxycholic acid in alloxan-induced pancreatic islet cell injury. Folia Endocrinol. Jpn. 53:1191-1201, 1977.

h Watkins, J.B., Tercyak, A.M., Szczepanik, P.A., and Klein, P.D. Bile salt kinetics in cystic fibrosis (CF): Influence of pancreatic enzyme replacement. Gastroenterology 68:1087, 1975.

i Watkins, J.B. and Perman, J.A. Bile acid metabolism in infants and children. Clin. Gastroenterol. 6:201-218, 1977.

j Watson, W.C. Chenodeoxycholic acid: Cost. N. Eng. J. Med. 920:406, 1974 (Letter to Editor).

k Watt, S.M. and Simmonds, W.J. The specificity of bile salts in the intestinal absorption of micellar cholesterol in the rat. Clin. Exptl. Pharm. Physiol. 3:305-322, 1976.

l Watts, J.McK., Jablonski, P., and Toouli, J. Medical treatment of gallstones. Drugs 10:342-350, 1975.

m Watts, J.McK., Jablonski, P., and Toouli, J. The effect of added bran to the diet on the saturation of bile in people without gallstones. Am. J. Surg. 135:321-324, 1978.

n Way, L.W., Admirand, W.H., and Dunphy, J.E. Management of cholelithiasis. Ann. Surg. 176:347-359, 1972.

o Way, L.W. In vitro dissolution of cholesterol gallstones. Surg. Forum 24:412-414, 1973.

a Way, L.W. Retained common duct stones. Surg. Clin. N. Am. 53:1139-1147, 1973.

b Way, L.W. Symposium "Duct Stone Disease". Contemporary Surgery 18:83-118, 1981.

c Weber, A.M., Roy, C.C., Morin, C.L., and Lasalle, R. Malabsorption of bile acids in children with cystic fibrosis. N. Engl. J. Med. 289:1001-1005, 1973.

d Weber, A.M., Roy, C.C., Lepage, G., Chartrand, L., and Lasalle, R. Interruption of the enterohepatic circulation (EHC) of bile acids (BA) in cystic fibrosis (CF). Gastroenterology 68:1066, 1975 (abstract).

e Weber, M. and Paumgartner, G. Surgical, endoscopical and medical treatment of gallstones. Ther. Umsch. 35:738-741, 1978.

f Webling, D.D'A. and Holdsworth, E.S. Bile and the absorption of strontium and iron. Biochem. J. 100:661, 1966.

g Webling, D.D'A. and Holdsworth, E.S. Bile salts and calcium absorption. Biochem. J. 100:652-660, 1966.

h Webster, K.H., Lancaster, M.C., Hofmann, A.F., Wease, D.F., and Baggenstoss, A.H. Influence of primary bile acid feeding on cholesterol metabolism and hepatic function in the Rhesus monkey. Mayo Clin. Proc. 50:134-138, 1975.

i Weinbeck, M. and Strohmeyer, G. Dissolution of gallstones. Med. Welt 28:123-125, 1977.

j Weiner, I.M. and Lack, L. Absorption of bile salts from the small intestine in vivo. Am. J. Physiol. 202:155-157, 1962.

k Weiner, I.M., Glasser, J.E., and Lack, L. Renal excretion of bile acids: Taurocholic, glycocholic and cholic acid. Am. J. Phys. 207:964-970, 1964.

l Weiner, I.M. and Lack, L. Bile salt absorption: Enterohepatic circulation. <u>In</u> Handbook of Physiology. Section 6: Alimentary Canal, CF Code, ed. American Physiological Society, Washington, D.C., 1968, pp 1439-1455.

m Weis, E.E. and Barth, C.A. The extracorporeal bile duct: A new model for determination of bile flow and bile composition in the intact rat. J. Lipid Res. 19:856-862, 1978.

n Weis, E.E. and Barth, C.A. Inhibition of cholesterol synthesis in rat liver by physiological doses of taurocholate. Europ. J. Biochem. 18:2289-2294, 1980.

o Weis, H.J. and Dietschy, J.M. Failure of bile acids to control hepatic cholesterogenesis: Evidence for endogenous cholesterol feedback. J. Clin. Invest. 48:2398-2408, 1969.

a Weis, H.J. and Dietschy, J.M. Adaptive responses in hepatic and intestinal cholesterogenesis following ileal resection in the rat. Europ. J. Clin. Invest. 4:33, 1974.

b Weis, H.J. Klinischer Ueberblick ueber die bisherigen Ergebnisse der Therapie mit Chenodesoxycholsaure und die Frage der Dosierung. Z. Gastroenterol. 13:304-308, 1975.

c Weis, H.J. Medikamentose von Gallensteinen. Dtsch. Arzteblatt 36:2464-2466, 1975.

d Weis, H.J., Baas, E.U., Holtermuller, K.H., and Weihrauch, T.R. Klinische Erfahrungen der medikamentosen Auflosung von Gallensteinen. 82. Tagung der Dtsch. Ges. Inn. Med., Wiesbaden, April, 1976.

e Weis, H.J. Cholecystectomy or drug litholysis of bile calculi? Dtsch. Med. Wschr. 104:603-605, 1979.

f Weis, H.J., Holtermuller, K.H., Stiehl, A., and Czygan, P. Clinical experience in bile composition in patients taking ursodeoxycholic acid for gallstone dissolution. _In_ Biological Effects of Bile Acids. G Paumgartner, A Stiehl, and W Gerok, _eds_. MTP Press, Lancaster, 1979, pp 99-102.

g Weis, H.J. Indikationen zur medikamentosen Gallenstein Auflosung. Fortschr. Med. 98:1235-1239, 1980.

h Weis, H.J., Holtermueller, K.H., and Gilsdorf, P. Gallstone dissolution with chenodeoxycholic acid. Klin. Wschr. 58:313-320, 1980.

i Weis, H.J. Medikamentose Auflosung von Gallensteinen. Therapiewoche 31: 6226-6227, 1981.

j Weis, H.J. Cholelitholyse. Indikationen und Ergebnisse. Med. Welt 33: 94-95, 1982.

k Weis, H.J. Die medikamentose Auflosung von Gallenblasensteinen. Therapiewoche 32:959-962, 1982.

l Wenckert, A. and Robertson, B. The natural course of gallstone disease. Eleven-year review of 871 nonoperated cases. Gastroenterology 50:376-381, 1966.

m Wenger, J. and Heymsfield, S. Adsorption of bile by aluminum hydroxide: A rationale for use in regurgitation gastritis. Gastroenterology 64:821, 1973 (abstract).

n van der Werf, S., Huijbregts, A.W.M., Lamers, H.L.M., van Berge Hengouwen, G.P., and van Tongeren, J.H.M. Age dependent differences in human bile acid metabolism and 7_a_-dehydroxlyation. Europ. J. Clin. Invest. 11:425-431, 1981.

a van der Werf, S.D.J., Nagengast, F.M., van Berge Henegouwen, G.P., Huijbregts, A.W.M., and van Tongeren, J.H.M. Colonic absorption of secondary bile acids in patients with adenomatous polyps and in matched controls. Lancet 1:759-761, 1982.

b Westergaard, H. and Dietschy, J.M. Delineation of the dimensions and permeability characteristics of the two major diffusion barriers to passive mucosal uptake in the rabbit intestine. J. Clin. Invest. 54:718-732, 1974.

c Westergaard, H. and Dietschy, J.M. The mechanism whereby bile acid micelles increase the rate of fatty acid and cholesterol uptake into the intestinal mucosal cell. J. Clin. Invest. 58:97-108, 1976.

d Westra, P., Houwertjes, M.C., Wesseling, H., and Meijer, D.K. Bile salts and neuromuscular blocking agents. Brit. J. Anaesth. 53:407-415, 1981.

e Wheeler, H.O. and Ramos, O.L. Determinants of the flow and composition of bile in the unanesthetized dog during constant infusions of sodium taurocholate. J. Clin. Invest. 39:161-170, 1960.

f Wheeler, H.O. Determinants of the flow and composition of bile. Gastroenterology 40:584-586, 1961.

g Wheeler, H.O. The flow and ionic composition of bile. Arch. Int. Med. 108:156-162, 1961.

h Wheeler, H.O. Electrolyte transport and bile formation. Med. Clin. N. Am. 47:607, 1963.

i Wheeler, H.O. Transport of electrolytes and water across wall of rabbit gallbladder. Am. J. Physiol. 205:427, 1963.

j Wheeler, H.O. The function of the biliary tract. In Progress in Liver Diseases. H Popper and F Schaffner, eds. Grune & Stratton, New York, 1965, p 15.

k Wheeler, H.O. Inorganic ions in bile. In The Biliary System. W Taylor, ed. Blackwell, Oxford, 1965, p 481.

l Wheeler, H.O. and Mancusi-Ungoro, P.L. Role of bile ducts during secretin choleresis in dogs. Am. J. Physiol. 210:1153-1159, 1966.

m Wheeler, H.O. Water and electrolytes in bile. In Handbook of Physiology. Section 6, Alimentary Canal. CF Code and W Heidel, eds. Am. Physiol. Soc., Washington, D.C., Vol V, 1968, p 2409.

n Wheeler, H.O., Ross, E.D., and Bradley, S.E. Canalicular bile production in dogs. Am. J. Physiol. 214:866-874, 1968.

o Wheeler, H.O. Concentrating function of the gallbladder. Am. J. Med. 51:588-595, 1971.

a Wheeler, H.O. Secretion of bile acids by the liver and their role in the formation of hepatic bile. Arch. Intern. Med. 130:533-541, 1972.

b Wheeler, H.O. and King, K.K. Biliary excretion of lecithin and cholesterol in the dog. J. Clin. Invest. 51:1337-1350, 1972.

c Wheeler, H.O. Biliary excretion of bile acids, lecithin, and cholesterol in hamsters with gallstones. Gastroenterology 65:92-103, 1973.

d Wheeler, H.O. Pathogenesis of gallstones. Surg. Clin. N. Am. 53:963-972, 1973.

e Wheeler, H.O., May, R.J., and Loeb, P.M. Determinants of biliary lipid excretion. In The Liver. Quantitative Aspects of Structure and Function. Karger, Basel, 1973, pp 368.

f Wheeler, H.O. Principles of biliary secretion. In Jaundice. CA Goresky, MM Fisher, eds. Plenum Publishing Corp., New York, 1975, pp 195.

g Wheeler, H.O. Secretion of bile. In Diseases of the Liver. L Schiff, ed. Lippincott, Philadelphia, Fourth Ed., 1975, pp 87.

h Whipple, G.H. The origin and significance of the constituents of the bile. Physiol. Rev. 2:440-459, 1922.

i White, B.A., Cacciapuoti, A.F., Fricke, R.J., Whitehead, T.R., Mosbach, E.H., and Hylemon, P.B. Cofactor requirements for 7a-dehydroxylation of cholic and chenodeoxycholic acid in cell extracts of the intestinal anaerobic bacterium, Eubacterium species V.P.I. 13708. J. Lipid Res. 22: 891-898, 1981.

j White, B.A., Fricke, R.J., and Hylemon, P.B. 7b-Dehydroxylation of ursodeoxycholic acid by whole cells and cell extracts of the intestinal anaerobic bacterium, Eubacterium species V.P.I. 12708. J. Lipid Res. 23: 145-153, 1982.

k White, T.T., Tournut, R.A., Scharplatz, D., Kavlie, H., Olson, A.D., and Hopton, D.S. The effect of vagotomy on biliary secretions and bile salt pools in dogs. Ann. Surg. 179:406-411, 1974.

l Whiting, M.J. and Watts, J.M. Serum bile acid profiling for monitoring gallstone dissolution therapy. Gut 20:A930, 1979 (abstract).

m Whiting, M., Jarvinen, V., and Watts, J. Chemical composition of gallstones resistant to dissolution therapy with chenodeoxycholic acid. Gut 21:1077-1081, 1980.

n Whiting, M.J. and Watts, J.M. Prediction of the bile acid composition of bile from serum bile acid analysis during gallstone dissolution therapy. Gastroenterology 78:220-225, 1980.

a Whiting, M., Down, R., and Watts, J. Precision and accuracy in the measurement of the cholesterol saturation index of duodenal bile. Gastroenterology 80:533-538, 1981.

b Whitlock, R.T. and Wheeler, H.O. Coupled transport of solute and water across rabbit gallbladder epithelium. J. Clin. Invest. 43:2249-2265, 1964.

c Whitney, J. and Thaler, M. Compartmentation of bile acids (BA) during fetal and post natal development. Gastroenterology 79:1130, 1980 (abstract).

d Whyte, H.M., Nestel, P.J., and Pryke, E.S. Bile acid and cholesterol excretion with carbohydrate-rich diets. J. Lab. Clin. Med. 81:818-828, 1973.

e Wicks, A.C.B., Yeats, J., and Heaton, K.W. Bran and bile: Time-course of changes in normal young men given a standard dose. Scand. J. Gastroenterol. 13:289-292, 1978.

f Wieland, H. and Reverey, G. Untersuchungen ueber die Gallensauren. XXI. Zur Kenntnis der menschlichen Galle. Z. Physiol. Chem. 140:186, 1924.

g Wilbur, B.G., Gomez, F.C., and Tompkins, R.K. Canine gallbladder bile. Effects of proximal vagotomy, truncal vagotomy and truncal vagotomy with pyloroplasty. Arch. Surg. 110:792-796, 1975.

h Williams, C.N. Progressive familial cholestatic cirrhosis and bile acid metabolism. J. Pediat. 81:493-500, 1972.

i Williams, C.N., Macdonald, I.A., and Park-Dincsoy, H. Bile acid pools in primary biliary cirrhosis. Gastroenterology 67:836, 1974 (abstract).

j Williams, C.N. Bile-acid metabolism and the liver. Clin. Biochem. 9:149-152, 1976.

k Williams, C.N., Mores, J.W.I., MacDonald, I.A., Kotoor, R., and Riding, M.D. Increased lithogenicity of bile on fasting in normal subjects. Dig. Dis. & Sci. 22:189-194, 1977.

l Williams, G., Maton, P.N., Murphy, G.M., and Dowling, R.H. Will ursodeoxycholic acid (UDCA) replace chenodeoxycholic acid (CDCA) as the medical treatment of choice for gallstone dissolution? Gut 19:A974, 1978 (abstract).

m Williams, G., Tanida, N., Maton, P.N., Murphy, G.M., and Dowling, R.H. Ursodeoxycholic acid (UDCA) therapy of gallstones. Is correction of biliary cholesterol saturation index according to percentage UDCA in bile necessary for prediction of gallstone dissolution? Clin. Sci. 57:23p, 1979 (abstract).

a Williams, G., Tanida, N., Maton, P.N., Murphy, G.M., and Dowling, R.H. The biliary cholesterol saturation index (SI) in ursodeoxycholic acid (UDCA) rich bile: Is the Carey correction necessary when predicting gallstone dissolution? Vth Internat'l Symposium on Bile Acids, Cortina d'Ampezzo, 1979, pp 56 (abstract).

b Williams, G., Mathews, L., Breuer, N.F., Murphy, G.M., and Dowling, R.H. Effect of ursodeoxycholic acid (UDCA) on primary bile acid kinetics in gallstone patients. Clin. Sci. 58:15p, 1980 (abstract).

c Williams, R.C., Showalter, R., and Kern, F., Jr. In vivo effect of bile salts and cholestyramine on intestinal anaerobic bacteria. Gastroenterology 69:483-491, 1975.

d Williamson, B.W.A. and Percy-Robb, I.W. Contribution of biliary lipids to calcium binding in bile. Gastroenterology 78:696-702, 1980.

e Willson, R.A., Webster, K.H., Hofmann, A.F., and Summerskill, W.H.J. Towards an artificial liver: In vitro removal of unbound and protein bound plasma compounds related to hepatic failure. Gastroenterology 62:1191-1199, 1972.

f Willson, R.A., Hofmann, A.F., and Kuster, G.G.R. Toward an artificial liver. II. Removal of cholephilic anions from dogs with biliary obstruction by hemoperfusion through charged and uncharged resins. Gastroenterology 66:95-107, 1974.

g Wilson, F.A. and Dietschy, J.M. Approach to the malabsorption syndromes associated with disordered bile acid metabolism. Arch. Intern. Med. 130:584-594, 1972.

h Wilson, F.A. and Dietschy, J.M. Characterization of bile acid absorption across the unstirred water layer and brush border of the rat jejunum. J. Clin. Invest. 51:3015-3025, 1972.

i Wilson, J.D. Relation between dietary cholesterol and bile acid excretion in the rat. Am. J. Physiol. 203:1029-1032, 1962.

j Wilson, J.D., Bentley, W.H., and Crowley, G.T. Regulation of bile acid formation in intact animals. In Bile Acid Metabolism. Schiff, Carey, and Dietschy, eds. Thomas, Springfield, 1968, pp 140-148.

k Wilson, J.D. The measurement of the exchangeable pools of cholesterol in the baboon. J. Clin. Invest. 49:655-665, 1970.

l Wilson, J.D. The role of bile acids in the overall regulation of steroid metabolism. Arch. Intern. Med. 130:493-505, 1972.

m Windaus, A., Bohne, A., and Schwarzkopf, E. Ueber die Chenodesoxycholsaure. Z. Physiol. Chem. 140:177, 1924.

a Wingate, D.L. The effect of glycine-conjugated bile acids on net water and glucose transport, and transmural potential difference across isolated rat jejunum. J. Physiol. 229:43P-44P, 1973 (abstract).

b Wingate, D.L., Krag, E., Mekhjian, H.S., and Phillips, S.F. Relationships between ion and water movement in the human jejunum, ileum and colon during perfusion with bile acids. Clin. Sci. Mol. Med. 45:593-606, 1973.

c Wingate, D.L., Phillips, S.F., and Hofmann, A.F. The effect of glycine conjugated bile acids with or without lecithin on water and glucose absorption in the perfused human jejunum. J. Clin. Invest. 52:1230-1236, 1973.

d Wingate, D.L. The effect of glycine-conjugated bile acids on net transport transmural potential difference, and lactate production in isolated rat jejunum and ileum. J. Physiol. 242:189-207, 1974.

e Wingate, D.L., Hyams, A., and Phillips, S.F. Luminal distention as a possible consequence of experimental intestinal perfusion. Gut 15:728-732, 1974.

f Wingate, D.L. Bile acids and bulk flow. In Ion Transport Across the Intestine. JW Robinson, ed. MTP Press, Lancaster, 1976.

g Winkler, K., Keiding, S., and Tygstrup, N. Clearance as a quantitative measure of liver function. In The Liver. Quantitative Aspects of Structure and Function. G Paumgartner and R Preisig, eds. Karger, Basel, 1973, pp 144-155.

h Winternitz, M., Deutsch, J., and Bruell, Z. Klinisch drauchbare Bestimmungsmethode der Blutumlaufszeit mittels Decholininjektion (kurze mitteilung). Klin. Med. 27:986, 1931.

i Wise, L. and Stein, T. The effect of jejunoileal bypass on bile composition and the formation of biliary calculi. Ann. Surg. 187:57-62, 1978.

j Wiss, O and Wiss, V. The degradation of labelled lanosterol by homogenate of rat liver: Evidence for the formation of lithocholic acid from lanosterol without cholesterol as intermediate. Biochem. Biophys. Res. Comm. 83:857-862, 1978.

k Witzel, L., Wiederholt, J., and Wolbergs, E. Dissolution of gallstones by perfusion with Capmul via a catheter introduced endoscopically into the bile duct. N. Engl. J. Med. 303:465, 1980 (letter).

l Witzel, L., Wiederholt, J., and Wolbergs, E. Dissolution of retained duct stones by perfusion with monooctanoin via a Teflon catheter introduced endoscopically. Gastrointest. Endos. 27:63-65, 1981.

m Wolfson, M., Miyai, K., and Javitt, N.B. Ursodeoxycholic acid toxicity in rabbits. Gastroenterology 73:1255, 1977 (abstract).

a Wollenweber, J., Kottke, B.A., and Owen, C.A., Jr. Quantitative thin-layer chromatography of chenodeoxycholic acid and deoxycholic acid in human duodenal contents. J. Chromatog. 24:99-105, 1966.

b Wolpers, C. Spontanauflosung von Gallenblasensteinen. Dtsch. med. Wschr. 93:2525-2532, 1968.

c Wolpers, C. and Blaschke, R. Electron microscopy of human gallstones. 29th Ann. Proc. Electron Microscopy Soc., Boston, 1971 (abstract).

d Wolpers, C. Gallensteine: Pathogenese und Therapie. Niedersachsisches Arzteblatt 4:136-137, 1974.

e Wolpers, C. Morphologie der Gallensteine. Leber Magen Darm 4:43-57, 1974.

f Wolpers, C. Cholesterin-Steine auflosbar. Chenodesoxycholsaure greift besonders junge, kleine Konkremente an. Praxis Kurier Nr. 23, pp 10, 1975.

g Wolpers, C. Gallensauremedikation: Jungere Steine reagieren gut. Arztl. Praxis 27:2296, 1975.

h Wolpers, C. Die Gallensaurentherapie der Cholelithiasis. 84. Tagung Nordwestdeutsche Ges. Inn. Med. Hamburg, Feb., 1975 (abstract).

i Wolpers, C. Die Gallensteine (Arten, Bildung, Spontanauflosung). In Gallenblase - Pankreas. Boecker, ed. Thieme, Stuttgart, 1975, pp 22-27.

j Wolpers, C. Medikamentose Cholelitholyse. Multiple "junge" Cholesterinesteine in 50% verkleinert. Med. Tribune Nr. 20, pp 49, 1975.

k Wolpers, C. and Mockel, G. Gallensteinentfernung. Die unblutige Methode. Euromed No. 6, pp 252-253, 1975.

l Wolpers, C. Auswahl der Gallensteintrager zur Litholyse. Leber Magen Darm 6:43-46, 1976.

m Wolpers, C. The natural history of gallstone formation. In Interdisciplinary Trends in Surgery, Edizioni. Minerva Medica, 1979.

n Wolpers, C. Cholanorm (Chenodesoxycholsaure). Int. Praxis 1:141-151, 1981.

o Wolpers, C. Lytische Therapie der Cholezystolithiasis. Inn. Med. 14: 14-19, 1981.

p Wolpers, C. Aus der Praxis: So lose ich seit 8 Jahren Gallenstine auf. Med. Tribune (Schweiz) 41:9, 1981.

q Wolpers, C. Lytische Therapie der Cholezystolithiasis. Der Informierte Arzt 9:14-19, 1981.

a Wolpers, C. Polypoid lesions of the gallbladder and the formation of human gallstones. Hepato-Gastroenterology, Supplement 1981 (abstract).

b Womack, N.A. The development of gallstones. Surg. Gyn. Obst. 133:937-945, 1971.

c Wood, J.R., Saverymuttu, S.M., Morton, I.K.M., and Reuben, M.J.G. Effects of sodium chenodeoxycholate, sodium cholate, and their glycine conjugates on fluid transport by the isolated guinea-pig gallbladder. 6th Internat'l Congress of Pharm., Helsinki, 1975 (abstract).

d Wood, P.D., Shioda, R., Estrich, D.L., and Splitter, S.D. Effect of cholestyramine on composition of duodenal bile in obese human subjects. Metabolism 21:107-116, 1972.

e Woodbury, J. and Kern, F., Jr. Fecal excretion of bile acids: A new technique for studying bile acid kinetics in patients with ileal resection. J. Clin. Invest. 50:2531-2540, 1971.

f Woodford, F.P. Enlargement of taurocholate micelles by added cholesterol and monoolein: Self-diffusion measurements. J. Lipid Res. 10:539-545, 1969.

g Wosiewitz, U. and Schroebler, S. Solubilization of unconjugated bilirubin by bile salts. Experientia 35:717-718, 1979.

h Wosiewitz, U., Schenk, J., Sabinksi, F., and Schmack, B. Choledocholithiasis nach Cholezystektomie/Choledochotomie. Z. Gastroenterol. XIX (9), 1981 (abstract).

i Wurbs, D., Phillips, J., and Classen, M. Experiences with the long standing nasobiliary tube in biliary diseases. Endoscopy 12:219-223, 1980.

j Yahiro, K., Setoguchi, T., and Katsuki, T. Effect of cecum and appendix on 7a-dehydroxylation and 7b-epimerization of chenodeoxycholic acid in the rabbit. J. Lipid Res. 21:215-222, 1980.

k Yamaga, N. Isolation of allochenodeoxycholic acid from bile of carp Yonago. Acta Med. 15:18, 1971 (Japanese).

l Yamanishi, Y., Kishimoto, Y., Kawasaki, H., Hirayama, C., and Ikawa, S. Oral ursodeoxycholic acid tolerance test in patients with digestive disease. Gastroenterol. Jpn. 16:472-477, 1981.

m Yamasaki, L., Wakutani, T., Yakimoto, H., and Simizu, K. On the transformation of dehydrocholic acid into deoxycholic acid in the rabbit. J. Biochem. 46:809-811, 1959.

n Yamatake, Y., Ishikawa, S., and Yanaura, S. Effects of some bile acids on hepatic blood flow in dogs - with reference to biliary excretion. Japan. J. Pharm. 26:273-275, 1976.

a Yanagisawa, J., Itoh, M., Ishibashi, M., Miyazaki, H., and Nakayama, F. Microanalysis of bile acid in human liver tissue by selected ion monitoring. Anal. Biochem. 104:75-86, 1980.

b Yanaura, S. and Ishikawa, S. Choleretic properties of ursodeoxycholic acid and chenodeoxycholic acid in dogs. Japan J. Pharmacol. 28:383-389, 1978.

c Yellin, T.O., Klaiber, M.S., and Webb, E. Lithogenic effects of cholic acid and chenodeoxycholic acid in the cholesterol fed mouse. Biochim. Biophys. Acta 320:478-485, 1973.

d Yeomans, N.D., Williams, D.R., Mackinnon, M.A., McLeish, A.R., and Smallwood, R.A. Effect of cigarette smoking on duodenogastric reflux of bile acids. Aust. N.Z. J. Med. 11:347-350, 1981.

e Yokomura, T. Effect of antibiotics on bile acid composition of bile. Japan. J. Gastroenterol. 71:755-763, 1974 (Japanese).

f Yoon, D-S., Shim, B-S., and Kil, T-S. Bile-specific protein components in human hepatic bile. J. Lab. Clin. Med. 67:640-649, 1966.

g Yoshida, T., McCormick, W.C., III., Swell, L., and Vlahcevic, Z.R. Bile acid metabolism in cirrhosis. IV. Characterization of the abnormality in deoxycholic acid metabolism. Gastroenterology 68:335-341, 1975.

h Yoshimuta, S. Factors affecting solubility of cholesterol in bile. Fukuoka Acta Med. 51:510-528, 1960.

i Young, D.L. and Hanson, K.C. Effect of bile salts on hepatic phosphatidylcholine synthesis and transport into rat bile. J. Lipid Res. 13:244-252, 1972.

j Yousef, I.M., Kakis, G., and Fisher, M.M. Bile acid metabolism in mammals. III. Sex difference in the bile acid composition of rat bile. Canad. J. Biochem. 50:402-408, 1972.

k Yousef, I.M., Magnusson, R., Price, V.M., and Fisher, M.M. Bile acid metabolism in mammals. V. Studies on the sex difference in the response of the isolated perfused rat liver to chenodeoxycholic acid. Canad. J. Physiol. Pharmacol. 51:418-423, 1973.

l Yousef, I.M., Yousef, M.K., and Bradley, W.G. Bile acid composition in some desert rodents. Proc. Soc. Exptl. Biol. Med. 143:596-601, 1973.

m Yousef, I.M., Kakis, G., and Fisher, M.M. Bile acid metabolism in mammals. VI. Effect of ethionine on bile acids of rat bile. Lipids 9:407-414, 1974.

n Yousef, I.M., Kukis, A., and Fisher, M.M. Isotope derivatives assay of plasma bile acids by radio-gas chromatography. Gastroenterology 67:838, 1974 (abstract).

a Yousef, I.M., Bloxam, D.L., Phillips, M.J., and Fisher, M.M. Liver cell plasma membrane lipids and the origin of biliary phospholipid. Canad. J. Biochem. 53:989-997, 1975.

b Yousef, I.M. and Fisher, M.M. Bile acid metabolism in mammals. VIII. The biliary secretion of cholyl arginine. Canad. J. Physiol. Pharm. 53:880-887, 1975.

c Yousef, I.M. and Fisher, M.M. Bile acid metabolism in mammals. IX. Conversion of chenodeoxycholic acid to cholic acid by isolated perfused rat liver. Lipids 10:571-573, 1975.

d Yousef, I.M., Fisher, M.M. Piekarski, J., and Holub, B.J. Activity of phospholipid-synthesizing enzymes in rat liver plasma membranes and the source of biliary lecithin. Lipids 12:140-144, 1977.

e Yousef, I.M., Tuchweber, B., Vonk, R.J., Masse, D., Audet, M., and Roy, C.C. Lithcholate cholestasis--sulfated glycolithocholate-induced intraheptic cholestasis in rats. Gastroenterology 80:233-241, 1981.

f Zaidman, I., Sorgi, M., Garnica, E., Monserat, R., Santana, M., Paradisi, C.E., Isern, A.M., and Palao, R. El tratamiento de la litiasis vesicular von acido quenodesoxicolico. IV. Congreso de la Sociedad Latinoamericana de Hepatologia. Caracas, Oct., 1974, pp 42 (abstract).

g Zaki, F.G., Carey, J.B., Jr., Hoffbauer, F.W., and Nokolo, C. Biliary reaction and choledocholithiasis induced in the rat by lithocholic acid. J. Lab. Clin. Med. 69:737-748, 1967.

h Zheng, R., Wang, Z.L., Yuan, L., and Li, N.K. Absorption, distribution and excretion of ^{3}H-chenodeoxycholic acid (CDCA) in mice. Yao Hsueh Hsueh Pao 16:235-237, 1981.

i Ziboh, V.A., Matschiner, J.T., Doisey, E.A., Jr., Hsia, S.L., Elliott, W.H., Thayer, S.A., and Doisy, E.A. Bile acids. XIV. Metabolism of chenodeoxycholic acid-24-C^{14} in surgically jaundiced mice. J. Biol. Chem. 236:387-390, 1961.

j Ziboh, V.A., Hsia, S.L., Matschiner, J.T., Doisy, E.A., Jr., Elliott, W.H., Thayer, S.A., and Doisy, E.A. Bile acids. XVIII. Further studies on the metabolism of chenodeoxycholic acid-24-C^{14} in surgically jaundiced mice. J. Biol. Chem. 238:3588-3590, 1963.

k Ziller, S.A., Mitra, M.N., and Elliott, W.H. A two-step synthesis of allochenodeoxycholic acid. Chem. Indust. 24:999-1000, 1967.

l Ziller, S.A., Doisy, E.A., and Elliott, W.H. Bile acids. XXV. Allochenodeoxycholic acid, a metabolite of 5a-cholestan-3b-ol in the hyperthyroid rat. J. Biol. Chem. 243:5280-5288, 1968.

m Zimmerer, R.O., Jr. and Lindenbaum, S. Enthalpy of bile salt-lecithin mixed micelle formation. J. Pharm. Sci. 68:581-585, 1979.

a Zimmerman, H.J. Chenodeoxycholic acid and the liver: good news--bad news. Hepatology 2:288-289, 1982.

b Zimmon, D.S., Kerner, M.B., Aaron, B.M., Raicht, R.F., Mosbach, E.H., and Kessler, R.E. The effect of a hydrocholeretic agent (Zanchol) on biliary lipids in post-cholecystectomy patients. Gastroenterology 70:640-643, 1976.

c Zouboulis-Vafiadis, I., Dumont, M., and Erlinger, S. Conjugation is the rate-limiting step in the hepatic transport of ursodeoxycholic acid in the rat. IV Internat'l Gstaad Symposium, 1981 (abstract).

d Zuin, M., Dioguardi, M.L., Festorazzi, S., Racca, V., and Podda, M. Is the saturation index predictive for gallstone dissolution during treatment with ursodeoxycholic acid? Gastroenterology 78:1327, 1980 (abstract).

e Zurier, R.B., Hashim, S.A., Van Itallie, T.B. Effect of medium chain triglyceride on cholestyramine induced steatorrhea in man. Gastroenterology 49:490-495, 1965.

Author Index

Subject Index